Health First!

An essential manual
for protecting your most vital asset

by William C. Rawls, Jr., M.D.

Copyright © 2009 William C. Rawls, Jr. M.D.
HEALTH FIRST!, An Essential Manual for Protecting Your Most Vital Asset

First Do No Harm Health Systems, Inc.
3106 Arendell Street
Morehead City, N. C. 28557

Printed in the United States of America
Bookmasters, Inc.

ISBN 978-0-9823225-0-5

LCCN 2009901564

This book is dedicated to my patients.

INTRODUCTION

My first clinical rotation in medical school was on the nephrology (kidney disease) service. Most of the patients were very ill and large quantities of potent drugs were necessary to keep them alive. Quality of life was quite low. It was decidedly not the type of medicine I wanted to pursue as a career. My interest, as a physician, was in keeping patients from getting to that point.

By my fourth year of medical school I had made a decision to pursue a career in obstetrics. Obstetrics dealt with bringing life into the world. It was generally bright and uplifting, and did not involve heavy drug use. Four years of postgraduate training in obstetrics and gynecology was both challenging and stimulating. Though much of obstetrics deals with healthy individuals, pregnant patients do get sick and helping them get well is an important part of the job. Training in gynecology also included a large cancer service, offering exposure to the full spectrum of medical care. The overall approach, however, was much less drug oriented and much more wellness oriented than other specialties of medicine. The Ob/Gyn specialty fit my personality well.

The first ten years in private practice were some of the most exciting in my life. At a young age, I could easily balance long nights on call with a busy practice and at the same time have a normal family life and contribute to my community. By mid-forties, however, worsening insomnia and fatigue, presumed to be related to years of night call, was beginning to erode my health. At first I turned to colleagues practicing conventional medicine for help, but quickly found that all drugs available for insomnia, even the newest ones, were accompanied by significant side effects. For several years I existed in a compromised state, using medications on nights not on call to get enough sleep to last through the nights when I was on call. I finally made the difficult decision to leave obstetrics behind, changing my practice of medicine and my life forever, but not necessarily in a negative way.

Throughout my career I considered health and wellness to be of paramount importance, but as I shifted away from obstetrics and toward primary care, these concepts became the central focus of my practice and my entire life. It was like going back to medical school again, learning completely different approaches to treat the same old problems. I bought new textbooks and learned everything that I could about nutrition. I read everything available in the lay press about herbal remedies and then searched the academic literature to determine what was real and what was not. I attended conferences on holistic and alternative medicine, but retained my ability to apply objective scientific scrutiny. I volunteered at a local free clinic to familiarize myself with the conventional medicine approach to everyday primary care problems, but at the same time searched for better solutions.

All the while, I was working to regain my own health. Everything I learned, I applied to myself. By necessity, my life became very regimented. Moderate exercise, meditation and yoga were daily routines. I became a self-taught expert in nutrition and only allowed healthy foods in my diet. I found supplements that actually helped the sleep problem, without the risk of side effects and dependence. My health and my energy level gradually rebounded.

During the transition, I decided to leave a large Ob/Gyn practice and start an independent practice based on concepts of wellness. While this entailed significant stress in itself, I felt a calling to spread my new-found message. For individuals whose needs were not met by conventional therapy, my new practice would provide an alternative. Motivated individuals who wanted to regain their health, as I had, could find resources to do so. Patients who were not able to tolerate drug therapy could find non-drug alternatives and combinations of nutraceuticals that would work just as well.

Writing a health book was not part of my original intent; it simply evolved while everything else was going on. While brief office visits work in the conventional medical setting, they do not provide enough time to guide major changes in someone's life. I found written information to be an essential part of patient education. Most of the available "canned" health information was not satisfactory, so I started writing it myself.

Initially my writing consisted mainly of short essays about specific topics, to be passed along to patients at individual office visits. Gradually, the topics came together to explain the concepts of why disease occurs, and more importantly, what to do about it. As it coalesced into book form, I added personal insights and patient experiences to convey sometimes dry information in a pleasant manner.

For the past three years the book has existed as a living document, primarily used as a manual for an eight week health improvement course in the office. Maintained as computer text, the book could be edited with every question asked and every new concept that came along. With each edit it evolved to be more complete. This final edition, finally ready for print, is truly a definitive resource for achieving optimal wellness and longevity.

The book is designed to provide a practical and comprehensive foundation for health optimization. It was specifically not intended to be a self-diagnosis/self-help book for self-treatment of medical problems—there are plenty of those on the market, some of which are potentially harmful. People turn to self-help books because they are not getting the answers they want at their doctors' offices. Personally, I feel that illness is best treated under the guidance of a qualified healthcare practitioner, but patients need and want more than just prescriptions. It is time for the healthcare profession to evolve beyond this level.

In my office, the health program and the book provide core information for general health improvement. This is complemented by counseling and a set of monographs I wrote called "Health Briefs," which serve to guide the patient in treatment of a specific illness. The entire system is designed to empower the patient to gain control over personal health and overcome disease. Therapy is focused on maximal healing with the lowest possible potential for toxicity.

Of course, I need to note that all patients referenced in the book were fictitious, each a conglomeration of different patients, used to convey ideas. None of the names used here correspond to the names of those individuals.

The knowledge I have to offer does not consist of miracle cures, as I believe those are few and far between. The miracle is in life itself; all the rest is instinct. Most of us inherently know what is good for us, but we tend to ignore it or lose tract of it. Sometimes we need a beacon to guide us back to what really matters in life. Just writing this book has been a beacon for me. I hope it will be for you.

Your personal starting point, from a health point of view, does not really matter. If you have a significant illness, seek the guidance of a qualified healthcare provider, but at the same time, take control of your own health by following the guidelines in this book. Anyone, at any level should be able to gain benefit. If you follow any of the recommendations in this book, you will regain lost health. If you follow most of the recommendations in this book, you will maximize your potential for achieving a fulfilling and healthy life. *I am confident that most health problems can be overcome by improved health habits. Better health is within anyone's grasp!*

The first four chapters of the book are devoted to constructing a model of how and why disease occurs and how it is balanced by the natural healing potential of the body. Understanding these concepts is very important. They are the backbone for making real change. The approach is "holistic" but certainly complementary to any medical therapy you may be receiving.

The remainder of the book is divided into three sections labeled "pillars." Pillar I includes five chapters devoted to everything you would ever want to know about food and nourishment. Pillar II discusses toxins and detoxification. Pillar III focuses on synchrony of the mind and body. This concept is useful for developing a practical approach to exercise and stress modification.

There is a lot of information in the book, but it is designed to be a complete resource without reading like an encyclopedia. It does not have to be read from front to back, cover to cover, to be best utilized. Some sections of the book present and discuss concepts, while others stand alone as reliable references on important health topics. Throughout the book there are suggestions for lab tests that correlate with specific topics (noted in bold italics). These are summarized in an appendix and can be ordered under the direction of your personal healthcare provider. Specific guidelines for what classifies as healthy food can be found in chapter eight. Chapter nine applies the guidelines by teaching concepts of healthy cooking. If stress management is an issue, you may want to turn directly to chapter fourteen. As you are reading the book, consider following the detoxification protocol found at the end of chapter eleven. It is an excellent way to break into a healthier lifestyle!

Your body is your vehicle for experiencing this life.
How well you take care of your body will greatly influence the quality of
that experience.

CONTENTS

CHAPTER 1
Health of America

Flying across the country offers a perfect opportunity for people watching. A cross-section of America, young and old, all sizes and shapes, different races and certainly different levels of health, sandwiched within the confines of a jet airliner. For a four hour period I will be sharing time and direction with this group of individuals. With any luck, our flight will go well and we will arrive on time at Denver International Airport.

I pass the time studying the people around me. We are all alike, but dissimilar at the same time. The greatest thing we share in common, besides our destination, is a genetic code that is similar enough to define us all as being one species. Beyond this, we are different. This remarkable code allows for such an infinite number of variations that, with the exception of the identical twin girls in row 24, the genetic makeup of each individual on this plane is unique. Different shapes, different sizes, different skin tones, and different hair color. Differences that can sometimes be covered up but not truly changed.

Many of our individual differences can be traced to birth, but many others have been shaped by our environment over time. Choices make us who we are. Choices—possibly even more than our genes—define how healthy we will be throughout our lives. Human nature tends to drive us toward choices that are not always the best for our health. There is a good chance that fewer than half of the individuals around me consume fresh fruits and vegetables with any regularity and a good chance that they survive mostly on a processed form of the corn and wheat harvested from the fields that lie below us. To be candid, most of them are overweight. Of the ones under the age of thirty, most have never had major health problems and, therefore, take their health completely for granted, but a large portion of those over forty have had their lives limited or shaped in some way by changing health.

The flight attendant leans over to pass me a bottle of water, a cup of ice and a package that the airline describes as a "snack." The water tastes like plastic, and I assume it has been sitting out in the sun on the tarmac before being placed inside the plane, but I am thirsty so I drink it anyway. Inside the box there is a small sandwich made with white bread, plastic-looking yellow cheese and what I think may be ham. Also included are a napkin, a plastic knife, fork and spoon set, a package of mayonnaise, a small clump of grapes and a chocolate bar.

I notice the people around me have no problem consuming their snack, but I have learned to be more particular about what goes into my mouth. With the exception of the grapes and chocolate, the other food items do not pass my scrutiny for healthy food and get tossed back into the box. Knowing what to expect from airline food, I came prepared with a whole grain sandwich, an apple, and some fresh mixed nuts, choices that I think will be better for my health.

The luxury of having time to contemplate our health is a fairly recent phenomenon. One hundred years ago people in America had little opportunity to consider the matter. Consuming healthy food was not nearly as much a concern as simply having something to eat. For much of the population, having enough to eat meant back-breaking labor from dusk till dawn. Life was not easy; risks of trauma, infection and malnutrition were high.

My great grandfather was a horse-and-buggy doctor of that era. Compared to today, essentially no health care system existed in his time. All of the technology available to him was packed into a small black bag, and the nearest hospital was far, far away. The lack of adequate healthcare meant that people regularly died of diseases that could be easily treated today. Shockingly, 25% of children perished before their first year of life, and infections and accidents claimed the lives of many young adults long before they had an opportunity to develop the chronic diseases that we now commonly associate with aging.

Our present day healthcare system has done a wonderful job of relieving us of many of those past-day maladies, but the question as to whether the overall health potential of the average middle-aged American has been improved is still unanswered. A higher percentage of people are living past middle age, but are they reaching their peak life expectancy *and* their peak health expectancy? Disease is still with us, but it seems to be changing. The diseases more commonly associated with aging seem to be on the rise in younger individuals. Conditions such as diabetes, arthritis, heart disease, and most threatening of all, cancer, are becoming almost ordinary in forty- and even thirty-year-olds.

This surprising bit of reality comes at a time when our country seems to have an acute focus on health. A whopping 15% of our economy is devoted exclusively to health care. Advertisements by pharmaceutical companies now dominate television, and virtually every magazine at the newsstand regularly features articles on health. Longevity and vitality appear to be for sale. Clever displays hawk endless varieties of vitamin drinks, "healthy" snack bars, and processed "health" foods. In terms of money spent, the United States should be the healthiest place on the planet.

Even so, the majority of Americans are far from reaching their maximum health potential. The sad fact of the matter is that even with all the hype over diet and health, more people than ever are either unwilling or unsure of how to take control of their own health. The pressures of modern life tend to perpetuate unhealthy lifestyles. Though healthy food choices are widely available, people regularly eat on the run, choosing foods that are more convenient than nutritious. With most jobs being indoors, physical activity has become optional and the perceived stress of living is at an all-time high. The industrial machine that has made America great has also left us with an unparalleled mix of toxins in the environment.

Instead of focusing on health, diet and lifestyle changes are instead focused on weight loss and the treatment of disease has been left almost exclusively in the hands of pharmaceutical companies. Instead of eradicating disease, modern pharmaceuticals and surgery are allowing people to *live with* disease. Ironically, the overall health potential of the average person today may actually be declining, despite some of the best healthcare in the world.

Modern pharmaceuticals prolong life and decrease symptoms, but rarely prevent or eliminate disease. The actual incidence of disease, including cancer, is on the rise. Until we begin to address the causes of disease, instead of just treating the symptoms, the incidence of chronic disease will likely continue to rise.

We are each interested in our own personal health. Conventional medicine does offer answers and hope for some people, but there is more to health than just a prescription. All of the healthcare options at our disposal are nothing without the healing potential that lies within each of us. *The key to maximizing this healing potential is making good health choices.*

The pilot breaks in over the loudspeaker to announce our landing in Denver. Everyone on the plane seems to breathe a collective sigh of relief and individually each person prepares for landing. Finally, at the gate with the seatbelt sign off, we squash ourselves into the aisle in anticipation of the door opening. As we file out, it feels good to stretch, and some of the collective stress from being cooped up in a confined space rolls off my shoulders. Next stop is baggage claim, then on to the rental car agency and out onto the highway.

It is still early afternoon, and the traffic is not too heavy. Denver is a great city, but with the summer smog stacking up against the Rockies, I'm glad to be heading into mountains above it all. Through the haze I can make out the snow-capped peaks near Rocky Mountain National Park in the distance. I look forward to the peace, quiet, rest and relaxation that I know higher elevations will bring. For me, this is a very important health choice.

CHAPTER 2
Health and Disease in the Balance

Hiking is a favorite pastime, and Rocky Mountain National Park is a favorite place. Though I live on the coast, the Rockies offer a perfect place to "get away from it all." The park includes some of the highest mountains in the lower forty-eight. The rugged terrain and thin air challenge my abilities and test my limits. Though the trails do not change from year-to-year, my ability to conquer them certainly has.

The last time I hiked the Rockies was about three years prior, with two teenagers. Even in this short time period, I can tell a difference. My energy level is just not the same. The resilience of my younger years seems to have ebbed, and sleep does not come as easily as it once did. Certainly my condition would not be described as disease or even poor health, but it is not perfect either. I guess you could call it aging, but I'm not quite willing to accept that reality. I commonly see these same symptoms in many patients over age forty. Tiredness and loss of energy are some of the most common complaints I hear. In fact, I would say most patient's complaints are non-specific and do not amount to enough to be classified as classic textbook disease processes.

In western medicine we typically define a disease process as a collection of symptoms resulting from a derangement of the normal processes of the body. Standard training in medical school typically focuses on evaluating signs and symptoms of disease to arrive at a diagnosis, followed by treatment, usually with drugs or surgery. Goals of achieving optimal long-term health often remain secondary concerns. The seemingly most important part of evaluating disease, discovering the root causes, is most often glossed over. When the focus of therapy is directed predominantly toward relieving the signs and symptoms of disease, discovering root causes becomes somewhat irrelevant.

The western medical approach works best when patients are comfortably classified with a diagnosis. A firm diagnosis allows a specific treatment protocol, much easier for the physician and patient alike. A very large amount of our healthcare resources are devoted to defining a specific diagnosis. Even so, a significant number of patients present with non-specific symptoms that elude the label of an absolute diagnosis, complicating treatment and often leaving the patient frustrated. Over the years of practicing medicine I have been gradually shifting away from this "classify and categorize" approach toward more of a "cause and effect" approach.

Disease does not just "happen," and understanding the actual causes of disease offers insight for achieving optimal long-term health.

Disease can come on suddenly, as with an infection or accident, but most of the time disease is insidious, with symptoms occurring long before a diagnosis is evident. Looking for causes, even before a diagnosis is made, offers a whole new approach to healing. Interestingly, once you start looking for causes, you will find they are similar for many, if not most, diseases. Looking at disease in this fashion is actually simpler and alleviates the constraints of an absolute diagnosis. Primary therapy to counteract the forces of disease can begin immediately for any situation, even before symptoms begin to occur.

The next chapter is devoted to defining the causes of disease, but for now, we can collectively refer to these combined factors simply as the "forces of disease." We are continually exposed to these forces, and gradual, cumulative damage to the body is inevitable. If it were not for the healing systems of the body always at work repairing any damage that occurs, our day-to-day survival would be somewhat limited. Considering the abuse the human body receives over a lifetime (much of it self-induced), the magnitude of the healing potential of the human body is absolutely astounding.

From the day we take our first breath, a tug of war begins between the forces of disease and the healing systems of the body. This struggle will last a lifetime. If these two forces are held in balance, an equilibrium is reached that can be referred to as "good health." Early in life good health is easy to maintain because little damage has accumulated and the healing systems of the body are in prime working order. Up until age thirty most people can live anyway they want to and still expect to feel good most of the time (Figure 1). Staying out all night, smoking cigarettes, eating fast food and living life on the edge does not impact health significantly at that point.

FIGURE 1

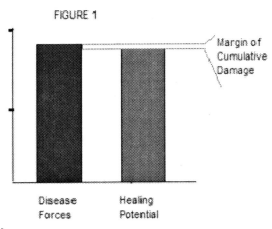

The invincibility of youth does not last forever. Without careful attention, damage caused by the forces of disease begins to add up, and the healing capacity of the body becomes compromised and cannot keep pace. As the gap widens between these two forces, the difference can be referred to as "cumulative damage." (Figure 2). Initially this discrepancy shows up as non-specific symptoms such as fatigue and loss of energy, irritability, weight gain, irregular periods, and other such complaints—because of genetic variation, symptoms may be different for different individuals. As the discrepancy becomes more pronounced, overt disease develops that can be classified, categorized, and located within the pages of a medical textbook (Figure 3).

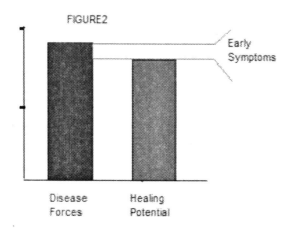

Most of us, by early- to mid-forties, will have some early symptoms of disease and will be modeled by Figure 2. By age fifty, many will be on medications and will look more like Figure 3. The whole situation is a progressive downhill slide, unless you change the way you look at disease. Understanding the underlying causes of disease allows an opportunity to regain the equilibrium of good health by appropriate lifestyle and dietary modifications. By lessening the forces of disease, the healing potential of the body will be given an opportunity to rebound—maybe not to the level of our youth, but enough to restore and maintain good health (Figure 4).

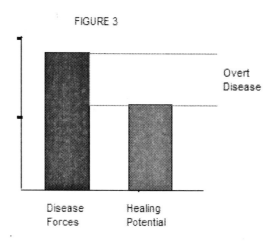

Compromises are in order, but isn't good health worth it?

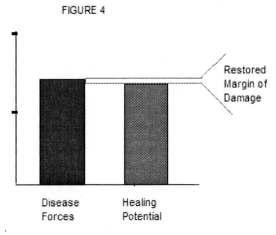

FIGURE 4

Restored Margin of Damage

Disease Forces

Healing Potential

I think about these concepts as I break through the tree line and head across the side of a mountain along a moderately steep, rocky trail. I still have some of my youthful resilience left but would like to have the energy to continue with activities of this sort for many years into the future. I can handle compromise. I have already made some changes in my diet and lifestyle and am willing to make more. Having the health to enjoy life is worth the tradeoff. With maturity and knowledge gained over the years, I can even do some things I would not have been able to accomplish in my youth. With the right compromises I can envision the possibility of my senior years being savored rather than just endured (Figure 5).

The trail leads to a saddle between two mountaintops. The vastness has the feel of being infinite. Looking out from the saddle to the east I see a small glacier made of leftover snow pack. The base lies at my feet and extends down into a valley between two shear rock faces. In the valley below, elk appear to be so close that I could touch them, yet they are a mile or more away. The air is so

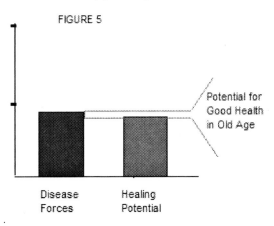

FIGURE 5

Potential for Good Health in Old Age

Disease Forces

Healing Potential

clean and dry that the views seem surreal. It is interesting how being part of such a huge expanse can bring one's personal life into focus.

Coming to grips with my own health and wellness has been important on a personal level, but it has also influenced the way I practice medicine. It started with a goal to do more than just pass out prescriptions. Addressing the causes of disease certainly makes more sense than just treating symptoms alone. I was aware that other providers across the country had incorporated alternative therapies and less toxic natural therapies into their practices with very good results, but I also knew that of all the ways that I could help my patients, none was more important than teaching them how to help themselves.

CHAPTER 3

A New Style of Healthcare

Making an effort to understand the causes of disease offers a whole new approach to the treatment of disease. Virtually all diseases can be traced back to common origins. The trick is doing something about them. Offering patients better health choices requiring substantial lifestyle changes, admittedly, is not an easy sell. Changing the way people live is such a difficult task that conventional medicine generally pays little attention to the concept. Treating symptoms is easier. I can tell you from experience that handing a patient drug samples and a prescription with a reassuring pat on the back generally goes over much better than providing good sound advice alone. The act of giving someone some "thing" feels good to the doctor and the patient alike and somehow, by itself, helps to make the situation better.

Unfortunately, the "make the situation better" part is short-lived, as side effects are common and drugs are mainly designed to treat symptoms. *Treating symptoms alone generally does not cure disease.* Symptoms worsen as the forces of disease add cumulative damage to the body, often with more drugs soon to follow. Frequently the drugs become part of the problem. For the early part of my career I practiced in this fashion. I would listen to patients' symptoms, fit them into the diagnostic category matching the proper medical code, and compassionately write out prescriptions to relieve their suffering. Sometimes it actually worked. Often, however, patients would have significant side effects to medications, would stop taking their medications all together, or would just become more ill.

As my practice evolved, I found myself asking patients about what they ate and how much stress affected their lives. I constructed a questionnaire to help me hone in on the contribution of the different factors of disease to a patient's symptom complex. This process often allowed me to bring that person "on board" in the healing process. With proper direction, the patient could take an active role in improving his or her own well-being. For a motivated individual, lifestyle and dietary changes could be—and should be—first-line therapy. Over time, this concept became as important to me as handing out a prescription.

I do understand that alleviating symptoms is an important part of therapy when someone is sick. Symptoms can be not only quite bothersome, but also frightening, and thus a barrier to healing; however, relieving symptoms should not be limited to conventional pharmaceuticals alone. Appropriate combinations of natural supplements can be as effective as drug therapy, usually with lower potential for toxicity. Yoga, meditation therapy, physical therapy, massage therapy, and acupuncture have stood the test of time as valuable healing modalities. Alleviating symptoms, while at the same time helping the patient make better health choices, is an important step toward making the patient well.

As I began to develop a reputation for offering more than just drugs, patients who had not tolerated conventional medications and therapy began to show up on my doorstep searching for other options. Often frustrated and dissatisfied, they tended to be very motivated to try whatever I had to offer. Sarah was one of those patients.

Sarah had been waiting for a diagnosis for over six weeks. She had been to see three different physicians and no one had been able to give her absolute answers. The problem started a little over a year ago when she went to her primary care provider with complaints of acid reflux and anxiety. Prescriptions were given for a medication to stop acid production in her stomach and something to calm her nerves. Both medications worked, and Sarah was able to continue with life; however, her symptoms began to reoccur and other symptoms began to develop.

The burning in her throat was only kept at bay if she took the medication every day. Gas, bloating, and abdominal cramping, which previously had been only minor annoyances, were now becoming a major concern. An evaluation by a gastroenterologist included a CT scan, colonoscopy and other tests. Except for mild esophageal irritation and early signs of an ulcer, all of the studies were negative. She was told to continue the antacid medication and was given an anti-spasm medication. In retrospect, she related that she did feel better after the endoscopies, which had included complete bowel preps, but the respite was short lived.

Her ability to handle day-to-day stress slowly began to deteriorate. Worsening anxiety often left her agitated by the end of the day. Her first panic attack was a real shock. Under the advice of her primary care provider she stepped up taking the anti-anxiety medication to several times each day. She found that she could not sleep at night without it. An anti-hypertensive drug was added to manage rising blood pressure. Routine blood tests discovered a mildly elevated fasting blood sugar, suggesting that she may also be developing adult onset diabetes. With each week she became increasingly fatigued, often to the point that working a full day was nearly impossible.

Most recently Sarah was being seen by a neurologist for symptoms of burning, tingling and numbness in her hands and feet associated with muscle pain and spasm. These symptoms were the most disconcerting of all. In her mind, a disease such as multiple sclerosis was a real concern. She had undergone a battery of tests and was now waiting for results.

By the time I saw Sarah as a patient, she was taking six different medications and felt worse than ever. At age 43 she was not happy with life and was quite sure that she had some terrible illness, yet to be diagnosed. In the past I would have had little to offer but sympathy, but by looking at her situation from a different point of view, I definitely had some positive advice. Often a thorough medical evaluation is necessary, but therapy should not await a diagnosis. Therapy in the form of reducing the causative factors of disease can begin immediately. As the healing potential of the patient recovers, symptoms often improve, even before a final diagnosis is made.

A prerequisite for using this approach is recognizing that chronic diseases involve the whole body. This is not always readily apparent. A condition as seemly simple as a fungal infection of the toe is a red flag that the entire immune system is not functioning properly. Treating only the toe and not addressing widespread immune dysfunction is an open door for other chronic conditions that will inevitably show up.

If you distinguish that chronic disease is a reflection of dysfunction in the body's healing systems, then it should not be a surprise to find so many individuals with more than one chronic disease process. Chronic sinusitis and gastrointestinal problems often go hand-in-hand. Hypertension, arthritis, diabetes and elevated cholesterol rarely show up as isolated conditions, as a majority of patients in primary care waiting rooms across America can attest. This fact alone would suggest that chronic diseases have common origins.

Many individuals, including some health care providers, have the misconception that the origins of most diseases are difficult to define; that disease just happens, and the best way to deal with disease is by treating its symptoms. This is far from being the case, as all things that occur in the natural world have causes, including disease. When I was first exploring this concept, I came upon the last chapter of my 30 year old biochemistry text (the part we never got to) which delineated the known causes of disease. A surprisingly short list of categories was offered. With further reading and research, I have refined the list a bit, but the point is that ***all diseases have common roots within a small number of well-defined categories of causes:***

1. **Oxidative stress:** exposure to free radicals generated by metabolic processes and immune system function is the most important factor in aging.
2. **Exposure to toxins:** sources suggest that upwards of 200,000 man-made chemicals have made their way into the environment over the past one hundred years.
3. **Malnutrition:** our food supply, characterized by excessive glucose and abnormal fat, is also profoundly deficient in nutrients and fiber.

4. **Emotional stress:** emotional stress plays a role in most disease processes.
5. **Physical stress:** basic wear and tear, cold and heat.
6. **Microbes:** bacteria, viruses, fungi, and protozoa have been factors of disease since life began.
7. **Radiation:** both ionizing and non-ionizing radiation have adverse effects on tissues of the human body.

GENETICS: the deciding factor. *Because we all have genes that are unique, exposure to the same sets of risk factors results in different diseases for different individuals.*

What a radical concept! *It implies that not only do all diseases have common causes but they also have common roots in prevention and treatment.* This profound bit of insight certainly begs the question: why does modern medicine seem to be ignoring this important information? The answer lies in human nature itself. Treating disease by removing the causes requires effort, whereas taking a pill is a much easier way to control symptoms. Also, the causes of disease are very much a part of life itself and eliminating them would be impossible. Lessening their impact, however, *is* an option—one to which more of us should be paying attention. *Understanding these causative factors offers a unique opportunity to alter our destiny.* We can, in essence, cut disease off at the pass just by making intelligent choices in the way we conduct our lives.

Before I could help Sarah with changes that she was going to have to make to alter her own destiny, I needed her to understand these basic concepts. Even when an absolute diagnosis seems elusive, identifying causative factors can open an avenue toward healing. Knowing everything there is to know about the causes of disease is not necessary, but a basic understanding of these factors does answer many questions that patients have about illness. Gaining this type of knowledge offers the patient control and alleviates fear. This, in itself, is a positive healing force.

Understanding basic information about the causes of disease is an absolute necessity for understanding health. Just as it would be unwise to enter a battle without obtaining intelligence information about the enemy, it would be unwise to try to improve your health without knowing about the forces working in opposition to that goal.

THE SEVEN BASIC CAUSES OF DISEASE

Any discussion about the causes of disease must start with a living cell. There are thousands of different types of cells in the human body, but they all share some common features. A living cell can be thought of three-dimensionally as a blob of gel surrounded by a thin membrane holding it all together. Suspended in the middle, almost like an egg yolk, is the nucleus. The nucleus contains chromosomes that hold DNA, the blueprint for all vital functions of the cell. Also suspended within the gel that we call "cytoplasm" are the functional parts of the cell. *All functions of the cell require energy; yet, paradoxically, this basic necessity of life is the root of one of the main causes of aging and disease.*

1 OXIDATIVE STRESS

Oxidative stress, a term unfamiliar to most people, is possibly the most significant overall factor in aging. The most ubiquitous factor of disease, oxidative stress, is continuously present in all living things and is definitely one to know something about. Cancer, atherosclerosis, arthritis, and inflammatory conditions all have direct links to oxidative stress; in fact, most disease processes have some link to oxidative stress. What is this peculiar-sounding term? The answer is right under your nose.

Take in a deep breath. About 20% of the air you just inhaled is composed of oxygen. Oxygen, a necessity of life that we sometimes take for granted, is actually a potently toxic substance. It is so toxic, in fact, that it took life on earth a couple of billion years to figure out how to use it in energy production.

All living things derive energy by breaking down molecules containing hydrogen and carbon. Fat and sugar are examples of hydrocarbon molecules. When the chemical bonds of hydrocarbon molecules are broken, a small amount of energy is released. Production of energy from this basic chemical reaction was enough to get life started here on earth, but only allowed a marginal foothold. More energy was a necessity for life to truly thrive—oxygen was the key ingredient. Throwing oxygen into the mix was like throwing gasoline onto a fire; an organism could produce ten times the amount of energy from the same amount of hydrocarbon. This little metabolic trick turned out to be the real key to the success of life on earth....but it came with a price.

In high school science class you learned that plants use energy from the sun to make glucose and animal cells, in turn, can use glucose as a primary energy source or can turn it into fat for storage of energy. The basic chemical reaction of combining glucose or fat with oxygen to release energy with the end products of water and carbon dioxide completes one of the most important cycles of life.

$$C_6H_{12}O_6 \text{ (glucose)} + O_2 \rightarrow CO_2 + H_2O + \text{ENERGY!}$$

For this seemly simple reaction to occur, the oxygen molecule must break apart into two very reactive components. These reactive components are "electron greedy" and pluck electrons off of molecules such as glucose. When exposed to these reactive components, the glucose molecule becomes unstable, and the chemical bonds are easily broken, thus releasing energy.

The reactive oxygen components belong to a wider group of chemical substances generically referred to as "free radicals." Free radicals occur in most kinds of chemical reactions and, of course, there are many chemical reactions occurring in the human body at any given second. The fact that free radicals propel a chemical reaction in a forward direction is necessary for life to occur, but with any given reaction, there is always collateral damage. These reactive chemical substances steal electrons from other adjacent molecules, thus damaging and weakening vital components of a living cell.

The process of free radicals "stealing" electrons from other molecules is called oxidation, and it occurs in nature almost continuously. Rust is an example of oxidation. To visualize the process of oxidation in action, cut an apple in half and leave it on the counter. Oxidation is represented by the brown color that rapidly forms when the cut surface is exposed to oxygen in the air. The peel would normally protect the apple from oxidation.

Take another apple, cut it in half, and rub lime juice all over the cut surface. Notice the apple does not turn brown as rapidly. The vitamin C in the lime acts as an antioxidant that protects the tissue from oxidation. Vitamin C and a host of other antioxidants protect us internally from oxidation. We could not survive without antioxidants.

Within living cells, energy production is confined to small, oval-shaped structures called "mitochondria" that are strategically distributed throughout the cytoplasm. Think of them as microscopic power plants, constantly churning out raw energy. Free radicals are an obligatory byproduct of this intense energy production. Not being completely contained within the mitochondria, free radicals shoot off like sparks in every direction. Like microscopic firecrackers going off inside the cell, they have the propensity to damage all structures, including cell membranes, proteins that compose the functional parts of the cell, and very importantly, our DNA. No structures, however, take more of the brunt of the damage than the mitochondria themselves. *A gradual decline in energy production by damaged mitochondria is one reason we slow down as we age.*

Though all cells of the body are exposed to the damaging effects of free radicals, some carry more of a burden than others. The cells of metabolically active tissues require more energy and, therefore, have a higher propensity for damage. Everything from muscle atrophy as we grow older to dementia in the elderly is at least partially a result of damage by free radicals. This same process very likely contributes to hormonal decline as we age. Damage to our DNA from continual exposure to free radicals almost certainly plays a role in the development of cancer. *Estimates suggest that the DNA within each cell in the body receives an average of 100 "hits" from free radicals each day.*

The good news is that our cells have very effective, innate repair mechanisms that have evolved over time. Enzymatic processes are constantly repairing breaks in DNA, repairing damaged machinery and filling in defects in cell membranes. These are the most basic healing functions of the body. Healing processes can, however, become overwhelmed by free radical production. Cell survival is very dependent on a diverse group of substances known as *anti-oxidants*. These chemicals have the ability to neutralize free radicals before they have an opportunity to damage vital elements of the cell. Cells have the ability to generate anti-oxidants, but dietary sources of anti-oxidants are also vitally important.

Free radical production is not limited to the inside of cells. Other types of free radicals can be found within the body. Free radicals are actually generated by cells of the immune system to do away with offending substances and invaders. This process occurs in the bloodstream and spaces between cells. It is a vital part of the healing systems of the body. A certain amount of this "inflammatory process" is in our best interest, but an exaggerated inflammatory response is a root cause of many diseases, from arthritis to atherosclerosis.

Free radicals can come directly from dietary sources. The most notorious of the dietary offenders, oxidized fat, is commonly found in processed food products of all types, processed meats, and food products that have become spoiled. Oxidized fats are especially concerning because they have the propensity to set off chain reactions in other fats, from cholesterol-containing lipoproteins in the bloodstream to cell membranes of all the cells in the body.

In the constant tug-of-war between these opposing forces, damage from free radicals always holds a little bit of an upper hand. This net balance in favor of free radical damage is termed *oxidative stress*. Oxidative stress is a potent force of disease. Minimizing oxidative stress is the key to slowing the process of aging. Fortunately for us, there are lots of different types of anti-oxidants, both naturally occurring inside the body and available from dietary sources.

Turning back our biological clock is impossible and oxidative stress is as much a part of life as breathing oxygen itself, but the burden of oxidative stress can be influenced by choice of diet and how we live our lives. Fresh vegetables and fruit are loaded with anti-oxidants and can definitely shift the balance in our favor. Unfortunately, only a minority of Americans take advantage of this simple opportunity to protect themselves from this significant factor in aging and disease. Even worse, the average American diet actually contributes to oxidative stress. Fats and oils used in processed foods, refined using high heat and chemicals, can become potent free radicals. That hotdog may taste good, but the contents are potentially deadly.

Blood tests are now available to check your "anti-oxidant potential," but testing is rarely necessary for individuals following a healthy diet. An enormous variety of different anti-oxidants can be obtained from natural food sources. Testing for excessive inflammation in the blood stream may, however, be worthwhile as it is a root cause of atherosclerosis. Ask your healthcare provider about having blood testing for "C-reactive protein."

2 TOXINS AND ALLERGENS

Well off the coast of Nova Scotia lies Sable Island, an isolated sand spit created by eddies between the Labrador Current and the Gulf Stream. At this remote outpost, a weather station monitors climatic changes and airborne toxins. Recently, Cruising World magazine featured a sailing trip to Sable Island. These quotes from the article poignantly illustrate the degree of concern we face as a culture:

> *"...on an island that seems so remote and pristine were instruments measuring ever-increasing levels of industrial aerosols, chemical insecticides and herbicides, methane, carbon dioxide, and other human-generated carcinogens, pollutants, and greenhouse gases."*

> *"Because of its location at the edge of the continent, Sable is in a unique location for making such measurements," stated the keeper of the station. "When the winds are easterly, we measure only traces of these substances. But when they blow from the west, well, then many of the measurements go off the scale, and Sable might as well be at the end of a huge, continental sewer pipe."*

Though some substances considered toxic to humans occur in nature, our world is gradually becoming saturated by toxic substances created by man. The conveniences of modern life have come with a price. The evolution of an industrial society has brought with it the introduction of an unprecedented amount of man-made chemicals into the environment, all having at least some potential for toxicity. Most sources suggest the list of man-made chemicals now tops 200,000, the majority of which were non-existent one hundred years ago. Initially, as man-made chemicals made their way into the air, the water, and across the surface of the land, it seemed the environment was like a huge sponge that could absorb it all, but eventually the level of toxins started to add up. We first saw it with fish kills along the coast and declining bird populations, but there is little doubt that toxins in the environment also contribute to human disease.

In some respects we have become more "toxin aware" over the past fifty years, as open industrial waste-sites are less prevalent and many cities are making vigorous efforts to clean up their act, yet environmental toxins have become more pervasive than ever before. Our thirst for energy is high, and present regulations are not sufficient to protect the environment from pollutants released when millions of tons of coal are burned each year to produce electricity. Automobiles are designed to pollute less, but more people own cars and commute long distances. Chemical use in agriculture is still quite prevalent. *Everything* is made of plastic. Not only is the manufacture of plastics toxic, but plastics also leach toxins into the environment continually for a lifetime. Toxins of many varieties can be found in our food, in the water we drink and in the air we breathe...where we work, where we play, and in our homes.

Toxins have made their way into our environment insidiously. Rarely are concentrations of specific toxins high enough to be implicated in a specific disease process, yet common sense and a steadily rising cancer rate would suggest a cause for concern. We have come to accept toxins as being part of our everyday world, but our complacency means that the ever-increasing concentration of toxins in the environment is a real contributor to disease and adds up in ways that you would not expect.

When humans living in industrial areas of the world are randomly tested for toxins, the findings are alarming. A stew of chemicals including styrene (found in Styrofoam, plastic containers and computers), trichloroethylene (dry cleaning), dioxins (bleaching agents), PFC's (nonstick cookware), phthalates (plastic, vinyl, nail polish), PCB's, pesticides, xylene (plastics) and many others are routinely discovered. When laboratory animals are subjected to these chemicals individually, cancers and terrible diseases result—imagine the effect if they are all mixed together. (www.pollutioninpeople.org).

It is now common knowledge that larger fish such as swordfish are contaminated with mercury, but have you ever considered why? Certainly the ocean is not saturated with mercury, but it has to come from somewhere. Surprisingly, for fish in the Atlantic Ocean, the source is coal-fired power plants on the North American continent. Coal is high in mercury. Mercury and many other pollutants carried in the smoke precipitate onto the land and are washed into estuaries by rain or precipitate directly onto the surface of the ocean. Micro-organisms take up the pollutants, and in turn, are eaten by larger animals. With each step up the food chain mercury is further concentrated in the animal's tissues. The cycle continues until the highest concentrations are found in the largest animals in the ocean. This food chain phenomenon is not limited to fish. Many airborne pollutants end up in our water and food supply via this mechanism. Toxins accumulate in fatty tissues of *all* animals, including and especially humans.

Toxic heavy metals including aluminum, antimony, beryllium, bismuth, cadmium, lead, mercury, thallium, uranium are much more prevalent in the environment today than ever before. Mining brings these elements to the surface from deep in the earth. Living organisms, having never been exposed to these elements to any significant degree, are at significant risk. Illnesses in children associated with exposure to lead and birth defects in newborns associated high levels of mercury in humans are cause for grave concern. Warning about consumption of certain fish is now a standard part of pre-conceptual counseling.

We deal with a similar phenomenon in agriculture. Chemicals used in agriculture are certainly toxic to pests and their use in production of grains, vegetables, and fruit should be of concern, but because concentrations of pesticide residue are not high, regulatory agencies such as the FDA suggest that traces of man-made chemicals found in our produce are not enough to worry about....but *should* we worry?

Most of the chemicals used in agriculture are fat soluble, and plants generally have very little fat. It is true that toxic chemicals mostly end up as a residue on the surface of the vegetable or present in small amounts within the oil-containing germ of grains. The actual measurable concentration of chemicals is low. Even so, environmental toxins found in our food are very real contributors to disease. The key to the concern lies in the fact that most toxic chemicals are fat soluble, and, even when consumed in minute amounts, these substances accumulate and concentrate within the fatty tissues of any living organism that consumes them. *The more fatty tissue, the higher the level of concern.*

Livestock and poultry fed a continuous diet of toxin-tainted grain, concentrate these subtle amounts of chemicals into their fatty tissues. Mostly confined to tight quarters with little ability to move around, these animals have a higher tendency to retain toxins. Hormones, which are also fat soluble, are widely used in this industry. The result is meat that is excessively fatty and may contain concerning levels of toxic chemicals. Often these chemicals are hormonally active. Humans, being right up there at the top of the food chain, in essence get a double dose of toxins when they consume meat from animals raised in this fashion.

Ever wonder about the association between breast cancer and consumption of red meat? Think about it: any toxins or hormonally active substances found in the fat of that nice juicy hamburger or steak are further concentrated in the fatty tissues of the individual consuming it. Hormonally sensitive breast tissue is predominantly fat and that's where toxins may end up.

Most of the time the role toxins play in chronic disease is only a piece of the puzzle, but occasionally it can be a major factor. Not infrequently, I have been able to provide direction and hope to individuals with chronic disease just by asking questions that others had not asked. I can remember one patient who owned a cleaning business and was exposed to potent chlorinated chemicals on a daily basis. Chronic fatigue and chronic sinus infections had developed insidiously over several years. She had been through the gamut of antibiotics, anti-inflammatory medications, and antihistamines with a progressively worsening condition. While seeing her for a routine exam, I suggested that avoiding chemical exposure was the only way she would ever get well. A complete lifestyle change is a tough recommendation, but after several years of no improvement, she finally sold the business. Once free of the toxins, her symptoms gradually resolved completely.

There have been numerous patients since then: the farmer with chronic sinus abscesses who was regularly exposed to chemical pesticides; a manicurist who spent her days inhaling nail polish and could not get rid of vaginal yeast infections; and numerous patients with headaches and other odd complaints who work in retail businesses where the air is always saturated with the smell of plastic. None of them had had improvement with conventional medical therapy. Resolution of these problems could only be expected with removal of the inciting factors. We would all do well to be more "toxin aware," as sometimes even the most obvious sources of toxins do not seem so obvious.

Exposure to toxins is sometimes self-inflicted. Smoking cigarettes and chewing tobacco are at top on the list. Alcohol is definitely a toxin (admittedly, in moderate amounts this toxic effect seems to be balanced by other, beneficial ingredients in wine and beer.) It goes without saying that illicit street drugs are harmful. Though pharmaceuticals are delivered in non-toxic and often beneficial doses, most have the potential for toxicity. Many, if not most drugs poison enzymes in the body to achieve a desired result. All drugs have the potential for side effects. Many drugs have the potential for tolerance, dependence, and withdrawal syndromes. *Ironically, many drugs used therapeutically for treatment of chronic disease are known to suppress the immune system, certainly not in keeping with an intended goal of therapy meant to improve health.*

Often the only difference between a beneficial drug and a toxin is the dose. Therapeutic medications have great value, but their potential for toxicity must be respected.

Because toxins come from so many diverse sources, they exert their negative effects in different ways. All biochemical reactions within the body can be, in effect, "poisoned" by different toxins. Toxins can directly damage DNA. Some toxins generate free radicals or are free radicals themselves, increasing our burden of oxidative stress. This is a major factor in diseases such as atherosclerosis and arthritis. Many toxins derived from pesticides and plastics have the potential to mimic hormones in the human body, providing a direct link to hormonally active cancers such as breast, uterine and prostate.

It is estimated that at least half of man-made toxins have the ability to affect hormone systems in the human body in some way.

Occasionally, as in the case of therapeutic drugs, these effects are desirable, but most often they are unwanted or harmful. Toxins tax the healing systems of the body and cause damage to the immune system allowing increased susceptibility to disease. The effects are subtle, but cumulative over time; measuring the exact contribution toxins make to disease is virtually impossible.

Fortunately for us, the body does have the ability to eliminate toxins via a very sophisticated detoxification system. As we have come to know, most toxins are fat soluble. To be eliminated by the kidneys and intestinal tract they must be converted into water soluble substances. This process occurs almost exclusively in the liver. Eliminating toxins is dirty business. The detoxification process produces free radicals that over time cause damage to the cells of the liver. As we age, this affects not only our ability to remove toxins, but other functions of the liver as well.

Be kind to your liver. Become more "toxin aware" by minimizing everyday sources of toxins. Not smoking cigarettes and acquiring adequate protection from occupational exposure to toxins goes without saying. Regular consumption of antioxidants provided by a diet high in fresh vegetables and fruit helps protect liver function. Vegetables from the cruciferous family such as cabbage and broccoli are especially protective of liver function. Dietary fiber provided by vegetables, fruit and whole grains is essential for adequate toxin removal. Drinking plenty of water helps flush things through. Exercise facilitates removal of toxins via increased blood flow and sweat is a route of elimination for some toxins.

Testing for a number of different types of toxins via hair samples or blood tests is available and can be considered by individuals with chronic disease or who have higher than average exposure. Testing for heavy metals is also available, but the testing is more complex. Individuals retain toxins

differently depending upon the person's genetics, liver function and amount of body fat.

ALLERGENS

Allergens can be simply defined as substances that induce allergic reactions. Allergic reactions are hyper-reactive responses of the immune system, causing symptoms. People can have allergic reactions to many different substances. Substances defined as allergens are generally nontoxic to the majority of individuals, who lack sensitivity to that substance. In contrast, toxins are substances that cause harm to *all* living things, to one degree or another.

Types of allergies and the degree of reactions vary widely. The most common allergic reactions occur to airborne substances such as dust, mold, pollen, and animal dander. Allergic reactions of the skin can be manifested directly (as with poison ivy) or can be a reflection of an internal allergic response (as in the case of a drug reaction or a bee sting). Typical symptoms of allergic reactions include watery eyes, runny nose, sneezing, itching and swelling of the skin and mucous membranes. Severe reactions include difficulty breathing and shock. Onset of symptoms associated with an allergic reaction is immediate.

Allergic reactions to foods can be severe, but true food allergies are not actually all that common. True food allergies must be differentiated from food sensitivities, which are relatively common. Food sensitivities are generally associated with gastrointestinal dysfunction and immune hyper-stimulation. Typically, multiple foods are involved. Unlike symptoms of true allergy which are immediate, symptoms of food sensitivities are highly variable, nonspecific and generally delayed for hours or even days from the time the food is consumed.

Almost anything can cause an allergic reaction. Everyone has allergies to something. Mine is a most convenient allergy—contact of my skin with raw shrimp causes an immediate and intense allergic reaction with itching and swelling, but as long as someone else heads, peels, cleans, and cooks them for me, I can eat all I want. My son's allergy is even more convenient— his reaction to poison ivy is severe enough to get him out of most of the yard work.

In some rare individuals, allergies can be life-threatening. Even brief exposure can mean a trip to the hospital or death. For most individuals, however, allergies are a non-life-threatening irritation. In average people, allergies become a significant problem only when the immune system becomes dysfunctional. Other factors of disease including poor diet, toxins, stress and microbes can contribute to immune dysfunction. Immune dysfunction contributes to other disease processes such as atherosclerosis and arthritis—everything is interrelated.

The obvious way to avoid an allergic reaction is by avoiding the offending allergen, but when the immune system is in a hyper-reactive state, exposure to a single trigger can set off a cascade of reactions. Allergy testing can be beneficial for identifying specific allergens, but better health practices in general are beneficial for calming a hyper-stimulated immune system and reducing the intensity and frequency of allergic reactions.

3 POOR NUTRITION

You can tell a lot about a person's health just by examining what he or she eats. As much as the wrong foods can cause ill health, the right foods can be protective from damage resulting from other factors of disease. Ironically, here in one of the wealthiest countries on the planet, many (if not most) people are suffering from malnutrition. Not the protein-deficiency malnutrition found in the third world, but a form that is self-imposed. The prefix "mal" literally translates to mean "bad" and the types of "bad" nutrition that we suffer from result mainly from excesses rather than deficiencies. The average American diet contains gross excesses of sugar and abnormal fat. This shift in balance caused by excessive food processing occurs at the expense of fiber and nutrients found in natural foods that are so vital for good health.

When it comes to food, you can almost think of it as being living or dead. Living food, as you would expect, appears in its original form—a stick of broccoli, a carrot or fresh shrimp. Living food provides for much more than a source of energy. Minerals, fiber, healthy fats, natural enzymes and all of the nutrients essential for good health can be found in forms that are easily and naturally assimilated by the body. These vital nutrients are hard to duplicate.

A tasteless, hard pear, if left in the windowsill long enough, will ripen into a soft, sweet delicacy. During ripening, the deeper flesh is protected from oxidation by the tough outer skin. Ripening occurs as enzymes present in the fruit break down the hard tissue into sugar. When we consume the pear, natural enzymes aid digestion.

There are many types of enzymes present in different types of living food. Beyond digestion, the body has the ability to absorb certain enzymes for use in other ways. Enzymes that break down proteins, called proteases, have anti-inflammatory properties and may protect against atherosclerosis. Processed food is totally devoid of natural enzymes.

All the qualities that make living food desirable (highly absorbable nutrients, just the right balance of sugars and favorable fats, antioxidants and digestive enzymes) also make living food highly susceptible to spoilage. Food preservation, especially when it includes chemical preservatives, decreases the nutritional value of food. Living food is best when consumed at the peak of freshness. Fortunately, we live in a time when fresh food is more available than ever before.

The average American diet contains little food that resembles its natural origins. Food that has been pounded, pulverized, over-cooked and over-processed could certainly be classified as dead. Dead food has no resemblance to the original food source and almost exclusively comes in a synthetically derived form—always with an over-abundance of starch, sugar and fat, designed only to appeal to our senses of smell and taste. If there are any significant nutrients present, they are usually synthetically derived additives that never match the nutrient potential of real food. Most often this type of food comes in a package or a box that is also designed to appeal to our senses.

"Factory farms" and industrial food production could easily be targeted as the source of our dietary woes, but we can only blame ourselves. The commercial food industry only gives us what we want. We have a natural craving for foods that are high in sugar and fat because the immediate need for energy is preferential over other nutritional requirements. This is quite a change from how it has been for most of human history. For many thousands of years humans were relegated to a very high fiber, high nutrient, low energy diet—not by choice, but by availability. With the advent of choice, our natural cravings pushed us to consume a diet very in high energy, but otherwise deficient in vital nutrients and fiber.

Reliance on high-energy, processed foods is the root cause of the American epidemic of obesity that has evolved over the past fifty years. Excessive body fat is associated with increased risk of heart disease, increased wear and tear on joints and ligaments, increased risk of certain types of cancer and increased risk of chronic disease in general. Often "central" obesity is accompanied by an alarming collection of signs and symptoms including *elevated fasting blood glucose, hypertension, decreased HDL cholesterol and increased blood triglycerides.* This condition, referred to as *insulin resistance syndrome, metabolic syndrome* or *syndrome* X, now affects somewhere between 25% and 50% of the population.

Obesity, once established, is not an easy problem to overcome. The first and most important goal in any successful weight-loss strategy is regaining lost health. The advice and guidelines in this book are designed to address this primary goal. Actual weight loss will occur gradually over time just by staying with good health practices. The weight loss process can be augmented with therapy designed to rectify hormonal imbalances and increase metabolism. For optimal results, therapy should be directed by a qualified healthcare provider. In cases of extreme obesity surgical procedures are often indicated and can be life-altering.

The shift in our food supply has occurred within a period of only a hundred years—almost overnight in relative terms, and certainly not enough time for the human body to adapt to such a drastic change. Though it is more convenient for a busy American lifestyle, the overall costs in terms of human health are enormous. Our total healthcare expenditure would be dramatically reduced if the American populace simply started making better food choices.

An ideal diet should consist predominantly of whole vegetables and whole seeds (grains, nuts, and beans), followed by whole fruits and rounded out with a variety of free range meats, seafood, and carefully chosen oils. Better choices in food slow the absorption of glucose, strengthen cell membranes, decrease inflammation, provide fiber for optimal digestion and toxin removal, and provide for optimal nutrients and minerals. Though most Americans are regularly making poor food choices, good food choices are more available than ever before. We are truly living in the "Golden age of food"—if you take the time to look for it.

4 EMOTIONAL STRESS

It was the first day of summer when Mary returned with a chronic cough. She had been battling respiratory infections through the winter and spring, receiving numerous courses of antibiotics. With each course of antibiotics she would come down with a vaginal yeast infection and come to see me. "Why do I keep getting this stuff?" she complained. Her evaluation had so far had included a normal chest X-ray and a negative tuberculosis test. Allergies did not seem to be a factor and I could not ascertain that she had been exposed an unusual burden of toxins. Something was, however, having an adverse effect on her immune system and my next question brought out the reason. When asked how much she was sleeping, she answered, "about five hours on a good night." Emotionally it had been a terrible year for her and she rated her stress level as being extremely high. When these issues were addressed her condition gradually began to improve.

Day-to-day living causes a certain amount of emotional stress that is not detrimental from a health point of view. Stress can be a motivational factor that gets us going on to the next thing in life. Emotional stress only becomes a problem when it begins to rob the healing potential of the body. For many individuals this is every day. Well recognized as the root of anxiety and depression, emotional stress can aggravate virtually all disease processes. When patients ask if emotional stress could be playing a role in their particular problem, my answer is always a definitive "yes." Understanding and managing stress is an important adjunct in the treatment of *all* diseases.

For simplification, we can think of the body as having an "alert mode" and a "healing mode." Classically, the "alert mode" would be induced by a confrontation or threat such as having a dog run out in front of your car. With a surge of adrenaline, pulse quickens, eyes become wide, breathing rate increases, and muscles tense. All resources of the body are directed toward dealing with that threat. Other general maintenance functions, such as digesting food, normal immune functions, and daily maintenance and repair are placed on hold. Assuming the brakes work and the dog is fast, the threat passes, the mind relaxes, and the body goes back to normal affairs.

In an average American life, however, confrontations of some sort are seemingly a minute-by-minute affair. We never get a break. Excessive daily stress constantly places us in alert mode and prevents day-to-day repair and maintenance from occurring. The link between stress and diseases such as hypertension, autoimmune diseases, atherosclerosis and even cancer should be obvious. With a stressful lifestyle, we unknowingly place normal gastrointestinal function at a level of low priority while at the same time bolting down unhealthy food on the run. Is it any wonder that drugs for gastro-intestinal maladies are some of the best-sellers on pharmacy shelves?

The body is continually in the process of damage control and general maintenance, but it needs resources to do so. The energy and resources of the body are most devoted toward healing when they are not taxed in other ways. This "healing mode," as I like to refer to it, occurs when the body and mind are completely relaxed. Healing occurs most intensely during deeper stages of sleep. As we age, chronic disruptions in hormonal systems prevent the body from relaxing properly and sleep becomes less efficient.

Ironically, at a time in life when we would seem to need sleep the most, restful sleep is hard to gain. Learning tools to encourage spontaneous relaxation of the body and the mind become immensely important as we age.

5 PHYSICAL STRESS

Another type of stress that is part of day-to-day life is basic *wear and tear*. The daily grinding down of bones, joints, and teeth is to a certain extent unavoidable, but here again, there are ways to lessen some of the impact. First and foremost, staying at a healthy weight prevents undue stress on joints and ligaments. A healthy diet certainly contributes to maintaining healthy joints, ligaments, and bones. The right combination of dietary fats can actually decrease the inflammation of joints associated with arthritis. Exercise done appropriately with proper stretching ahead of time and practicing disciplines such as yoga lessen the effects of wear and tear on the body.

Physical stress can tax the healing systems of the body as much as any other stress. Extremes in temperature can be quite debilitating. Excessive cold is something that few of us are threatened with today, but cold temperatures have been an ever present concern to those who have ventured toward the most northern and southern regions of the globe.

I have always been fascinated with the story of Ernest Shackleton, who, in 1914, set out with a crew of 28 men on an attempt to cross the Antarctic continent by dogsled. Early on, their ship was trapped in an ice flow and crushed. The band of intrepid adventurers spent nine months moving with the ice flow until they escaped to desolate Elephant Island via three remaining lifeboats. Shackleton, with a crew of five men, sailed one of the lifeboats across 800 miles of inhospitable southern ocean to seek rescue. He survived the harrowing journey and returned months later to find all crew members alive.

Shackleton's adventure was one of a number of expeditions to the northern and southern poles that occurred during that time in history. What sets his experience apart was that the crew survived horrendous conditions for an astoundingly long period of time with no loss of life and minimal loss of limb. Different from other expeditions, they decided early on to supplement their food supply with seal blubber. Toward the end, this made up a large portion of their diet. Seal blubber contains very high amounts of omega-3 fatty acids, and I, for one, believe that diet was a key factor in their survival. Their blood was like antifreeze! Today the harvest of seals is appropriately banned and seal blubber probably contains much higher levels of toxins than it did in 1914, but regularly consuming other sources of omega 3 fatty acids certainly makes sense for many health reasons.

Most of us would rather be hot than cold, but extreme heat, especially dry heat can be quite threatening. Excessive heat and dehydration are becoming more of a concern as the world heats up. In 2003 Europe experienced the hottest summer on record. The loss of 35,000 lives could be attributed to either the heat itself or crop shortfalls associated with the drought. As the population of the world continues to expand and the atmosphere becomes hotter, severe heat waves and shortages of food production across the globe are something with which we will all have to contend.

Trauma, another physical stress, affects all of us during our lifetimes to one degree or another, but is less of a threat than in days gone by. Before about 1920, trauma was a major contributor to decreased life expectancy. Today, trauma and accidents are minor factors. As much as I would like to attribute this shift to people having better sense, we owe it all to "big brother." Rules, regulations, and government bureaucracies make us wear our seat belts, force manufacturers of automobiles and machines to make safer products, and in general, make our world a safer place. Even so, being ever careful and ever vigilant is a wise practice.

6 MICROBES

Microbes rule the world. They always have and they always will. Historically, infectious diseases have caused more death and devastation over the years than war and all of the other causes of disease combined. Even today, infectious diseases are the leading cause of death worldwide. Modern antibiotics and vaccines have made inroads into cutting the loss of life, but this is chiefly in developed countries. The plague and the pox have given way to AIDS and influenza as causes of worldwide devastation. Gonorrhea, syphilis, and the common cold have never left us. Lyme disease is now widespread across North America and Europe.

Interestingly, the most successful microbes are not the most lethal. Success in the microbe world is defined by the ability to propagate and flourish. Killing or severely disabling the host can be counterproductive. Take your average common cold virus. The virus infects, propagates rapidly, and quickly spreads to another host before the initial host's immune system catches up with it. The minimally disabled host organism actively participates in viral spread. Cold viruses may be the most successful microbes on earth.

Though the production of vaccines in the late nineteenth century and effective antibiotics in the mid-twentieth century can be recognized as major contributors to increased life expectancy, we can mainly thank government bureaucracies and social services for the improved health we enjoy today. Improved sanitation and health standards have done more to protect us from infectious disease than anything else has. As much as I hate to sign over a portion of my paycheck every month to Uncle Sam, the cost of this part of our "social good" is worth paying.

A visit to a third world country is a real eye-opener. Well beyond the lack of funds to buy antibiotics and vaccines, the lack of sanitation and public health in third world countries translates into poor health for most of the population. Standards that we take for granted such as indoor plumbing, public restrooms, restaurant grading, and garbage collection are often rare. Health standards, in the way that we know them, do not exist. As a result, diseases such as cholera are still common. Tuberculosis and malaria are present now as much as ever before.

In developed countries, microbes have seemingly taken a back seat to other causes of disease, but be assured, they are still there—seen and unseen. Microbes contribute to disease in ways that you would not expect. There is evidence that diseases like juvenile-onset diabetes, multiple sclerosis, and cervical cancer are initiated by viral infections and malfunctions in the immune system. Many cases of chronic fatigue syndrome have been found to have an association with a history of Lyme disease and other microbial illnesses. Some speculate that all autoimmune diseases may have microbial origins.

Some of the most successful microbes are those that go unnoticed. Again, the goal of a successful microbe is not to kill or even severely disable the host. They propagate and flourish in the background, producing chemical substances that inhibit or control the immune system and neurological system, all the while remaining completely concealed. To us, these chemical substances are toxins and though they make us feel miserable, they may not significantly shorten our lifespan. At some point we may find that many diseases have roots to microbes that are presently concealed from our detection.

As much as microbes can be the enemy, certain microbes are our allies in many ways. Favorable bacteria inhabiting our skin and internal passageways prevent infections from pathogenic microbes. We actually could not survive without the help of the normal flora of bacteria within our gastrointestinal tract. These bacteria aid in digestion, convert vitamins into active forms, and help us rid ourselves of toxins.

Poor dietary habits and overuse of antibiotics can contribute to overgrowth of pathologic strains of bacteria in places where we depend on friendly bacteria. Toxins produced by abnormal bacteria not only cause problems in the gastrointestinal tract but also have effects that are far reaching. In understanding this connection, it is not surprising to find studies that link excessive antibiotic use to breast cancer. Even diseases such as depression and autism have links to bowel function altered by bacterial imbalances.

There are two main strategies for preventing disease caused by microbial infections: avoiding exposure and maintaining a healthy immune system. Accumulated knowledge of how bacteria, viruses, fungi, and parasites function allows us a better chance to avoid crossing paths, but complete avoidance is, of course, impossible. Our best chance of staying healthy in a world dominated by microbes is to keep our defenses up. Free radicals, toxins, and excessive stress tax the immune system. Good nutrition, regular exercise, and stress reduction best support a healthy immune system.

7 ENERGY

$E=MC^2$, the common equation that defines that all matter is made of energy. We are beings of energy—most specifically a type of energy called electromagnetic energy. Our energy fields can actually be sensed by certain gifted individuals and are the basis of several forms of traditional medicine. Acupuncture uses well-placed needles in the skin and tissues to affect these energy fields in a positive way to rid us of certain symptoms. Modern medicine studies our energy fields for diagnosis of certain problems. An EKG measures the dynamic energy fields produced by the heart to diagnose many types of cardiac malfunction. An EEG machine measures electrical waves produced by the brain. An instrument called an MRI measures the electromagnetic energy of tissues to produce a picture of our internal organs. This unique technology is able to do this without causing any known damage.

MRI does not cause internal damage because electromagnetic energy is "non-ionizing." In other words, radiation from electromagnetic sources does not have the ability to strike and damage the internal components of our cells. Even so, a very difficult question to answer is how much our own energy fields are affected by energy fields around us. Most of us now exist in an environment saturated with conflicting sources of electromagnetic energy such as computers, hair dryers, and other electrical devices. How many times have you felt "out of sorts" after sitting beside a computer all day? The magnitude of this problem is unknown and difficult to evaluate, but probably does play a role in disease.

Other, more concerning forms of energy include X-rays, gamma rays, and UV rays. These types of radiation definitely have the ability to do damage to our tissues. Referred to as "ionizing" radiation, they act very much like free radicals. They have the ability to pass through the body and "hit" microscopic structures, causing damage. They also have the ability to create free radicals. Some forms of ionizing radiation such as X-rays and gamma rays can pass completely through the body, whereas, others such as UV radiation only pass "skin deep." Exposure to some ionizing radiation is unavoidable. We are constantly exposed to "background" radiation from the depths of the universe and from the sun.

The ionizing rays of the sun penetrate the skin and strike other molecules, generating free radicals. Free radical damage to cells and structures within the skin is a direct link to wrinkling, aging of the skin, and skin cancer. Sunscreen may be the best protection, but, surprisingly, a diet rich in anti-oxidants may be almost as valuable. I once heard a story about a fellow who had a habit of consuming a large container of juiced carrots and vegetables every day. They say he had a strange orange glow about him, but he was able to cruise the entire Caribbean in a small sailboat without a drop of sunscreen.

Exposure to some background radiation will always be unavoidable, but I wonder about how much effect nuclear testing and the use of nuclear reactors around the world have added to our daily exposure. As individuals we have very little say in the matter, but common sense would suggest that living within the vicinity of a nuclear power plant or a nuclear testing site would not be a wise choice. Supporting politicians who oppose nuclear testing also makes sense.

Some ionizing radiation comes from the earth. Most of it fits into the category of background radiation, which we can do nothing about. One type that all homeowners should be aware of, however, is radon gas. This radioactive gas is emitted from the soil in some locations. The gas collects in basements and crawlspaces and can be a threat. Testing kits are commercially available and protecting yourself is a matter of installing a simple barrier. If you live in an area where radon gas is a problem, testing your home would be wise.

Concern over sun exposure is not enough to compel me to forgo a life outdoors. As with all things in life, there is a good and a bad side to sun exposure. Exposure to the rays of the sun means exposure to ionizing radiation, but sun exposure is necessary for vitamin D production and is well-recognized for its value in cultivating an increased sense of wellbeing. Vitamin D is not only important for strong bones, but is vital for many functions within the body, including a properly functioning immune system. Wintertime colds and flu may be as much related to decreased production of vitamin D from lack of exposure to sunshine as to indoor confinement with other people. As for me, I will drink my carrot juice, eat vegetables regularly, and have my days in the sun as often as I can get them.

As we shun the sun and apply sunscreen liberally (sunscreen blocks as much as 95% of vitamin D production), America may be headed toward an epidemic of vitamin D deficiency. Many experts are recommending vitamin D levels at yearly physical exams, along with appropriate supplementation.

GENETICS, THE DECIDING FACTOR

Anyone who has seen the size of an average medical textbook would be obligated to wonder how so many diseases could come from such a short list of causes. The answer lies in our genes: Our individual genetic blueprints are so diversely different that an almost infinite number of diseases can come from a lifetime of exposure to a limited number of stress factors. This means that people vary in their susceptibility to different diseases. One person may consume flour and sugar for a lifetime and never develop diabetes, while another with the same diet will be destined to be on insulin by age fifty. Some people develop heart disease from smoking cigarettes and others will develop emphysema. Still, the list of causes is the same.

We each inherit a unique set of genes, different from any other set of genes that have ever existed (unless you are an identical twin, of course!). Our genes, however, are not perfect. They carry a mix of variations that have been passed down through the ages from all of our ancestors. Some of these "defects" may have actually been adaptations that worked very well for our ancient ancestors, but are of disadvantage in our modern world today. For example, individuals who rapidly absorb glucose and turn it into fat may have had ancestors who also had this trait and were, during lean times, resistant to starvation. *Good or bad, our genes are the hand we draw and how we play that hand is up to us.*

Our genetic blueprint codes for all of the biochemical functions within the body. Because these functions are so remarkably complex, there is a significant amount of room for variability and error. Though we cannot change our genes, we can sometimes work around genetic defects.

We all have adaptations in our genes that affect our risk of disease, but good habits can often overcome "bad genes."

On a basic level, nutritional modifications can alleviate the risk of disease by addressing the biochemical restrictions introduced by these genes. For example, most Native Americans have innate intolerance to high glucose diets. For thousands of years their ancestors existed on food containing almost no sugar or grain; however, this population of people has very high rates of diabetes when exposed to the average diets of today. Respect for their genetic history would suggest that this population should always follow a very low-sugar diet similar to that of their ancestors.

Sometimes specific mutations occur in genes that affect the biochemistry of that individual. Some people are born with PKU disease, the inability to metabolize the amino acid phenylalanine. When exposed to dietary phenylalanine they develop neurological disturbances and epilepsy. Removal of dietary phenylalanine allows completely normal life. There are many other examples of similar types of genetic diseases that can be alleviated by understanding the genetic defect and others still that could be treated with nutritional changes if we better understood the underlying problem. Autism is a common affliction for which there is no known cure, but many patients respond positively to specific nutritional therapies.

The strategy of being able to turn on, turn off, or bypass completely certain genes through dietary changes, nutritional supplements or specifically designed drug therapy is very interesting science. This is the future of medicine. Newer and more targeted drugs that act at the level of the gene, as opposed to blocking biochemical reactions to impede symptoms, offer a whole new avenue in the treatment of disease.

In the future you may be able to walk into a clinic and have a blood test that defines your entire genetic profile; the risk for each disease laid out in black and white. Certainly knowing your personal risk of specific diseases would be beneficial, but if most diseases have the same origins, why wait until that information is available? *No matter what our genetic background happens to be, the choices we make in life will determine how much we get out of life. We all have the choice of being healthy if we desire.*

At this point you may be adding up a mental list of factors that may be contributing to your personal risk of chronic disease—if not, you should be. Everyone has a threshold for chronic disease, defined by exposure to the forces of disease and genetic makeup. Symptoms do not occur until that threshold is crossed. You may go for years without symptoms while cumulative damage is adding up, then, almost suddenly, symptoms occur— different symptoms, seemingly unrelated symptoms. You may find yourself searching for a diagnosis, but your ultimate health will depend on whether you search for causes.

CHOICES

In some ways illness can be thought of as a state of mind. We make choices that make us ill. We are driven to make these choices by learned behavior from observing those around us and by human nature itself. We must free ourselves from poor health choices and learn to make better choices. Only when we accept these choices as being a necessity of good health and better life can we experience all that life has to offer.

The forces of disease represent the obstacles that prevent us from having a full, happy, and disease free life. Freedom from these obstacles is achieved by making better choices.

What about Sarah, my patient with GI and other symptoms? As she began to change her thinking, her situation appeared in a different light. Sarah now felt reassured that she probably did not have some terrible illness and that she would be able to overcome her problem. With my encouragement, she decided to proceed with on-going evaluations with other physicians, just in case, but her approach was much calmer. Sarah was starting to see how important it was for her to start making her own choices. She understood that being well was simply a matter of choice. Now, with a motivated patient, I sent her out the door with more extensive information to read about the causes of disease and a lifestyle questionnaire to complete before her next visit.

CHAPTER 4
Factors in Healing

A scan of Sarah's questionnaire quickly revealed the source of her original symptoms. Her diet mainly consisted of processed and packaged food eaten on the run, her general health habits were poor, and her stress management skills were terrible, even on good days. Problems with a difficult teenager, conflicts in her marriage, and coping with an unsatisfying job had left her in a state of constant anxiety.

Her stomach was the first to suffer. Perpetually being placed on standby by chronic stress, her GI tract was left in a state of dysfunction. Slow gastric emptying distended her stomach and allowed stomach acid to splash back up into the esophagus, causing constant burning in her throat. Compounding the problem, Sarah regularly ate foods that adversely affected the ability of her body to heal itself. The linings of the stomach and esophagus (called mucosa) began to break down, allowing the acid to do further damage. Ulceration was the result. Once ulcers are present, an infection commonly occurs with a bacterium called *H. pylori*. Many experts have concluded that stomach ulcers are caused by this bacterium, but we also know that many normal people carry these bacteria without having ulcers, suggesting that it is a secondary infection.

There seems to be a widely-held belief that stomach acid is the root of the problem and most conventional medical therapy is geared toward eliminating acid production completely. In the short term this strategy is effective. Healing of the mucosal lining occurs, but without addressing the original inciting factors, the medications have to be taken perpetually. Pharmaceutical companies are acutely aware of this fact, and competition for the newest and best acid-reducing medication is high.

Somewhere along the way, everyone seems to have neglected to remember that stomach acid has purpose. Without acid, proteins are not broken down properly and the initial stages of digestion are not activated. Foreign microbes pass through unharmed. Food stagnates along the tract and digestion becomes even more dysfunctional. Bacterial imbalances in the colon can occur, leaving the patient with symptoms of gaseous distention and constipation alternating with loose stools. The possibility that long term use of these medications may adversely affect bone density and risk of cardiovascular disease makes them even more concerning. Even though Sarah's reflux symptoms were kept in check, the longer she took this medication, the worse her other digestive symptoms became.

Sarah had noticed that after the colonoscopy her symptoms improved for several days. This was not a mere coincidence. Preparation for the procedure included two days of a liquid-only diet along with complete flushing of the gastrointestinal tract with laxatives. The flush expelled the buildup of toxin-producing bacteria in the colon. It took several days for overgrowths of abnormal bacteria to again occur. This is the same experience many people have after using "colon cleanse" products. These products do not remove toxins from the body as much as relieve bacterial overgrowth in the colon. Unless dietary habits are changed, the effects are usually transient. Overuse of laxative-containing products poses the risk of damage to the colon.

Sarah's treatment for anxiety was similarly shortsighted. The brain and nervous system include a delicate balance of inhibitory (calming) and stimulatory (exciting) chemical messengers called neurotransmitters. The high adrenaline associated with a stressful lifestyle, in a way, uses up the inhibitory neurotransmitters, leaving the nervous system in a state of perpetual excitation. The common name for this state of imbalance is anxiety.

Anxiety is often treated with a class of drugs called benzodiazepines. In this country, Xanax and Valium are the most commonly used brand names. These medications are extremely effective for treating anxiety, but only in the short term. They work by replacing the normal inhibitory neurotransmitters, thus setting the nervous system back in balance. Unfortunately, they also suppress synthesis of the natural calming chemicals of the nervous system. This results in the brain and nervous system becoming dependent on the drug to remain calm.

Compounding the problem is the fact that the body's normal response to a drug is to break it down. The liver recognizes any type of foreign chemical as being a toxin and produces enzymes to get rid of it. The longer a foreign chemical such as a drug is around, the more rapidly enzymes are made to eliminate it. As removal of the drug accelerates, the original symptoms being suppressed by the drug gradually return. This can occur with any type of medication, from anti-hypertensives to antihistamines. In the case of benzodiazepines, the brain and nervous system are left in a perpetually excited state. The situation often spins out of control and peculiar symptoms occur, such as the ones Sarah was experiencing.

When evaluating a patient like Sarah, I not only consider symptoms, but also routinely go down the list of stress factors that contribute to disease. Often specific modifications can be recommended that help the patient reduce offending stress factors and encourage healing. Sarah's situation appears less complex when broken down into categories of causes.

Emotional stress is the disease category that initiated her symptoms and catapulted her into her present condition. To achieve a full recovery, Sarah would have to expend a greater amount of effort learning better stress management skills. Stress combined with poor dietary and eating habits compromises gastric function and can lead to esophageal erosion. Stress also increases acid production, resulting in mucosal damage to the stomach and esophagus.

Routinely eating processed food on the run added to her burden of oxidative stress and increased inflammation, adversely affecting immune system function and increasing her risk of all known diseases, including and especially cancer. As with many chronic conditions, poor diet is a major contributor to poor healing. Her eating habits did not necessarily create her problems, but compounded all of them.

In Sarah's case the drugs were actually causing most of her secondary symptoms. This is not uncommon. Side effects of medications often mimic symptoms of actual disease. Distinguishing between the two is sometimes challenging. In the case of benzodiazepines, stopping the medications suddenly causes worsening of the side effects, complicating the picture even further. All synthetic medications have the potential for side effects and many have the potential to suppress immune system function. While drug therapy is sometimes indicated and necessary, it usually represents a compromise in care. All synthetic drugs should be used judiciously.

I discussed other disease factors with Sarah. She had not been infected with any unusual microbe, it seemed, but toxins produced by bacterial imbalances within her gastrointestinal tract had certainly contributed to her symptoms. Regarding radiation, she would be classified as having only average exposure. As with all of us, her genes defined her susceptibility to disease. She appeared to be more sensitive than average to imbalances of her inhibitory neurotransmitters and she seemed to develop tolerance to medications very easily.

Once she understood what was going on, Sarah was very motivated to make changes in her life, but often change does not come easily. It would take over a year of hard work and effort for her to regain good health. The first step was placing her on a slow taper to discontinue the benzodiazepine medication. To counteract the negative effects of the medication and reduce her symptoms, she was started on several natural supplements that carried no risk of habituation. This helped her cope and facilitated coming off the medication.

When it came to a healthful diet, Sarah was starting at ground zero. For most individuals used to an average American diet consisting mainly of processed foods, healthy foods are downright unpalatable. For Sarah, making changes to a better diet was a real challenge. Vegetables had never been much a part of her diet, and nothing tasted good unless it was sweet or coated in fat. In the beginning she had to force changes, but as her diet improved she realized that she felt better and, unexpectedly, the new foods actually began to taste "normal."

Along with better eating habits, Sarah was started on several supplements to protect the mucosal lining and encourage healing of her esophageal and stomach linings without disrupting the normal functions of the body. Nature often provides in ways that man cannot. Digestive enzymes were recommended to improve digestion of food. A probiotic supplement was initiated to reestablish the normal bacterial balance of the colon until yogurt and other fermented foods became dietary staples. With time, Sarah was able to taper and eventually stop the acid-reducing medication completely and her bowel function returned to normal.

An essential component of her recovery was learning better stress management skills. The anxiety she experienced every day was an impediment to getting off the benzodiazepine medication and a roadblock to better health in general. In our overmedicated, stressed-out world, this is a challenge for anyone. Regular exercise is a good place to start, as improved blood flow is good for everything, but Sarah would have to learn other skills that she could apply throughout the day. She took up yoga and worked one-on-one with an instructor who taught breathing and relaxation techniques. The relaxation training helped her learn to focus on the moment at hand and shield herself from the negativism of the world at large. All of these changes took time and she had to modify her schedule accordingly, but returning to her previous life was not an option.

As her health habits improved, so did her blood pressure. Most cases of what is commonly referred to as "essential" hypertension (implying that we do not know the causes) can be readily explained in simple terms. States of high adrenaline induced by chronic stress cause constriction of blood vessels and elevated heart rate. Poor diet usually plays a role, as insulin resistance contributes to derangements in adrenal hormone function (also being affected by stress) with the result of fluid imbalances and further constriction of blood vessels. Abnormal dietary fats contribute to inflammation in the bloodstream with consequential damage to blood vessel walls. Eventually, "hardening of the arteries" occurs and hypertension becomes irreversible. Fortunately, Sarah's condition had not progressed that far. In the end, she was able to stop the blood pressure medication and her blood glucose returned to normal.

After a year of concerted effort Sarah happily left the medications and all of her symptoms behind. Her energy level rebounded and she could get more done each day. Her life was far from being stress-free, but she could tolerate stress better with improved stress-management skills. She would never return to her old life. Interestingly, there were spin-offs that she did not expect. Her husband stopped smoking and improved his eating habits. Their relationship became more amiable and family relationships in general improved.

Sarah was lucky. She regained her health before reaching the point of finding a diagnosis. Her situation was relatively simple and intervention came early. Others are not so lucky. Sometimes cumulative damage has progressed to the point of a well-defined disease process and conventional therapy in the form of pharmaceuticals or surgery is mandatory. Even so, the kinds of changes that Sarah was willing to pursue should be first-line therapy for any disease process.

The body has an amazing propensity to heal itself, if given the opportunity. Doctors do not heal. Drugs do not heal. Only the body can heal itself.

Sometimes doctors do have an opportunity to point the body in the right direction, *but true healing can only come from within.* The first responsibility of any healthcare provider is to help the patient create a healing environment by providing information and therapies that promote healing. A part of this process may include alleviating symptoms and correcting hormonal imbalances with conventional medicines and alternative therapies, but the urge to go for the "quick fix" should be resisted. Therapies should always be directed toward helping the patient actually heal.

As a surgeon, I am frequently humbled by the realization that my skills and training would be nothing without the profound healing potential of the human body. Almost as soon as an incision is made, healing begins. Bleeding dries up almost as quickly as it started. The immune system works overtime to eradicate any microbes that have inevitably slipped through the "sterile field." The liver immediately detoxifies any drugs used to induce anesthesia. Before the procedure is finished the body begins to adapt to whatever changes have been made. By the next day the incision has sealed over. By one or two weeks later the patient is well on the way to recovery. All of this is of course quite dependent on the ability of the body to heal itself. The success or failure of a surgery is generally much less dependent on the skills of the surgeon than on the overall state of the patient's healing systems.

THE HEALING SYSTEMS OF THE BODY, IN BRIEF

Healing begins at a microscopic level within each and every living cell. Repair mechanisms are constantly at work rectifying damage caused by free radicals and toxins to DNA and other functional parts of the cell. Most of the time, equilibrium is reached and the cell remains viable, but sometimes cumulative damage is overwhelming and the cell begins to function improperly. At this point the cell must be destroyed before it begins the abnormal growth process that we know as cancer.

Our immune system is responsible for recognizing and obliterating these abnormal cells. Collectively, the immune system is the most elaborate part of our healing system. Not only is it responsible for scavenging potential cancer cells, but it also collects cells that are simply worn out and protects us from foreign invaders such as microbes or toxic substances. The immune system is composed of a complex network of cells and chemical messengers. It also includes the detoxification systems of the liver and the spleen. When everything is functioning properly, we go about our business in good health, totally unaware that our existence is being relentlessly threatened.

Much of disease occurs because the immune system is overwhelmed or has malfunctioned. Even though malfunctions in the immune system can occasionally be traced to specific genetic defects, most of the time the causes are environmental. All of the known factors of disease—nutritional deficiencies, excessive glucose and abnormal fats, oxidative stress, toxins, emotional and physical stress, microbes and radiation—play a role in adversely affecting immune function. *Though we cannot change our genes, we definitely have a say in controlling our exposure to these other primary factors.*

Dysfunction in the immune system can be manifested in several ways. Mobilization of the cells and chemicals of the immune system is part of the normal healing process. When this process is excessive and damaging, it is termed inflammation. *Chronic inflammation** is one of the main processes of disease. This exaggerated immune response is the basis of everything from arthritis to heart attacks and strokes. Chronic allergies also result from a hyperactive immune system. A malfunctioning immune system can turn on us and attack our own tissues in various ways resulting in a class of diseases referred to as the "autoimmune diseases"—but the most concerning malfunction of all is, of course, cancer.

I've heard it said that cancer is cause for concern and everything else is just an inconvenience. To some extent this statement is very accurate. Cancer is the diagnosis that nobody wants. Cancer is more threatening than any other disease process and despite all the money that has been poured into cancer research, we are still in the dark ages when it comes to treatment.

---

* *I am sometimes asked why inflammation is not listed as a cause of disease. The answer is a simple matter of cause and effect. Inflammation occurs as a result of the factors of disease and is therefore a process or manifestation of disease and not a cause in itself.*

I wish I could tell you that adopting a better diet and a healthier lifestyle would alone cure cancer, but life is never quite so simple. These factors can certainly help prevent cancer, but cannot alone provide a cure once cancer is established. Two basic things have to happen for cancer to occur. First, cells in the body have to become mutated in such a way that they become abnormal and their growth becomes unrestricted. This actually happens all the time, but one of the primary jobs of the immune system is to recognize these cells as being abnormal and remove them. The real problem occurs when a flaw in the immune system continues to recognize these abnormal cells as normal or "self" and their growth continues uninhibited. Once established, this process is hard to reverse.

Once a cancer is established, improved health practices are not enough alone to cure the cancer, but they are essential for helping the body heal and also are important for helping the patient survive therapy. Presently, the only effective therapies for cancer are surgical excision, chemotherapy, and radiation—all therapies that are potentially toxic to normal tissues as well as to the cancer. Improved health habits and detoxification are as important for surviving the therapy as the cancer. Any strategy for overcoming cancer should include comprehensive health revitalization.

None of the modalities for treating cancer available today are ideal and hopefully the future will provide clues of how to repair the immune system malfunction itself. Until then, the best strategy for dealing with cancer is prevention. With the majority of our resources focused on early detection and finding "the" cure for cancer, a superb opportunity for prevention is being missed. **In my opinion, if we devoted a decent portion of cancer research funding toward educating the public about preventative measures, we could decrease the rate of cancer by 50% or more!**

THE COAGULATION SYSTEM

Closely tied to the immune system is the coagulation system, the healing mechanism responsible for tissue repair. When we are injured, an elaborate sequence of chemical messengers and chemical cascades is initiated to clot blood, prevent bleeding, and begin mending of tissues. An excessive or abnormal response from the coagulation system can lead to abnormal clotting. Excessive coagulation is a contributing factor to heart attacks and strokes and is a risk factor for the formation of blood clots in the lower extremities. Heredity does play a role, but is far from being the exclusive cause. As the saying goes: genetics loads the gun, but choices in diet and lifestyle pull the trigger. In this case, the end of the smoking gun is often a cigarette; poor dietary habits are also central to the problem.

Stress contributes to atherosclerosis through effects on the coagulation system. Chronic emotional stress causes platelets, one of the main components of the coagulation system, to become extra "sticky." Increased platelet "clumping" accelerates plaque formation. Stress management and natural "blood thinners" such as omega 3 essential fatty acids are important therapeutic additions to counteract this effect.

Some people are "hyper-coagulators" and are at risk of thrombotic events (blood clots). Screening labs for genetic susceptibility include Leiden factor V, homocysteine, protein C deficiency, protein S deficiency and antithrombin. These tests should be considered in anyone with a family history of thrombotic events, especially if estrogen products are being considered.

HORMONE AND MESSENGER SYSTEMS OF THE BODY

The immune system, and all functions within the human body for that matter, could not function properly if all the different types of cells were going about their business independently. Synchronization of function requires elaborate communication systems which include the nervous system and hormonal systems of the body, cumulatively referred to as the neuro-endocrine system. Communication among the different systems of the body is essential for normal function, as a whole, and for healing to take place. These communication systems are so complex that we still do not completely understand them. What we do understand, however, is how easily they can become imbalanced.

Patients frequently ask to have their hormone levels checked, being quite sure the symptoms they are having must be related to some hormone being "out of whack." Often they are right on track, but do not realize that there are literally hundreds and possibly thousands of different types of chemical messengers in the body, and they are all interrelated. Even measuring something as seemingly straightforward as a thyroid hormone level is fraught with different interpretations by various experts and labs. Second-guessing and micromanaging these imbalances is challenging for even the best specialists in the field.

Central to the neurological and hormonal systems of the body is the hypothalamic-pituitary-endocrine connection (often called the Hypothalamic-Pituitary-Adrenal axis, HPA axis). If you strip away the thinking portion of the brain and leave only the reactive portions of the brain, this is what you have left. With the autonomic (automatic) nervous system, brain stem and peripheral nervous system included, it would be the near equivalent of the entire functioning brain, nervous system, and hormonal systems of a lower vertebrate such as a turtle. With only a limited portion of the brain devoted to higher thinking, a turtle can only respond to stimuli in a defined and predictable fashion. This portion of the brain and neuro-endocrine system allows the body to maintain balance in the face of constant change.

The *hypothalamus*, an almond sized structure at the base of the brain, and the autonomic nervous system together control body temperature, thirst, hunger, weight, glucose and fat metabolism, physical manifestations of mood, sleep, fatigue, night and day rhythms, blood pressure, heart rate, and gastrointestinal function. The *hypothalamus* can be thought of as the central thermostat of the body that maintains balance in the face of constant change. This balance is referred to as *homeostasis*.

Though small in size, the *hypothalamus* is central to all parts of the brain. It receives feedback from all of systems of the body, input from the sensory organs, and input from the higher thinking brain. Everything we think and feel influences the *hypothalamus*, and in turn, the *hypothalamus* influences all functions in the body. The *hypothalamus* exerts its influence by way of the *pituitary gland*, a small gland that hangs down from a stalk just below the hypothalamus. The pituitary gland, in response to hormones secreted from the *hypothalamus*, secretes hormones that regulate the *thyroid gland*, the outer portion of the *adrenal glands* (located on top of the kidneys), and the *reproductive glands* (ovaries and testes). The *pituitary gland* also regulates the balance of fluids within the body, stimulates uterine contractions in labor, induces breast milk, and secretes growth hormone.

The *autonomic nervous system* includes the reflexive or automatic parts of the nervous system. Examples would include the regular beating of the heart or the processes of digestion, functions that are beyond voluntary control. It also has a direct connection to the middle part of the adrenal glands where *adrenaline* is secreted. *Adrenaline* is the chemical messenger that gets us going in response to acute stress. Increased adrenaline secretion causes increased heart and blood pressure, increased muscle contractions, and increased mental acuity associated with the classic "fight or flight" response.

Maintaining balance in the face of continual change is what health is all about. Any of the factors of disease (stress and negative thinking are very high on the list) has the ability to induce imbalances in the system, resulting in many symptoms of disease. As all parts of the system are intimately interlinked, isolating and treating dysfunction in only one part of the system is often not effectual. A thyroid disorder is rarely a thyroid disorder by itself. Menstrual irregularly is rarely a problem with the ovaries alone. Even the symptoms of menopause, associated with the cessation of estrogen production by the ovaries, are manifested through imbalances in the entire hypothalamic-pituitary-endocrine connection.

Hormonal dysfunction is not a *cause* of disease, but a *manifestation* of disease. Emotional stress, oxidative stress, excessive dietary glucose, abnormal fat, toxins, radiation and microbes are the primary causes of disease. When these forces are acting on the body as a whole, glandular function becomes compromised. When stress factors that cause disease are minimized, some rebound in glandular function can be expected. How much rebound occurs is highly dependent upon the gland. Possibly the most sensitive gland in the body is the thyroid gland. The thyroid gland, responsible for managing metabolism, can be affected by any chronic disease process—therefore, supporting thyroid function is important whenever thyroid function is abnormal, especially in the face of chronic disease.

Traditionally, thyroid function has been evaluated indirectly by measuring thyroid stimulating hormone (TSH), produced by the pituitary gland to regulate thyroid function. A high TSH suggests inadequate thyroid function. Many practitioners also routinely measuring the active thyroid hormones, free T-4 and free T-3. Iodine, essential for normal thyroid function, is often deficient in average American diets and supplementation should be considered whenever abnormal thyroid function is present.

The thyroid gland is very sensitive to the factors of disease. If you have been diagnosed with a thyroid disorder, or any other glandular dysfunction for that matter, hormonal replacement may be necessary, but reducing the factors that caused the problem in the first place is essential.

Adrenal function and the reproductive hormones can also be adversely affected by the forces that cause chronic disease. The adrenal gland can be thought of as "stress central," because the main hormones produced by the adrenal gland direct where resources of the body will be allocated during stress. During prolonged periods of excessive physical or emotional stress, adrenal function can become compromised and the whole body suffers. Rest from stress is the ultimate solution, but support of glandular function through supplementation is sometimes indicated. The fluctuating and rhythmic nature of these hormones, however, makes evaluation and supplementation very challenging.

Adrenal and reproductive hormones fluctuate throughout the day, and therefore are more difficult to assess than thyroid function. Blood samples only offer a "snapshot in time" and are only indicated in certain situations. Salivary hormone levels offer a more general assessment of function and can be used as a rough guide but are less accurate overall than blood levels. Salivary levels of cortisol, a primary adrenal hormone, are considered the most reliable of any salivary assessments and are typically measured four times within a 24-hour period. Salivary measurements of other adrenal and reproductive hormones are less reliable because blood hormone levels are much lower, but sometimes can be beneficial as an imprecise guide for therapy.

The exception to all rules is menopause. Menopause happens. Even with the best of health habits, menopause still happens. It is a natural process, but has the potential to adversely affect all of the hormonal systems of the body. The hormonal changes that occur at menopause with the normal and natural cessation of reproductive function often throw a monkey wrench into the body's entire hormonal balance. Menopause is especially devastating when it occurs abruptly with surgical removal of the ovaries. Though hot flashes, night sweats, mood changes, and insomnia are classic, almost any symptom that occurs at this point in a woman's life can be attributed to menopause. In almost all individuals these hormonal imbalances gradually equilibrate over time, but in very symptomatic individuals, nutritional and herbal therapies with properly dosed, bio-identical hormone therapy can be safe, effective, and sometimes almost lifesaving.

Many well-meaning healthcare providers have a tendency to micromanage illness. Treating only symptoms with specific targeted drug therapy is often ineffective and can actually be an impediment to healing. Correcting hormonal imbalances is important, but overzealous hormone supplementation can actually impede restoration of normal glandular function. The goal of therapy should be support of glandular function, not suppression by over-supplementation.

We know that certain hormones such as insulin and thyroid are essential for life and must be maintained at normal levels throughout life. Other hormones, including reproductive hormones, melatonin and growth hormone, gradually decline with age, even in healthy individuals. Certainly any hormone found to be below normal for age in a symptomatic individual should be considered for replacement therapy, but whether to adjust all hormones to the level of a youthful adult is a subject of great debate.

A complete understanding of the complexities of the healing systems of the body is not a necessity to maximize the body's healing potential. From the intricate mechanisms constantly repairing damage created by free radicals, background radiation and toxins at the cellular level all the way up to destruction of threatening microbes by the immune system, our healing systems are constantly on guard and at work. By taking steps to minimize the impact of the forces of disease while at the same time providing ideal working conditions and proper nutrients for all the healing systems of the body, we can create an environment of optimal healing.

ACHIEVING OPTIMAL WELLNESS AND LONGEVITY

The irreversible, cumulative damage that we call aging is an inevitable consequence of being alive, but we can slow down the process by adopting improved health habits. The rate at which aging occurs is partially dependent on an individual's genetic makeup, but in most cases is more dependent on the degree of exposure to the forces of disease, which are, of course, quite modifiable. Ideally I would say that the sooner you figure this out in life, the better, but these concepts are hard to get across to young people who are healthy. Most people do not start becoming concerned about their personal health until it starts to falter.

Most of us are not aware that cumulative damage is occurring until after age 40. After the age of 40, the guarantee of good health is less and less secure. It all adds up. Minor complaints such as tiredness, difficulty losing weight, or elevated blood pressure are just the early warning signs. Symptoms foretell that change is coming, whether you like it or not.

None of us really likes change, especially when it comes to our health, and so often we look for the easy way out. We would rather find a quick fix or "magic bullet" that makes everything just right again, without making very much personal effort. The quick fix may include a drug, a regimen of vitamins, an herbal remedy or tonic, something off the TV or internet or even a surgical procedure, but these efforts alone rarely bring true health, harmony, or happiness in life.

Life is synonymous with change. Learning how to embrace change instead of resisting it is a key aspect of enjoying life. Cultivating an open mind and an open heart are the first steps. So often I see patients with changing or failing health for whom I know changes in diet and lifestyle are all that would be needed to completely rejuvenate their health, but resistance to lifestyle modifications remains a roadblock. They choose a quick fix for symptom relief as a first choice and never really get better.

Ironically, adapting to change and changing with change is the only way to slow down the inevitable and detrimental change that is associated with aging.

For anyone willing to make some compromises, there is hope! Much of the damage that has been accruing for years is reversible. Good health is available to anyone! The healing processes of the body are always there, just waiting to get back in the game.

Recognition is the first step in overcoming chronic disease. Once the factors that cause illness are defined, it becomes hard to ignore them. Even individuals who tend to resist change will find it hard to hold on to bad habits when these habits are recognized as an impediment to feeling well.

Our health and wellbeing are determined by the choices we make each day. The choices for creating an ideal healing environment are simple and straightforward, but not necessarily easy to master in the fast-paced world in which we live. Self discipline and compromises are necessary. The degree of compromise will depend on the condition of the healing systems of the body. Individuals with established illness may have to be rigidly particular about their health practices for a while, but be reassured that no matter what the degree of compromise, the benefits of renewed health will allow you to live life to its fullest.

Changing to a healthier lifestyle should not be equated with misery. "Healthier" means changing to different habits, but the changes can be pleasant—it all depends on whether change is approached with a positive attitude. With a positive attitude, better dietary and lifestyle habits are immediately complemented by feeling better and enjoying life more.

Guidance from other knowledgeable individuals is encouraged for help and support along this pathway. *Any and all disease processes* can be positively affected by paying better attention to the choices we make!

PILLARS OF OPTIMAL HEALTH AND HEALING

The three main pillars of health and healing include *nurturing the body, cleansing and protecting the body,* and *synchronization of the body and mind.* A fourth pillar includes all aspects of modern healthcare. All of the categories are interrelated and dependent on each other. Attention to each is necessary to create an optimal environment for health and healing. At the heart of each category is the matter of personal choice. As we make better choices, we can expect to be not only healthier, but also more successful in life's endeavors and more satisfied with life in general.

Pillar I Nourishment for the Body A healthy body cannot exist without proper nourishment. A diet high in fiber, nutrients, and minerals with just the right amount of sugar and the proper balance of fat is achieved by regularly consuming vegetables, whole seeds (grains, beans, and nuts), fruit, seafood, and meat raised in a healthy manner. There is little room in a healthy diet for commercially processed food.

Pillar II Body Purification Good food only goes so far in protecting the body. Learning where toxins exist in the environment and limiting your exposure to them, adopting good personal hygiene habits for avoidance of microbial infections, and maintaining gastrointestinal health for internal cleansing are all part of an optimal health strategy.

Pillar III Synchrony of the Body and Mind Exercise and the regular practice of relaxation methods for stress reduction are an essential part of good health, but when these forces are combined with exercises in brain synchrony, a powerful force of healing is created. Brain synchrony not only opens the door to wellness but is the key to happiness and harmony, in general.

Pillar IV Medical, Surgical, and Alternative Therapies The primary focus of healthcare should be complimentary and supportive. Medical, surgical and alternative therapies work best when directed toward reducing the pressures that cause disease and mending or compensating for cumulative damage. Treating symptoms is important, but should be a secondary and hopefully transient concern.

Cumulative damage to the body is inevitable and sooner or later we will all need extra help, in one form or another. Less invasive and micro-invasive surgery can not only be lifesaving, but also life rejuvenating. Well thought-out medical therapy using combinations of nutritional supplements and herbal therapies, combined with less toxic pharmaceutical therapy can support healing, improve longevity, and make life more pleasant in general. Alternative therapies such as acupuncture, massage therapy, yoga therapy, energy therapy, chiropractic care and others can promote healing and reduce the aches and pains that are part of being alive.

Conventional medicine tends to do a good job of taking care of the acutely ill, but does little to prevent chronic disease from occurring. Holistic providers and alternative healthcare providers do a better job of considering other factors of health, but still tend to retain control of the situation. To achieve optimal health and healing, you must take charge of your own well-being. No one is going to take as much interest in your health as you do. Even then, addressing only one pillar of health will not suffice. To achieve the balance of health that optimizes the healing potential of the body, the first three pillars must be addressed. Don't be caught in the "too little, too late" mode—start making changes now.

A PLAN FOR CHANGE

As you read the second half of this book, you will acquire the knowledge and skills necessary to cultivate a plan for change. In the next section, you will learn about all the reasons why you should change to a healthier diet and you will be offered tools to help you make it happen.

In our toxin-saturated world, becoming "toxin aware" is a good practice. The first chapter in Pillar II, Body Purification, offers practical advice for learning where hidden toxins exist and how to limit exposure. The second chapter discusses the elimination and detoxification processes and how these important facets of health can be optimized. At the end of chapter 11 you will find a thorough detoxification protocol to start you off in the right direction.

For many people, following a regular exercise routine and learning better stress management skills are significant hurdles to overcome. The chapters in Pillar III, Synchrony of Body and Mind, are designed to help you incorporate these important aspects of health and healing into everyday life.

Be patient as you read—everything will come together. Lifestyle changes do not happen overnight. Willpower comes in spurts, as the never-ending rotation of diet and exercise fads attests. Try one thing for a while until it becomes routine and then shift to something else. It does take some work and effort, but new routines will become habits over time. Unlike fads, which fade with the night, good health habits will last you a lifetime. Even people who have a tendency to see change as daunting can usually overcome obstacles and achieve their full health potential if they try hard enough. Once change becomes the accepted norm, life is always better.

Though each of the pillars is addressed independently, they must come together in practice. The conclusion pulls all of the principles discussed in the three pillars into a workable strategy for getting the most out of health and life. Suggestions are also made for formulating a strategy to overcome any type of chronic disease, where the same principles apply but must be practiced much more stringently.

If you are reading this and have a chronic illness, I would strongly encourage pursuing a thorough evaluation with an experienced healthcare provider—sometimes identifying and treating specific problems can augment your recovery—but do not wait for a diagnosis before beginning therapy! Mastering the principles outlined in the next three sections is your best bet for actually overcoming chronic disease. Whether your goal is losing ten pounds or overcoming a major illness, following the advice in this book will improve your situation.

The material in this book is complemented in my practice by a system of monographs called Health Briefs that are designed to provide information about specific therapy for individual health problems. The complete health program includes a complete evaluation customized for the individual patient, counseling, and appropriate Health Briefs for each situation. Information in the book is the cornerstone of the program; other parts of the evaluation can be pursued with any provider experienced in wellness medicine. The basic screening labs that accompany the health program and a schedule for the program are included as appendices in the back of this book.

REFLECTIONS ON CHANGE

On a personal level, I have certainly had to come to grips with change and compromise as much as anybody else. Life is not easy and by nature comes with challenges, though sometimes the most difficult parts are the ones that make life most interesting. Without challenges, life would be boring. Making good choices and accepting change is the best way to deal with the challenges of life. For the most part, I have come to accept change and in many ways have come to actually enjoy change. Maybe this is what maturity is all about.

The compromises that have become necessary with age have become a part of who I am. Regaining lost health has sometimes required effort and determination, but retrospectively, even that was not so bad. Life is now more settled, and I am more centered in many ways. I expect there will be more challenges in the future, and I hope to accept them gracefully. Some years down the road a simple life with a light diet of rice and vegetables, low stress, regular exercise, and daily meditation may be something to look forward to.

As a physician, my approach to the practice of medicine and healing has also changed and matured. Teaching and motivating patients about how to change or improve their own health is much more satisfying to me than handing out prescriptions. I have hopes that conventional medicine will mature in a similar way, and I have faith that modern science will provide us with better therapies for many diseases, including cancer. I am optimistic that change is on the horizon....that pharmaceuticals will lean more toward optimizing the healing potential of the body, rather than just treating symptoms....that surgery will become more and more micro-invasive.....that traditional will be used alongside conventional.....and that legitimate alternative and natural therapies will become a part of mainstream healthcare.

The human body has an amazing potential for healing, if given the right opportunity. The pressures from the forces of disease are great. Release the pressure, and the healing systems of the body will always respond.

PILLAR I
Nourishment for the Body

Nourishment is intimately tied to overall health.
The first step in adopting a healthier lifestyle is adopting a
healthier diet.

CHAPTER 5
Food...A Historical Perspective

One constant among all life forms is the need for nourishment. Nourishment, most commonly in the form we call food, includes not only fuel for energy, but also chemicals and minerals necessary for normal biochemical and physiologic functions of the body.

The first priority of survival for any living organism is obtaining adequate nourishment. Human history has been particularly influenced by this pursuit. Humans have been wandering around this planet for a surprisingly long period of time. Human habitation of the earth goes back much farther than written history. Fossil records document that our species, *Homo sapiens*, has existed for at least 90,000 years (most experts in DNA analysis would suggest a time span closer to 150,000 to 200,000 years). Appreciating how our distant ancient ancestors lived and what they ate to survive is essential for understanding the nature of many of the nutritional problems that we face today. Like it or not, we are all a function of how our species evolved.

Imagine the world about thirty thousand years ago. The North American continent would not yet have been populated, but some humans would have migrated out of Africa and into Europe and Asia. A typical pre-historic man probably looked like you or I except for being very short by our standards and much scruffier in appearance. Being human, he would not have had the prominent face and sloped brow of a Neanderthal, so commonly depicted as the average caveman. Very likely, his body was covered in scars, since life was hard for a prehistoric man. We would expect his skin to be dark in equatorial climates, but fitting him into any race category that we know today might be difficult.

The primary activity of humans of 30,000 years ago was collecting food. What a primitive man wanted from his food and what he actually got were two different things. Priorities of survival dictated the need for sources of energy to power the body and sources of protein to replace the daily turnover of amino acids. Primitive foods, however, were far from being high in energy. A prehistoric diet came packed with nutrients, minerals, and especially fiber but offered little in the way of sugars and fat; protein content was also minimal. Without these vital components of food, starvation was an ever-ominous threat. ***The drive to acquire enough sugar, fat, and protein for survival was stronger than any other, even stronger than the drive for sex.***

If we wanted to duplicate a "primitive-man diet," it might go something like this: an enormous variety of edible vegetable matter, fruits, seeds, fungi and nuts would be available for consumption, but none of it would resemble any food that we are used to today. We would find most of the food to be bitter or tasteless, with almost no sugar or fat. With the absence of refrigeration and food preservation as we know it today, a significant portion of the food would have been fermented or even spoiled. In fact, selective fermentation of food is an age-old method of preservation.

Nothing came in a package. Sauces, dressings, added sugar, or added fat, of course, did not exist. Cows did not exist, and no creatures on Earth drank milk past infancy. Oil for cooking and frying was rare. Wild honey might have been available as a natural sweetener—if one braved extracting it from the hive. Protein sources included an occasional bit of fish or a small mammal roasted on a spit, but this probably was not an everyday occurrence. The occasion of all the boys sitting around the campfire roasting rump of mastodon was probably quite rare, as was cooking food in general. Bird eggs, in season, might have been on the menu. All waking hours would be spent collecting enough food for basic survival. Exhaustion from the labor of it all would ensure a good night's sleep, night after night. In colder climates a primitive diet consisted mostly of animal sources, but in the warmer climates where most humans lived, vegetable matter was almost surely the most consistent food source.

Many plant substances are toxic and the fact that our primitive man knew which ones to pick was not by chance alone. Some knowledge was passed along from his parents and others in his group, but much of it was burned into his genes by thousands of years of natural selection. Plant substances that we consider food or use for medicinal purposes today are "familiar" to our genes and are generally well accepted. In this light, it should not come as a surprise to find that overly processed foods are commonly associated with disease and that synthetic drugs are often associated with side effects.

You can tell a lot about what types of foods an animal should be eating by examining its teeth. A typical herbivore, such as a horse, will have a few teeth up front specially designed for pulling grass and leaves from plants, with the remaining teeth consisting of molars for grinding vegetable matter into a pulp. A dedicated carnivore, such as a wolf, will display predominantly teeth for cutting and shredding meat.

Humans are omnivores. Examination of an adult human mouth will demonstrate two sets of incisors and one set of canines, intended specifically for tearing meat. Two sets of premolars and three sets of molars (one set are wisdom teeth) are designed for chewing vegetable matter. If the ratio of the types of teeth are considered, a normal human diet should consist of about 2/3's vegetable matter and 1/3 meat. If course, this was all well-defined before the processed food of the past century came on the scene.

Despite his instinctive knowledge of "safe" foods, our primitive man was primarily driven by the need for glucose and fat. If we brought a primitive man back today, he would immediately rush over to McDonalds like everybody else. There, as at most modern fast food restaurants and most groceries, he would find an abundance of the sugar and fat that were limited in his natural diet. The drive to consume these types of foods would be so strong that he would soon be overweight, lethargic, and in ill health like many people today. It would not be long before we would find him sitting in front of a television, wasting away the extra hours not needed for collecting food.

For the human body, glucose and fat are the primary fuels. Dietary proteins can also be used in a pinch, but are more readily suited for making up the structural components of the body than being used for producing energy. Of the three, glucose is the most important. Glucose, in the right amounts, is really good stuff. It provides instant energy. It burns cleanly with few by-products, making it the preferred fuel for the brain and muscles. ***The fact that taste of sweet tickles our taste buds like nothing else is no coincidence!***

We like fat just about as much. The aroma of sizzling fat from a thick steak on the grill is hard to forsake. Fat, as an energy source, is not as versatile as glucose and does not burn quite as cleanly, but it provides all-important energy for low-end power and endurance. The muscles of the heart use predominantly free fats in the blood as fuel. The muscles of endurance athletes such as long distance runners will convert from burning predominantly glucose to burning predominantly fat fairly rapidly as exercise progresses. Fat is also necessary for producing heat and providing insulation in a colder climate. Our basic primitive man living in prehistoric Europe or North America would have needed good sources of fat for survival.

In our present time of overabundance, the simple fact that only a small amount of glucose and fat are necessary for survival creates a significant dietary conundrum. Maybe in another 50,000 years humans could evolve to live only off of high concentrations of sugar and fat alone, but that does not help us right now. Like it or not, we have a strong dependence on all the other stuff that came with our ancestral foods. Though they do not affect our taste buds in nearly the same way, dietary fiber, enzymes, proteins, vitamins, minerals, bacteria from fermented food, and the host of beneficial chemicals found in plants are just as vital for our survival and well-being as sugar and fat. *The human body cannot function normally without them.*

The fact that we tend to ignore all the dietary "extras" is not a simple oversight, but is a result of how food sources of the world changed over time. Eventually humans grew tired of roaming the planet looking for food and figured out how to cultivate grain. Grains had glucose, fat, protein, fiber, nutrients, and minerals all rolled into one food source. Grains could be stored for the winter and transported long distances. No more wandering. Food actually began to taste better as grains, vegetables and fruit were cultivated to have more sugar. No need for hunting, either: domesticated animals could be fed grain and kept in one location. Humans thrived. Civilizations sprang up. The world changed. History was written.

The cultivation of grain itself was not necessarily a bad thing, as whole grains are fairly well balanced with carbohydrate (including fiber), protein, a little bit of oil, and some vitamins and minerals. The problem came when entire cultures became dependent on a crop of grain as a primary food source. Inevitable blights, droughts, and insect infestations commonly caused mass starvation and disease, a threat still common in the world today.

In spite of these problems, the advantages of grain cultivation were too much to ignore, and grain gradually became the dominant food source of the world: wheat in Europe, rice in Asia, millet in Africa and, to a lesser extent, corn in the Americas were the predominant grains. Even though grain did provide higher concentrations of glucose than were found in primitive diets, over several thousand years, most cultures adapted to it. Interestingly, there have been pockets of cultures around the world that have existed without dependence on grain. Descendants from these groups of humans—namely Native Americans, peoples from many parts of Africa, and Aborigines in Australia—never acclimated to the higher levels of glucose found in a grain-based diet and consequently have high rates of diabetes when exposed to the typical processed-grain diets today.

For several thousand years of recorded history the status of food changed very little, until about a hundred years ago with the onset of the processed food revolution. The catalyst that fueled this change was the discovery of the energy contained within petroleum. Shifting from plow and mule to tractors quickly altered the world's food production capacity. Suddenly food in the form of grain could be produced on a grand scale, the likes of which the world had never seen before. Petroleum also provided the means to transport large amounts of it to anywhere on the planet. North America became the bread basket of the world with production of staggering amounts of wheat and corn. The world changed again. Populations surged. Factories sprang up. The pace of life quickened, in America like nowhere else.

The pace of a new American lifestyle demanded food that was simple, easy to prepare, and cheap. Convenience became priority number one. The commercial food industry responded by lining the shelves and aisles of newly styled "supermarkets" with pre-processed and packaged foods. To improve efficiency and keep costs down, only a limited number of food sources were cultivated. Today, a surprisingly large proportion of our food comes predominantly from only two sources: wheat and corn. Industrial refinement pushed efficiency in food production to the outer limits and at the same time catered to those all-important tastes for sweet and fat. The cost was nutrition, but no one seemed to notice because everything tasted good.

The food processing and packaging industry has been very skillful in presenting a seemingly wide variety of unique products all derived from a limited number of food sources. Expert marketing is the key. Often more care and concern are given to the outside packaging than the food inside. Products are designed to appeal to our senses, especially capitalizing on those preferential tastes for sweet and fat—*giving people what they want always sells better than giving them what they need.* Today, packaged food products are so prevalent that many Americans rarely eat anything that doesn't come from a box or a wrapper.

When it comes to processed food, no ingredients are more ubiquitous than the "threatening three:" *refined white flour, high fructose corn syrup,* and *partially hydrogenated oils*—all derived predominantly from wheat and corn sources. These same ingredients are found in most packaged food products found on grocery store shelves today and they dominate the fast food industry. *We are eating the same stuff over and over again.* A look at the ingredients label found on a typical packaged food product will typically reveal at least one of the "threatening three" as well as preservatives, flavorings, and possibly added vitamins or minerals, but not very much in the way of good nutrition.

The dramatic rise in diabetes and metabolic syndrome over the past one hundred years has closely paralleled the increased consumption of processed corn and wheat products worldwide.

At present, we have such an abundance of grain that we not only have enough to feed ourselves but we have plenty left over to feed animals. In fact, the *majority* of grain and soybean production in this country goes toward industrial-scale livestock production. Grain is the ingredient that makes meat so tantalizing to our taste buds. I can remember growing up when meat tenderizer and a sharp knife were essential parts of eating a steak. Today, a steak cuts like butter and melts in your mouth. That exquisite taste is the result of abundant saturated fat from a corn-fed (a.k.a. "grain-finished") animal which ate, in its last months, an unnatural diet. Beyond having an unhealthy amount of fat, toxins (from the corn) that become part of the fat constitute an even graver concern associated with commercially-produced meat. It provides much more taste appeal but may compromise your health.

Turning back the clock to a different time in food history would seem to be a wise choice, but going back to a purely "primitive" diet is not a necessary move for good health. I can remember as a Boy Scout being turned loose in the woods for "survival weekends" with only a knife and a canteen. After several days scavenging for the "bounty of nature," we were always ready for a trip to McDonald's. We quickly discovered that surviving on a primitive diet is a hard way to get by. When the average American diet of today is compared to the average human diet of 30,000 years ago, we find two opposite extremes. *What we really need is something in-between.*

While most people allow their food choices to be dominated by the commercial food industry, they neglect to observe that we are truly living in the golden age of food. Fresh, nutritious, whole foods are more available than ever before. In the middle of December, I have access to locally grown collards, broccoli, cabbage, and winter squash; I can also enjoy fresh blackberries and strawberries imported from more southern climates, oranges and grapefruits from Florida, and many other fresh foods from around the country and even around the world. Though I do subscribe to the practice of buying locally whenever possible, the privilege of being able to supplement local seasonal foods with those from other places would certainly suggest we are living in the middle of the "Garden of Eden."

Even as petroleum supplies begin to decline and the world changes again, we should be able to maintain our Garden of Eden indefinitely if we make intelligent choices. Foods that are being transported by truck and plane could be transported just as well by train for a fraction of the cost. Better methods of preservation, such as flash-freezing meats and seafood on site, will allow slower and more energy-wise methods of transport.

The advent of refrigeration and freezing has allowed the nutritional value of food to be retained longer without preservatives. We should not have to resort to traditional methods of meat preservation such as drying, salting or use of chemicals. Many people still have a taste for sausage, ham, and other preserved meats, but these foods are not healthy food choices and should be consumed sparingly, if at all.

Fresh foods are more available than ever before, but we can make wise and healthy choices even with preserved foods. A hundred years ago, canning fruits and vegetables was a necessary part of every summer and fall routine just to have enough food for the winter. Today, refrigeration and freezing have answered that concern, but canned foods do offer convenience and economy. Canning is practical and involves the lowest expenditure of energy. Food is least expensive at peak harvest and that low cost can be retained within a can. Though many foods lose some nutritional value with canning, certain foods such as tomatoes, beans, certain fruits and fish do rather well in a can or a jar.

Cost containment can also be applied to most fruits by simply removing water. Because fruits are high in sugar, drying offers a satisfactory method of preservation. I, for one, enjoy dried blueberries, cranberries and cherries in my yogurt year-round, and my pasta primavera would not be the same without sun-dried tomatoes.

The difference between an unhealthy diet and a healthy diet is simply a matter of personal choice. Though evolution has left us with an insatiable appetite for sugar and fat coupled with a normal desire to consume significant quantities of food, it is possible not only to achieve but also to actually enjoy healthy dietary habits. Healthy food and—just as importantly, the knowledge to know what defines healthy food—are more available than ever before.

The "golden age of food" is truly upon us. Why squander it by making poor food choices?

CHAPTER 6
Food...A Scientific Perspective

The science behind food would have been of no interest to a primitive man. He did not take time to check labels for carbohydrate, fat and protein content; he simply ate anything that was edible, and as much of it as he could get. By necessity, he consumed a wide variety of foods, and his food came packed with vital nutrients, minerals and fiber. His greatest concern was obtaining enough glucose, fat and protein daily for basic survival. In the primitive world, acquiring energy from food trumped all other concerns.

If your diet consists of a wide variety of whole foods including vegetables, fruits, seeds, free-range meats, seafood, select dairy products and eggs, you may not be interested in the science behind your food, either, since your diet is contributing optimally to your health. On the other hand, if you were raised on a diet that included processed and packaged foods (as most of us born within the past seventy-five years have been), you may be interested to know how it has affected your health. Diseases such as diabetes, atherosclerosis and arthritis are directly related to diet and most specifically related to a processed-food diet.

CARBOHYDRATES

Carbohydrates include sugars and starches. Though there are many types of sugars in nature, the energy cycle common to plants and animals is built around the sugar glucose. This simple molecule makes life possible and while enough of it is essential, too much is a detriment to our health.

THE GLUCOSE PROBLEM

"Super-sized" American diets are super-saturated with glucose. The chief sources of excessive dietary glucose are sugar and starch found mostly in food products made from processed wheat and corn. From bread and bagels to donuts and pastries, processed white wheat flour makes up a large portion of the food American's consume on a daily basis. Starch, the main component of flour, is made of long chains of glucose linked together. By itself, starch is not very sweet, so many processed food products also contain some type of sweetener. Table sugar would do, but high fructose corn syrup is the sweetest of the sugars and is also the least expensive. The name is somewhat misleading, as it also contains a significant amount of glucose.

A simple concoction of flour, corn syrup, and fat tempts our taste buds like nothing else on earth—and with good reason! Of all the naturally occurring sugars in nature, glucose is preferred. Glucose is a very versatile fuel source. It burns cleanly with minimal free radical production and can be stored in the liver and muscles for immediate energy needs. Just as easily it can be converted into fat for long term energy storage needs. Glucose also can be converted into many other substances including certain amino acids (the building blocks of proteins) and is an integral part of many of the components of a living cell.

Glucose is a metabolic "must-have," but something that you do not need very much of to be healthy. In fact, having more than necessary is actually very toxic.

The toxicity of glucose relates to its inherent tendency to stick to proteins. Like carbon deposits built up on the pistons and cylinders of your car's engine, glucose sticks to proteins and gums up the vital machinery of the human body. Performance is adversely affected. This cumulative phenomenon occurs in all of us and is a major factor in aging, but it becomes a greater concern when blood glucose levels start to rise. Accelerated atherosclerosis, arthritis, leg ulcers and eye damage found in diabetics are all a direct result of this process. "Protein sticking" has an adverse effect on all the systems of the body, including and especially the immune system.

The degree of "protein sticking" (technically called "glycosylation") can be detected easily by measuring the amount of glucose stuck to hemoglobin molecules (hemoglobin is the stuff that carries oxygen in your blood). This test, called a Hemoglobin A-1-C, is useful for measuring the level of blood sugar control in a diabetic, but is also a useful measure of the degree of glucose toxicity in a non-diabetic individual. The normal range is 3% to 6%. A diabetic with poor control may have values of 8 or greater and with good control, a value of about 6%. Most "normal" patients have levels of 5.5 to 6%, evidence of a very concerning trend in America. Ideally I like to see a value of 5% in healthy individuals.

Marie is a breast cancer survivor. She was diagnosed three years ago and after completing therapy was given a good prognosis for survival. While seeing her for a routine PAP smear, she mentioned that she had been started on a medication by her internist for adult-onset diabetes. Even after being on the medication for several months her hemoglobin A-1-C was still well above seven. Knowing that even mildly elevated glucose levels can adversely affect the immune system, I was concerned that this condition may ultimately affect her survival from breast cancer. I recommended much more aggressive therapy including not only dietary changes, but also additional medical therapy to lower blood glucose levels even further. The drug I had in mind consisted of an insulin-

like compound that occurs naturally in the body. It works effectively without upsetting other systems in the body.

Most tissues of the body can use glucose for fuel, but the brain uses it almost exclusively. For this reason, the level of glucose in the bloodstream must be very tightly regulated. Too little, and the brain screams for more; too much, and the toxic effects of glucose quickly become apparent. This "glucose thermostat" is maintained by a complex series of hormones with the most important one being insulin.

When you take a bite out of a confection such as a donut, the starch and sugar are broken down into pure glucose almost before you taste the sweetness. The glucose is rapidly absorbed through the small intestine, sending a surge of glucose into your bloodstream that sets off alarm bells. In response, the hormone insulin (secreted by special cells in the pancreas) is immediately released. *Insulin sends a special message to the cells of your liver and muscle, allowing these tissues to take up the extra glucose, thus rapidly lowering your blood glucose back to normal.* Without insulin, this vital function could not occur and blood glucose would continue to rise until you were quite ill.

A donut every now and then is okay, but eating a high starch and sugar diet on a daily basis can only lead to dire consequences. After being subjected to unremitting surges of glucose followed by compulsory surges in insulin, the cells of the liver and muscles finally say, "Enough is enough, and no more!" Like teenagers ignoring nagging parents, they just stop listening. The body cannot have this, of course, because high levels of glucose are toxic, so the pancreas is pushed to secrete ever higher amounts of insulin to force cells into accepting more glucose. The chronically elevated insulin levels that result create a vicious cycle that is referred to as *insulin resistance*. *Impaired glucose metabolism* is a more general term also used to describe the same process.

With time, the insulin-producing cells of the pancreas gradually lose their ability to keep up the obligatory surges of insulin and the "glucose thermostat" starts to rise--initially to a *pre-diabetic* level, but eventually to a level classified as *Type 2* diabetes, generally requiring medications or injections of insulin. The incidence of insulin resistance and Type 2 diabetes in this country is astoundingly high and still on the rise.

Basic screening for Type II diabetes can be done by measuring a simple "fasting blood glucose level." A value over 110 mg/dL is considered pre-diabetic, but I become concerned about the possibility of loss of pancreatic reserves with anything over 100 mg/dL. Overt diabetes is suspected with a value over 130 mg/dL.

For optimal health, fasting blood glucose should be maintained below 94 and hemoglobin A-1-C should be less than 6.0. Fasting blood glucose consistently >100 mg/dL suggests that the pancreas has lost half of its ability to produce insulin—permanently. This is a case where active therapy beyond dietary changes alone should be considered to compensate for cumulative damage.

Not all of the sugar and starch in that donut is immediately burned for energy. The leftovers are stored for later use as *glycogen*, a substance similar to starch. Glycogen storage occurs in both liver and muscle tissue. This is very practical, as when we go for periods without eating, glycogen can be readily converted back into glucose to bring blood levels back to normal. During intense exercise we depend on our glycogen stores, but they can become depleted. When runners talk about "hitting a wall," they have used up all of their glycogen.

Interestingly, chronically high insulin levels block the body's ability to break down glycogen. Without the ability to break down glycogen, blood glucose levels quickly crash if an insulin-resistant individual goes without eating or attempts vigorous exercise. In other words, if you live on a steady diet of donuts, white bread, potato chips and the like, the body loses its ability to compensate if blood glucose is not constantly replenished. This phenomenon, referred to as *hypoglycemia* (low blood sugar), translates into an insatiable hunger, craving for carbohydrates, and exercise intolerance. When you include the additional effect elevated insulin has of blocking fat from being removed from fat stores, chronic obesity is inevitable.

The feeling of shakiness and hunger commonly associated with hypoglycemia can occur at normal blood glucose levels in insulin-resistant individuals. With insulin resistance the "glucose thermostat" is altered such that higher levels of glucose are required to maintain normalcy. A person with insulin resistance may start feeling uncomfortable at a blood glucose level of 95 or even 100, and will maintain blood glucose above that level. A normal person may not notice changes until the blood glucose is well below 80, and normally maintains blood glucose in the range between 80 and 90. This translates into a much higher level of tissue damage for the insulin-resistant individual, even though that person is not diabetic.

Any person with insulin resistance should be acutely aware of the fact that exercise allows glucose to enter cells without insulin. Regular exercise is one of the best ways to reverse the effects of insulin resistance and may help alter the set-point of the "glucose thermostat" in a positive way.

Screening for impaired glucose metabolism is not as straightforward as screening for diabetes. In the early stages of insulin resistance, fasting blood glucose may be perfectly normal. A person with fasting blood glucose of 83 could still be insulin-resistant. As cells of the body become more resistant to insulin and the pancreas becomes more stressed, the "glucose thermostat" gradually rises toward a concerning level. Formal testing for insulin resistance includes hourly measurements of glucose and insulin levels for three hours after consuming 100 grams of glucose (called a glucose tolerance test—3 hour GTT). Formal testing is not always necessary; any person who displays a triad of weight gain, carbohydrate craving, and episodes of hypoglycemia while following an average American diet can be assumed to have impaired glucose metabolism, no matter what the lab values show.

The adverse effects of insulin resistance are not limited solely to weight gain and concern for diabetes. Chronically elevated insulin levels not only throw a monkey wrench into the entire glucose-regulating system, but also have a negative influence on all of the hormone systems of the body. This cascade of dysfunction impacts the adrenal hormones, the male and female reproductive hormones, and definitely affects the way the brain functions. Either directly or indirectly, both insulin and glucose may play a role in inducing cancer.

Once insulin resistance is established, it takes a *long time* to reverse. Often, insulin-resistant individuals expect immediate weight loss and reversal of symptoms with dietary and lifestyle modifications. It just doesn't happen that way. Reversal of cellular changes takes months and sometimes years. Of more immediate concern is the need to tighten blood glucose control. Changing to a better diet and exercise are essential, but proper therapy can reduce the damaging effects of elevated glucose. Many supplements and medications are available to reverse insulin resistance. In certain situations, gastric bypass or gastric banding may be lifesaving for morbidly obese individuals with insulin resistance or diabetes.

Irene presented with complaints including irregular and sometimes heavy periods, weight gain across her middle abdomen, and acne. Other symptoms included carbohydrate craving and episodes of hypoglycemia. Her blood pressure was mildly elevated. She had been given a diagnosis of polycystic ovaries and was already on birth control pills to regulate her periods. Her mother was a nurse and had read that medications for diabetes could be helpful for treatment of polycystic ovaries. A series of lab tests ordered by another provider had confirmed the diagnosis of polycystic ovaries, but her hemoglobin A-1-C was only 4.7, suggesting that she was not diabetic. Irene's health questionnaire revealed very poor dietary habits and a very high stress level.

Often the diagnosis of insulin resistance remains elusive. Even though the hemoglobin A-1-C suggests that Irene's blood glucose levels have not been elevated, all the signs point to insulin resistance as the root cause of her symptoms. High glucose diets precipitate elevated insulin levels well before glucose levels start to rise. Elevated insulin levels have adverse effects on not only adrenal hormones but also reproductive hormones. Female reproductive hormones are shifted toward a male pattern, causing acne and irregular periods. The change in adrenal hormones contributes to central obesity and hypertension. A high stress level adds fuel to the fire, throwing off adrenal hormones even further.

My recommendations did include starting an anti-diabetic medication to normalize glucose metabolism as quickly as possible; more importantly, she was encouraged to follow strict dietary modifications limiting glucose consumption and was counseled about stress reduction. If she follows these recommendations, all of her symptoms should resolve completely and she should be able to stop the medication at some point, but she will have to stick with diet and lifestyle changes forever.

THE CHOLESTEROL CONNECTION

Like so many individuals, for many years I carried the belief that cholesterol problems came from consuming too much meat, eggs and dairy. Though diets high in saturated fat also tend to be high in cholesterol, this dietary cholesterol, except in rare incidences, is not the source of high blood cholesterol. Only 25% of cholesterol in the body comes from dietary sources; the remaining 75% is synthesized by the liver. Problems with cholesterol stem from the body's incessant ability to manufacture cholesterol and gradual loss of the ability to properly get rid of it.

As it turns out, having a cholesterol problem is more related to consuming a low fiber, high glucose diet than to eating too much fat! Here's why: By the third donut of the morning your glycogen stores are completely topped off for the day and not much energy is required for sitting at a desk. The extra glucose building up in your bloodstream has to go somewhere. That somewhere is the adipose tissue around your middle. Fatty tissue itself, however, does not readily convert glucose into fat; this process occurs mainly in the liver. *Newly formed fat must be transported from its origins in the liver to the adipose tissue of the body via the bloodstream.* This presents a problem. As you know, fat and water do not mix very well. To solve this dilemma, the liver is able to synthesize special particles called *lipo-proteins.* Lipo-proteins consist of a microscopic globule of fat enveloped with a layer of protein, allowing the particle to be soluble in the blood. Cholesterol is a necessary ingredient to keep the particle stable. *The liver regularly uses cholesterol to synthesize lipo-protein particles.*

Though cholesterol carries a negative image in many peoples' minds, cholesterol is vital for many functions within the human body. Not only does it stabilize lipoprotein particles, but it also stabilizes all of the cell membranes in the body. Cholesterol is the precursor for many hormones in the body and is an essential component of bile, necessary for the digestion of fat. The body considers cholesterol to be a precious substance and carefully re-circulates it. As we could never depend on dietary sources alone to provide all that we need, the body has a significant capacity to not only manufacture it, but also to conserve it. In fact, cholesterol inside the body only becomes a problem when it is not properly re-circulated.

A newly formed lipo-protein particle travels from the liver to adipose tissue via the bloodstream. On arrival at the adipose tissue, the fatty contents of the particle are disgorged into a fat cell. The leftover particle, now containing mainly cholesterol, is left floating around in the bloodstream. *This particle, referred to as LDL (low density lipo-protein), is the one your doctor is worried about.*

Much of the cholesterol found in LDL particles does end up back in the cholesterol re-circulation pathway, but not all of it. The liver acts like a net that captures vagrant LDL particles as they pass through the bloodstream. LDL particles, however, vary in size. Smaller particles tend to slip through the net and remain floating in the bloodstream, thus remaining a threat. Fortunately all is not lost, as a scavenger particle, called HDL, picks up cholesterol and adds it to smaller LDL particles, such that they can be "caught" by the liver and re-circulated. HDL particles are the good guys. *Risk of atherosclerosis is partially defined by the amounts of HDL particles as compared to small LDL particles.*

THE SILENT THREAT OF ATHEROSCLEROSIS

Risk, however, is not defined by quantities of small LDL particles alone. Small LDL particles left floating in the bloodstream *do not* become a problem unless they are "oxidized" by free radicals. Free radicals, as we know, are chemical substances that have the potential to do damage to living tissue. There are many varieties of free radicals. Certain types of toxins are free radicals or can generate free radicals in the bloodstream. Toxins in cigarette smoke would be a good example. Abnormal fats found in processed and fried foods are notorious for increasing the presence of free radicals in the bloodstream. Free radicals can also be produced by the inflammatory cells of the immune system as part of our defense mechanisms. *Any type of chronic inflammatory reaction in the body can contribute to the problem.* Chronic sinusitis, arthritis, inflammatory bowel disease and even periodontal (gum) disease can be associated with an increased risk of cardiovascular disease.

Dietary fats absorbed through the small intestines are transported via a different type of lipoprotein directly to tissues. Only a small portion of the fat from your diet contributes to atherosclerosis, and the contribution of dietary fat to the process very much depends on the type of fat consumed. Oxidized fat from processed foods, fried foods, processed meats and stale or partially spoiled foods is a primary culprit causing LDL oxidation.

Oxidized LDL particles have the ability to directly damage the internal lining of blood vessels. Blood vessels with fast-moving blood, such as those of the arteries of the heart, are at greatest risk. White blood cells try to control the problem by engorging these abnormal particles, but become so laden with oxidized LDL that they become adherent to the vessel wall, thus aggravating the injury.

The body tries to heal the injured vessel wall by laying down a type of scar tissue called fibrin. Platelets, the blood components responsible for the formation of blood clots, stick to the damaged surface, further compounding the problem. Stress, usually a part of a high-risk lifestyle, increases platelet "stickiness." (While running from a tiger, you would want your blood to clot easily in case you became slashed.) The addition of a little oxidized fat makes for the beginnings of a well-organized atherosclerotic plaque. Plaque formation can block the vessel entirely or break off and block the lumen of a smaller vessel, with the end result of a stroke or heart attack.

The process of atherosclerosis, as described above, is a major cause of premature morbidity and mortality in this country. As we age, cholesterol levels gradually rise and we must become increasingly vigilant about reducing the threat of atherosclerosis.

There are several components of a strategy to lower risk:

- *Decrease total cholesterol. The first step in lessening this preventable threat is dietary: avoid processed food to reduce consumption of excessive glucose and abnormal fats. Eat fiber-rich foods, which help remove cholesterol from the system. Certain supplements and pharmaceuticals have the ability to reduce cholesterol even further, but cholesterol should only be lowered to normal levels, <u>not</u> <u>below</u> normal levels. Cholesterol is essential for normal functions in the body and excessively low cholesterol is associated with many health concerns.* (**Avoid lowering your cholesterol excessively with drug therapy!**)

- *Increase favorable HDL particles. The three main strategies include following a regular exercise routine, enjoying a glass of wine or beer with meals, and supplemental doses of the vitamin niacin (under the care of a healthcare provider).*

- *Prevent oxidation of small LDL particles: Avoid foods with oxidized fat (fried or processed foods). Fruits and vegetables provide anti-oxidants that protect against* oxidative stress. Anti-oxidant supplements, such as grape seed/skin extract, provide additional protection.

- Prevent platelet aggregation and fibrin deposition: There are many types of blood thinners. Some safe ones to consider include fish oil or flax seed oil (which also provide anti-oxidant protection), garlic, and low dose aspirin (81mg enteric-coated). Effectively managing stress is also a key factor in decreasing platelet aggregation. Enzymes found in certain whole foods and fermented foods may play a role in degrading fibrin present in plaques. (**Essential fatty acid supplements may be as important as any drug for reducing the threat of atherosclerosis.**)

- Protect liver function by reducing exposure to toxins. Again, avoid processed foods, and become more "toxin aware" (see chapter 10). Vegetables, especially from the cruciferous family (broccoli, cabbage, cauliflower), artichoke and the herb milk thistle are especially protective of liver function. The damage that toxins cause to liver cells is a contributing factor to the gradual rise in blood cholesterol as we age.

- Treat insulin resistance and diabetes. The gradual rise of insulin and the set-point of the glucose thermostat parallel the gradual rise in cholesterol—the three are closely tied together.

TAKE HEART! Atherosclerosis is reversible! Atherosclerotic plaques will shrink with proper dietary changes, exercise, stress reduction, appropriate supplements and medications.

Most healthcare providers order a lipid panel, where cholesterol is broken down into different lipoprotein particles. Ever wondered what those numbers mean? Total cholesterol is less important than the values of the subcomponents. LDL cholesterol, the most concerning particles, should ideally have a value below 130 mg/dL. A normal HDL value is above 40, but the higher the better; values above 60 are more ideal. Risk of atherosclerosis is best evaluated by looking at the ratio between LDL and HDL. Ideally, the LDL/HDL ratio should be less than 4.5. For optimal health, the ratio should be less than 3.5. Supplements and sometimes carefully-chosen medications can be beneficial for achieving this goal.

More advanced testing measures the size of both LDL and HDL particles. Smaller particles of both HDL and LDL translate into higher risk.

Complete risk assessment includes measurement of C-reactive protein, an indicator of inflammation (and oxidative stress) in the bloodstream. For optimal health, the C-reactive protein level should be less than 1.0.

NOTE: *The primary method of treating atherosclerosis in conventional medicine today is with use of medications called statins. These medications effectively lower cholesterol, but are associated with significant side effects. Depletion of a vitamin-like substance called co-enzyme Q-10 is commonly associated with muscle pain and possibly increased risks of heart failure. Statins appear to inhibit the ability of the liver to process toxins, a factor that may contribute to increased cancer risks. There is a place for use of statin medications, but they should be used judiciously and at the lowest possible dose. As with most diseases, the risk of atherosclerosis should be addressed comprehensively instead of with drug therapy alone.*

FRUCTOSE: THE OTHER SIMPLE CARBOHYDRATE

Fructose, commonly known as fruit sugar, is also becoming a dietary concern. Fructose artificially added to processed foods and beverages is a greater problem than fructose naturally found in fruit. Because fructose is sweeter than glucose, it is heavily used in the commercial food industry. High fructose corn syrup long ago replaced sucrose (table sugar) as the predominant sweetener in processed foods. Many "health" drinks and foods are sweetened with concentrated fruit juices, which are predominantly concentrated fructose.

From a health point of view, excessive fructose may be more of a concern than glucose. Fructose has the same "protein sticking" problem that glucose has, but blood fructose levels are not as tightly controlled. Insulin has no influence over fructose levels. There are no mechanisms for direct storage of fructose in the body. It is not a preferred fuel for the brain. The only recourse the body has for getting rid of excessive fructose is turning it directly into fat. This process generates extra cholesterol synthesis and has the potential to contribute to atherosclerosis.

THE DISACCHARIDES

Sucrose: Ordinary table sugar is actually a "double sugar" made from a molecule of glucose bonded to a molecule of fructose. Enzymes in the intestine free the bond, releasing equal amounts of glucose and fructose. For this reason, sucrose does not deliver as much of a glucose load as starch. Even so, consumption of table sugar contributes to the daily total of simple carbohydrates and it should be used sparingly.

Lactose: Commonly known as "milk sugar," lactose is also a double sugar comprised of a molecule of glucose and a molecule of a sugar called galactose. Many adults lack the enzyme lactase, which is necessary to break down milk products. Without this enzyme, undigested lactose flushes through the intestinal tract, causing diarrhea and flatulence. Lactose-intolerant individuals should generally avoid all milk products with the exception of fermented products such as yogurt.

FAT

From a dietary point of view, fats are just as important as sugars for maintaining normal health. These molecules come in many different shapes and sizes, and they have numerous functions within the human body. In the case of dietary fats, the *amount* of fat is less important than the *type* of fat. While the right fats can add to your health in many ways, the wrong fats can make you very ill.

MISCONCEPTIONS ABOUT FAT

Consumption of not only excessive amounts of fat but also abnormal types of fat delineates another concerning aspect of processed-food diets. Fat plays a much larger role in the body than just providing an energy source. Many normal functions within the human body involve fats; the inventory of fats influences how well these functions will occur. The three different types of fat to know about include saturated fat, polyunsaturated fat and mono-unsaturated fat. Each category of fat comes in many forms, and the different forms serve different purposes within the body. The potential for harm, however, is often related to what was done to the oil or fat before consumption.

There is no doubt that baked goods plump up better and taste better when made with saturated fat. Your great-grandmother always used lard or butter to make biscuits, but biscuits may not have been an everyday affair because animal fats were expensive and did not keep well. A new age of cooking was ushered in when the Crisco Company introduced vegetable shortening in 1911. For a fraction of the cost of animal fat, liquid poly-unsaturated vegetable oil could be made into saturated fat by a process known as "hydrogenation." Margarine is made by this same process. Though margarine and vegetable shortening may look and taste very similar to their animal source equivalents, hydrogenation causes unnatural changes to the oil, leaving it of questionable value for human consumption.

If all of the fat we consumed each day was immediately burned, the source and type would actually not matter very much, but the role of fat in the human body goes well beyond energy production. The old saying, "you are what you eat" is very accurate when it comes to fat. All of the billions of cells in our bodies are individually surrounded by a membrane that is composed of a double layer of specialized fat. All together, this adds up to a significant amount of fat. Most of the lipids within your cell membranes come from fat that is consumed. *In fact, any type of fat that is consumed has the potential to end up in your cell membranes.*

Cell membranes deserve more attention than they get. Everything that the cell needs to function must come through the membrane. Some substances diffuse directly through the membrane and others are transported across by specialized proteins floating within the membrane. Other types of specialized proteins within the membrane act as receptors for hormones or other chemical messengers that direct functions within the cell. In short, cell membranes are vital for normal function of every cell within the body. *If your cell membranes are not up to par, you cannot expect to feel well.*

A diet high in *saturated fat* or *hydrogenated fat* creates cell membranes that are stiff (think of vegetable shortening). From a functional point of view, this is not how you want your cell membranes to be. Liquid fat (oil) makes the membrane more fluid, and therefore more functional, but there is a tradeoff. Poly-unsaturated fats are very susceptible to damage by free radicals. **Refined oils and hydrogenated oils contain fats that have already become free radicals and are therefore extremely damaging to cell membranes.** "Trans-fats" are polyunsaturated fats that have been shifted into an unnatural configuration by high heat or chemicals. *This abnormal configuration does not mesh well with other, normal lipids in the membrane and can disallow essential functions of that membrane.* These abnormal fats are certainly not something that you want in each of your trillions of cell membranes.

Deep frying, a central component of the American fast food scene, requires hot, liquid oil. The least expensive oils are derived from vegetable sources, most commonly corn, soybean or canola. Vegetable oil consists mainly of poly-unsaturated fat. Poly-unsaturated fats are very fragile and susceptible to damage by heat. Inexpensive vegetable oils are "refined" or extracted from the original source using high heat and harsh chemicals. This process damages the fat and creates abnormal fats that act as free radicals and become the infamous "trans-fats" that everyone is worried about. Pour this oil into a large vat and heat it to the temperature required for deep fat frying, and you have a real caldron of toxic substances on your hands.

Recently I was amused to read that several states have banned the use of trans-fats for deep fat frying in restaurants. Tran- fats do not occur readily in nature and are not present in vegetable oil before it is extracted from the plant. Tran- fats are created when the poly-unsaturated fat (oil) extracted from a plant such as corn is exposed to high heat during the extraction process. Exposure to high heat associated with deep fat frying actually creates trans-fats. Even if you start with "trans-fat- free" oil, trans-fats will be created during the deep fat frying process. Sometimes we do the most nonsensical things.

The type of fat that you do want to have in your cell membranes is a special class of poly-unsaturated fats called *mono-unsaturated* fats. These fats, commonly found in olive oil, nuts and avocados, are much more resistant to oxidation, but still maintain the fluidity necessary for good cell membrane function. The healthiest cell membranes are composed predominantly of mono-saturated fat with just a little touch of saturated fat thrown in for good measure.

Saturated fat is not all bad. It is extremely stable and resistant to damage by free radicals. This is a very desirable quality and having just the right amount of it in cell membranes is essential. Also, the link between saturated fat and atherosclerosis is not very strong. Fat, in general, is absorbed directly through the intestines and is transported through the bloodstream to other parts of the body by a different system of "lipo-proteins" than the one mentioned for glucose-derived fat transport. The body seems to know how to deal with these end-products more efficiently and they do not seem to be big players in atherosclerosis. The health concern associated with consumption of saturated fat in foods such as beef, pork, and dairy products has more to do with toxins dissolved in the fat and imbalances in a special group of fats called "essential fatty acids" than it has to do with the saturated fat itself.

Essential fatty acids (EFA's) are a special group of polyunsaturated fats termed "essential" because they cannot be synthesized by the body and must be obtained from dietary sources. Getting enough EFA's to survive is generally not a problem because they are abundant in the foods we eat, but getting the right ratio of the right types is a different story altogether. Essential fatty acids have many important functions in the human body, from contributing to healthy cell membranes to regulation of inflammation in the body.

The process of inflammation is intended to be part of a healing process. Our immune system is constantly correcting damage caused by free radicals, toxins, invading microbes and the like. This very complex system requires careful orchestration of specialized cells found in the bloodstream and other parts of the body. Various types of chemical messengers are used to organize an inflammatory response. Many of these chemical messengers are derived from essential fatty acids. A correct balance of different types of EFA's is important: With just the right balance of essential fatty acids, health is optimized; however, too much of one type of essential fatty acid may lead to an exaggerated inflammatory response occurs, which is damaging.

The types and amounts of essential fatty acids that we consume very much influence the inflammatory response in our bodies. The average American diet is very high in the essential fatty acids termed *Omega-6* but very low in *Omega-3*. Certain types of Omega-6 EFA's tend to heighten the inflammatory response while Omega-3 EFA's tend to moderate it. So, in terms of essential fatty acids, average American diets are very "pro-inflammatory." Grain-fed livestock and poultry are high in inflammation-inducing Omega-6 and very low in Omega-3. The opposite would be preferred (for the animal and for us). When these same animals are allowed to eat natural grasses (i.e. free-range) they have much higher levels of Omega-3's. Oily fish such as mackerel, tuna, salmon, and sardines are naturally high in these important essential fatty acids. Vegetarian sources of omega-3's include flax seed oil, borage oil, and walnuts.

The ratio of omega-6 to omega-3 fatty acids can be measured. For optimal health, the ratio for reduced inflammatory response is 4:1. The average ratio for most Americans is closer to 20:1. When omega-3 saturation testing becomes standardized, it may develop into an optimal test for predicting the incidence of both atherosclerosis and chronic disease.

Omega-3 EFA's have other benefits, too: for example, they help to prevent oxidation of "LDL" cholesterol. This may be more important in preventing arterial plaque formation than lowering the cholesterol. In addition, EFA's act as a mild blood thinner, which tends to protect against plaque formation. Diets higher in Omega-3 EFA's tend to lower one's risk of inflammatory diseases such as arthritis and atherosclerosis, and probably also decrease your risk of cancer. *A high-quality "fish oil" or essential fatty acid supplement is the one dietary supplement that everyone over the age of 40 should consider.*

PROTEINS

Proteins are responsible for a wide range of functions within the human body. They are, in essence, what makes us tick. Thousands of different types of proteins perform a mind-boggling number of functions within the human body.

These vital proteins include the following:

- *Enzymes, responsible for regulating all of the biochemical reactions necessary for life, are proteins. Often these enzymes require vital cofactors in the form of vitamins and minerals to function properly.*

- *Specialized proteins allow muscles to contract, skin to stretch, and hormones to work.*

- *Found in our blood, the hemoglobin molecule carries oxygen; other blood proteins are responsible for carrying nutrients and hormones throughout the body and also act as buffers to regulate blood pH.*

- *Antibodies and some other essential parts of the immune system are proteins that protect us from foreign invaders.*

- *Proteins are an integral part of all cell membranes. Some regulate the passage of substances in and out of the cell; other cell membrane proteins are receptors for chemical messengers.*

The most basic components of proteins are molecules called amino acids. There are about twenty amino acids used to make proteins in the body, but many other amino acids occur in nature. Nine amino acids are considered "essential," meaning they cannot be synthesized by the body and must be obtained from dietary sources.

One of the primary uses of amino acids is in protein synthesis. Long chains of amino acids are linked together to form the basic protein structure. The chain is then folded several times to create the final protein. The exact sequences of amino acids are coded for by DNA within our genes. *Mutations in our genes can result in improper coding and thus in formation of abnormal proteins.*

Amino acids can be linked to form shorter chains called peptides. Many of our hormones are peptides or polypeptides. Insulin is a good example of a polypeptide hormone. The sequence of the amino acids determines the function of the polypeptide.

Amino acids have other vital functions besides the formation of peptide chains and proteins. Amino acids themselves can be chemical messengers or can be modified into other chemical messengers within the body. Some of these amino acids are not ever found in proteins. The neurotransmitters epinephrine, dopamine, and serotonin found within the nervous system and brain are examples of chemical messengers made from amino acids. Thyroid hormones are modified amino acids. Certain amino acids are even precursors to the molecules that make up our DNA.

Another important function of amino acids is protection from free-radicals. Several amino acids containing sulfur groups can be converted into a chemical called *glutathione*. Glutathione is present in all cells and is a remarkably important antioxidant. *Glutathione* is especially important in liver cells where detoxification occurs. Adequate sources of these amino acids are necessary for glutathione synthesis. Also, Vitamin C and vitamin E are essential for regeneration of glutathione.

Proteins in the body continuously wear out and need to be replaced. Worn-out proteins are broken down into component amino acids, which are often reused. Protein, lost from the body via metabolism, urine, feces, and menstrual flow contributes to the constant turnover. Amino acids are also lost via metabolism for energy production or conversion into other vital chemicals. Our bodies use about 80 to 100 grams of protein each day. A moderate dietary intake of protein is necessary to replace daily protein and amino acid losses. Fortunately, in America, sources of quality dietary protein are readily available.

The quality of dietary protein is assessed by the assortment of amino acids contained. A complete protein source offers all of the essential amino acids. If a single essential amino acid is regularly missing from the diet, protein synthesis may be hampered.

Eggs are often the standard by which all other dietary proteins are graded. Eggs are considered a complete source of protein as they contain all of the necessary amino acids for protein synthesis including all of the essential amino acids. Eggs also contain vital minerals and many important chemicals substances. Other complete sources of protein include dairy products, meat, fish, and shellfish and soy beans. Adequate dietary protein can easily be obtained from vegetarian sources by combining foods. Certain plants may not be complete protein sources in themselves, but they may contain essential amino acids that others do not have. Varying foods such as brown rice with wheat, nuts, beans, or other seeds provides a complete source of protein.

The body has the ability to break down proteins to use as a primary energy source but only elects to do so in a pinch. It would be analogous to pealing the planks off a wooden ship to burn them in the engine room. Proteins from food sources, broken down into component amino acids in the intestines, can also be used as an energy source, but they are best used to make new proteins. Amino acids only become a primary energy source in the absence of sugars.[*] The body must actually expend more energy to use amino acids as an energy source. This is the premise behind weight loss using low-carbohydrate diets.

If by this point you have decided to exclude <u>all</u> dietary carbohydrates and join the throngs of individuals who have turned to strict low-carb diets, you should think twice. Without carbohydrates, fat and protein become the primary energy sources for the body. Fat is good for the "slow burn," but is a poor source of quick energy for activities such as thinking or running. The brain uses lots of energy and demands glucose. Often people complain of "brain fog" while following a low-carb diet for any length of time. Further, the fats consumed in low-carb diets tend to be unhealthy fats and contribute to oxidative stress and inflammation. High fat, high protein diets are directly linked to increased risks of arthritis, immune suppression and cancer.

Amino acids from broken-down or digested proteins can be used as a primary energy source, but are not designed to do so. Only part of the amino acid can be used for energy production and the left-over by-products are toxic. High protein diets are associated with

---

[*] The intestines do use certain amino acids as a primary fuel source, but this is a minor part of the total energy consumption of the body.

decreased absorption of calcium (and a concomitant increased risk of osteoporosis), an increased incidence of gout and an increased risk of kidney failure. When used as primary energy sources, protein and fat generate toxic by-products and excessive amounts of free radicals. (This is one of the problems with meat in general.)

VITAMINS AND MINERALS

Vitamins are chemical substances that must be obtained from dietary sources. Without these vital chemicals, key reactions in the body would not occur and life would not be possible. The classic vitamins include A, B, C, D, E, and K. While knowing all the details of each vitamin is not necessary, it is important to note that the letters represent "families" of chemicals and not just one single chemical. There are many different types of B vitamins and vitamin E comes in at least eight different forms (a fact that seems to be lost on many vitamin supplement manufacturers who supply only one synthetic form of each vitamin in their "once-a-daily's").

It is also important to note that the different vitamins are not related chemicals. Being distinctly different, they come from different food sources. This is one of the reasons why it is so vital to eat a wide variety of foods. All of the vitamins, with the exception of one, can be obtained from plant sources. Vitamin B-12 is synthesized only by bacteria and is acquired only by consuming meat products or through supplements.

Besides vitamins, there are many other key chemicals required for the body's vital reactions. These chemical substances differ from the classic vitamins in that the body has the ability to synthesize them; dietary sources are not essential. Even so, acquiring these substances from food sources saves the body work and energy—another good reason to follow a healthy diet. As we age, our bodies gradually lose the ability to produce some of these substances. Co-enzyme Q-10, a key chemical necessary for energy production, is one example. Some people over fifty will experience less daily fatigue when taking a co-enzyme Q-10 supplement.

A commonly asked question is why some vital substances can be synthesized by the body and others, termed essential, must be obtained from dietary sources. The answer probably has to do with availability of foods as humans evolved. Very likely, substances that we now call vitamins were so readily available from dietary sources that certain organisms simply gave up the ability to make them—why waste energy on something that is already there? A good example is vitamin C. Humans and other primates are the only higher animals that cannot synthesize vitamin C, evidence suggesting that the diets of primitive humans were very high in vitamin C.

Minerals from the earth are vital for all living organisms. Bones would not be possible without calcium and phosphorus. Our hemoglobin could not carry oxygen without iron. Thyroid hormones depend on iodine. Fluctuations in sodium and potassium ions are essential for many cellular functions. The immune system depends on both zinc and selenium. All the minerals required by the body for daily functions must be obtained from dietary sources and are readily present in a varied diet of whole foods.

Minerals are important for maintaining normal pH in the bloodstream and tissues of the body. Optimal pH for all chemical functions in the body is 7.4. Slightly alkaline pH keeps calcium and other minerals in bones and is associated with good health in general. The best way to maintain slightly alkaline pH is by regularly consuming vegetables and fruit. The regular dietary addition of unrefined sea salt may also help to maintain a slightly alkaline pH.

Processed foods, refined sugar, soft drinks and high protein diets push the body toward acidic pH. Beyond being associated with poor health in general, this may be a significant contributing factor to early loss of bone density and osteoporosis, which is now at near epidemic levels in the United States.

Though some minerals naturally found in the soil are beneficial for living organisms, others are actually poisonous. Metals including mercury, cadmium, aluminum, beryllium, lead and arsenic are quite toxic. These substances are not found to significant degree in natural foods and are by-products of industrialization and industrial food production. A healthy diet not only reduces exposure, but also helps the body rid itself of these toxic substances.

PHYTO-NUTRIENTS

Plants contain thousands of different types of chemical compounds that are commonly referred to as "phytochemicals." These chemical compounds are the ingredients that give a vegetable or fruit its distinct flavor; a factor that steers many people toward concoctions of fat and sugar which provide an intense taste of sweet, but offer little actual flavor. Anyone, however, can and should learn to enjoy these flavors, because they are important keys to enjoying a disease-free life.

Phytochemicals have many disease and cancer fighting attributes. Cruciferous vegetables (cabbage, broccoli, Brussels sprouts, cauliflower, kale are common examples) have been associated with diseases-fighting qualities since the beginning of recorded history and recently have been linked to reducing estrogen-related cancers. Berries contain chemicals with antioxidant, anti-inflammatory, anti-microbial and anti-cancer properties. Natural chemicals found in artichoke are potent antioxidants, lower cholesterol and at the same time, protect liver function. Green tea, soy and tomatoes are important anti-cancer foods. All culinary species have medicinal value. Turmeric, found in curries and ginger are known for potent anti-inflammatory properties. Both also have important cancer-preventing properties. Garlic and onions contribute to reducing many types of disease.

These are just a few important examples. Virtually all fruits and vegetables offer some disease-fighting value. The disease fighting capacity of a donut?—less than zero.

DIETARY FIBER

Dietary fiber includes all of the indigestible material in our food. Most of it comes from plant carbohydrates. Soluble fiber is made up of indigestible material that dissolves in water. Insoluble fiber makes up the bulk of stool and is not soluble in water. Both soluble and insoluble fiber are essential for normal health. Normal bowel function does not occur without adequate fiber. Fiber also aids in removal of toxins and excessive cholesterol, and it slows the absorption of glucose, helping to avoid insulin spikes. Though dietary fiber is not a source of energy or nutrients for us, certain types of fiber are a source of energy and nutrients for favorable bacteria in the large colon.

For optimal function, the waste disposal and detoxification systems of the body require a minimum of about 25 grams of dietary fiber every day. (An average American diet contains only about 5 to 10 grams.) Adequate dietary fiber, both soluble and insoluble, can easily be obtained by consuming a variety of vegetables, fruit, and whole grains.

Just the right amount of dietary glucose and other sugars found in whole foods are essential for good health. Healthy fats are essential to balance the cell membranes of the body. Adequate dietary protein must be present to offset daily turnover. Normal gastrointestinal function depends on fiber and vital chemical reactions would not occur without vital chemicals and minerals. Vegetables and fruits provide a host of disease-fighting phytochemicals. Mother Nature supplies the "right amounts" of each of these components in a well proportioned diet made up of a variety of fresh, whole foods.

CHAPTER 7
Getting to Know Your Food

Imagine an island.

With a moderate climate, the most likely location of the island would be in the Mediterranean or possibly off of New Zealand. The terrain of the island is mountainous in the central region with rolling hills and fertile valleys near the coast. Because of the central mountain range, the island is very wet on the side exposed to trade winds and dry on the opposite side. The air and water are clean. The growing season is long and a wide variety of fruits and vegetables can be produced year round. Coffee, tea, and cool weather crops are grown in the mountains. Vineyards and several wineries are located on the dry side. Olive trees grow locally and olive oil is a staple. Coconut trees are, of course, found along the beaches.

Small farms provide fresh eggs and unrefined dairy products. They also provide chicken, pork, and lamb in limited quantities. Beef is available, but rare. Seafood of all kinds is plentiful from the clean waters that surround the island. Fresh food is distributed at open-air markets found at several locations. At the markets you will also find fresh nuts, spices and fresh herbs. Small local groceries provide bulk goods such as basmati rice, beans and grain brought from the mainland. A stone mill will grind the grain into coarse flour for you to bake bread yourself, or you might patronize a bakery in the center of town that makes fresh whole grain breads daily. When planning a trip to the market, don't forget to bring your own containers, because nothing is encased in plastic.

Something to notice about the island is the absence of large grocery store chains. Processed and packaged foods, so common in America grocery stores, are too expensive to ship to the island and would go stale by the time they were sold. The islanders prefer food prepared fresh. Even the local restaurants and cafes prepare everything from scratch. Do not plan on fast food for lunch, as the midday meal is something to be savored.

I would have fared well being raised on such an island, but as it was, I grew up in the middle of the fast-food generation. For the longest time I thought Jimmy Buffet wrote "Cheeseburgers in Paradise" just for me—preferably two, with a whole plate of fries on the side. For most of my youth, I bought into the concept of fast food—hook, line, and sinker. And why not? Everything tasted good, didn't take any effort, and was available anytime you wanted it. Instant food, instant gratification. All that was necessary was a trip through the drive-thru, and a hot meal at home was as simple as browning a pound of hamburger and emptying the contents of a box into a skillet. Food was simple. Life was good.

As I crept into my thirties an expanding midline informed me that things were changing. Concern for a better diet was gradually forcing itself into my conscious thinking, but life was busy and change does not come easily. By mid-forties my blood pressure was creeping up a bit along with my blood glucose. A mid-morning snack and another one mid-afternoon had become a necessity to circumvent bouts of low blood sugar. This was occurring despite of the fact that I had become more nutritionally aware. My dietary habits had improved significantly, except for a cake and cookie addiction that I just could not shake. Starches and sugar had to go, but I was having a heck of a time giving them up.

Living on that island devoid of poor food choices would make switching to a healthier diet much easier, but life is never quite so simple. Finding healthier foods is not half as difficult as finding ways to incorporate them into daily life.

All of the healthy food choices available on the island can be readily found almost anywhere in America, but giving up all the unhealthy stuff is quite a challenge.

The first stage of my personal epicurean evolution included foods that *appeared* to be healthier versions of those to which I was already accustomed. Whole grains were emerging as a better choice, but my diet still consisted mainly of "healthier" forms of processed food. I call this my "granola bar and soy-burger phase". In an effort to be "totally healthy" I was not eating very much meat and was almost a vegetarian, though in retrospect my daily consumption of fresh vegetables was rather limited. This diet phase still contained a fair amount of "hidden" glucose and was heavy on grains. Because of their fat content I avoided foods that I now recognize as being healthy, such as nuts, eggs, and seafood. Gradually my nutritional education matured. Years of searching through both technical and non-technical information about nutrition all boiled down to basic common sense:

Healthy food, whether from vegetable or animal sources, is food that is closer to its natural origins.

Healthy food always starts with healthy soil. Topsoil, in its natural state, is a dynamic mixture of sand particles, water and organic matter. It is very much alive with a complex assortment of organisms including thousands of different types of bacteria, fungi, protozoa, insects and worms. Though these lowly creatures do not sound very exciting or important, they are vital for a natural cycle to take place. These living components of the soil constantly re-circulate dead and decaying matter from plants and animals, providing nutrients for new plant growth. This is an essential cycle of life. Any organic farmer will tell you this is the optimal way to provide nutrients for a healthy plant. Beyond the absence of toxic chemicals, organically grown food from living soil is much higher in nutrients that are important for our health.

Unfortunately, the vast majority of our food is *not* produced in living soil. Excessive tillage and pesticide use in modern agriculture destroys the living organisms within the soil. Without the natural decomposition of organic matter, a substantial amount of nutrients have to be artificially added back in the form of fertilizer. Mother Nature is hard to duplicate, and fertilizer never matches the nutrient capacity and delivery of dynamically living soil. The practice of growing monocultures of the same crops year after year depletes the soil even further. Raw food materials are then processed, pasteurized, homogenized, and pulverized into the nutritionally deficient commercial food products found on most grocery store shelves.

As I understood more about food, I realized my approach to food was going to have to change. It just did not make sense to regularly consume food that was obviously unhealthy, no matter how good it tasted. I decided that my shopping cart would no longer contain food items made with white flour, high fructose corn syrup and hydrogenated oil. I would not be visiting most of the aisles in the grocery store. Donuts and cakes I encountered daily would just have to go stale or be eaten by some other unfortunate soul. I would not be stopping at convenience marts or hording packaged snack foods to ward off bouts of low blood sugar. Fast food would be off-limits except for dire emergencies. *I would abstain.*

Compromises in life are often necessary. Food was going to cost a bit more, and I might have to make more effort to find quality food. Food products would have to be scrutinized carefully before being placed in the shopping cart. I would have to get to know the farmer down the road and search out local markets and vegetable stands. I might want to till a garden. Cooking more frequently would be a necessity. Tastes would have to change.

As with any change, changing to a better diet did not come easily, but change came with an almost unexpected transformation over a relatively short period of time. I immediately felt better. My taste buds gradually came alive as though they had been in a deep sleep. The sugar craving and episodes of hypoglycemia gradually subsided. My weight began to drop a bit. With time the new foods that at first tasted a bit odd became everyday staples and the processed stuff that I left behind began to seem as palatable as play-dough. A whole world of new foods opened up before my eyes. Healthy foods, combined with just the right amount of sugar, fat, and spices showed the potential of being quite appealing. An almost unlimited number of flavor sensations were possible. ***Healthy food became synonymous with tasty food.***

I have since come to think of my food only as "real" food—an apple as an apple. I do not want to know my food as a collection of processed flour, hydrogenated oil, high fructose corn syrup, polysorbate 80, red dye #53, and seasonings. What are those extras, anyway? The only label I want to see on my apple is one that defines where it came from and whether it is organic or not. Thinking of food in this fashion absolves me of the need for special equipment. I do not carry around a chart or calculator to figure out how much food to eat. I do not have a little book that tells me the "glycemic index" of the food I consume and I never count calories. A diet made up of a consistent variety of "real" food has the right amount of what you need on a daily basis and generalizations are quite sufficient. *Eating does not have to be academic to be healthy!*

This point was well illustrated the other day when I was leafing through a nutrition book dated to about 15 years ago. This particular book analyzed food by chemical components. An apple was rated as having moderate nutritional value with only average levels of vitamins and minerals which were all listed. There was no mention of quercetin, a chemical abundant in apples that reduces allergic reactions, or all of the beneficial cholesterol-lowering fiber that comes in an apple. Similarly, berries were not given high marks because of sugar content and moderate levels of vitamins. There was no mention of the potent anti-oxidants and immune-enhancing chemicals found in berries. They were not overlooked but were just not well-recognized at the time.

On a similar note, it seems that every year some new chemical is "discovered" from a natural food source and immediately hits store shelves as a supplement. Natural foods contain many different chemicals that are beneficial for our health. You do not have to wait until they are "discovered" to take advantage of these benefits. They are there all the time. We truly do live in the Garden of Eden, and you really do not have to look very hard to find it. Just pick from the wide variety of natural foods that are more abundantly available than ever before.

FOODS FROM PLANT SOURCES

An open-air market is one of my favorite places. Fruits and vegetables of all colors, shapes, and sizes, all presented at their peak of freshness, just waiting for someone to place them in a bag and carry them home for supper. And which ones should you choose? *Any* and *all* of them, of course! The reds, the blues, the oranges, the yellows, the purples, and especially the greens. The colors largely come from a group of chemicals called carotenoids. These substances are very potent anti-oxidants and are your best protection against oxidative stress, the chief factor in aging. You probably have heard of beta-carotene, lycopene, or lutein. They belong to the carotenoid family. There are over 600 different types of carotenoids, all of which have health benefits.

Beyond carotenoids, the fiber, vitamins, minerals, and other beneficial chemicals found in vegetables are important for preventing all types of disease, including cancer. Dietary fiber from vegetables, fruit, and whole grains not only improves gastrointestinal function, but also plays a large role in the removal of toxins and cholesterol from the body. Fruit pectin reduces fat absorption and removes heavy metals from the body. Enzymes present in natural foods have potent anti-inflammatory properties.

Admittedly, a plain stick of broccoli does not appear very interesting until you take a look at the health potential within. If everyone in the country were to eat a vegetable from the broccoli family at least once every day, the incidence of breast, prostate, and other cancers would drop dramatically! Now, that's something to get excited about. Cruciferous vegetables—which include not only broccoli but also cabbage, Brussels sprouts, kale, bok choy, and cauliflower—assist and improve the detoxification and removal of carcinogens by the liver. In addition, they increase the metabolism of hormones such as estrogen and hormonally-active toxins, an important function in preventing hormone-linked cancers.

The list of benefits from consuming vegetables goes on and on, but fortunately, you do not need to have a Ph.D. in biochemistry to take full advantage of their benefits. Mother Nature has done all of the research for you, and all you have to do is eat them regularly every day with as much variety as possible. For a truly healthy diet, I consider a regular assortment of vegetables to be more important than anything else.

Of the edible plants, the parts that can be consumed vary from species to species. Classically plants have roots, stems, leaves, an energy storage mechanism and some way to propagate. Many plants propagate by extending stems, but most often propagation involves a flower with resulting fruit and seeds. A seed contains all of the nutritional components necessary for starting a new plant. Various plant parts cover different aspects of adequate nutrition, and a healthy diet includes a mixture of many and diverse plants.

Which types of plants we consume is now very much dictated by agriculture. More than eight thousand years of food cultivation have selected for better tasting cultivars that provide a higher abundance of sugar, fat and protein, and other nutrients. Hybridization of food crops allows us to select out qualities of a plant we find desirable. New concepts of genetic manipulation allow desirable qualities of a plant to be targeted even more specifically and quickly.

The overall nutritional value of many edible plants has been increased. Several years ago, a display at our state fair documented the evolution of the sweet potato. The original from the late 1800's was a small, unappealing root with white meat, very different from the large, orange, anti-oxidant-filled potatoes in markets today. Many, if not most, cultivated fruits and vegetables have followed the same course of evolution.

Over-cultivation can, of course, go too far with the selection of sugar at the expense of other important nutrients and fiber. Many of our food crops have been cultivated to grow well in non-living soil to suit the constraints of modern agriculture. Here again, the trade-off is often at the expense of the nutritional value of the plant. Genetic manipulation of our food crops has the potential of taking this concern to an even higher level. *As a general rule, staying closer to what Mother Nature provides is the best way to make healthy food choices.*

VEGETABLE FRUITS AND "REAL" FRUITS

When it comes to the most desirable parts of plants, fruits are usually placed at the top of the list. Less sweet fruits such as tomatoes, squash, peppers, eggplants, pumpkins often get labeled as vegetables, but technically anything that comes from a flower is considered a fruit. For purposes of differentiation we can refer to these as "vegetable fruits" and to the better-recognized forms of fruit as simply "fruit." Vegetable fruits tend to be low in fat energy, moderately low in glucose energy, low in protein, but high in fiber, and very high in other important nutrients; these should be our daily staples.

The sweetness of the sugar held within is what makes "real" fruits so desirable. "Temperate" fruits are seasonal fruits grown in a climate with cold winters. They are moderate in sugar, low in fat, low in protein, high in fiber and very high in nutrients. Many members of this group contain potent anti-oxidants and immune enhancers. Examples include grapes, blueberries, strawberries, raspberries, apples, pears, peaches and cherries. Different types of melons also fit in this category.

"Tropical" fruits are grown year round in warmer climates. They are higher in natural sugars than temperate fruits but low in fat, low in protein, and high in fiber and other nutrients. Examples include: oranges, grapefruit, pineapples, star fruit, mangos, papaya and bananas.

Health Tip *Fruits, especially tropical fruits, are high in sugar, mostly fructose. Fructose, in excessive amounts, has the same "protein-sticking" effect as glucose and can raise cholesterol levels and contribute to increased body fat. Concentrated fructose found in fruit drinks is more of a problem than whole fruits, but excessive consumption of fruit should be avoided. Individuals in the process of trying to lose weight should especially limit quantities of tropical fruits and fruit juices.*

Variety is important with all foods. Too much of any one food is not a wise practice. A prime example is grapefruit. Grapefruit provides fiber and important nutrients including vitamin C, quercetin, and fruit pectin. Grapefruit also inhibits primary detoxification pathways in the liver, slowing metabolism of certain drugs, toxins and very importantly, estrogen. A recent study suggested that consuming one quart of grapefruit daily could increase postmenopausal breast cancer risk by 25-30%! (www.naturaldatabase.com)

STALKS, SHOOTS, STEMS AND LEAVES

Though they are often the least popular parts of the plant because of the absence of sugar and fat, stems, stalks and leaves were very much a part of ancestral diets and should be incorporated into our regular daily diet today. Low in energy and protein, but very high in fiber, nutrients, and especially minerals, these vegetable parts should make up the "bulk" of our diet. Examples include broccoli, cabbage, celery, rhubarb, kale, spinach, collards, chard, and bok choy.

Health Tip *Many Americans have the impression that a typical salad is health food. To the contrary, iceberg lettuce is probably one of the least nutritious foods on Earth and is certainly in the running for the most flavorless. The popularity of lettuce salad has more to do with the copious amounts of meat, cheese and salad dressing placed on top than it has to do with the lettuce itself. A better- quality, deep-green lettuce is a step in the right direction, but provides a smaller volume of actual food than you might expect. An entire bag of the "fancy" variety, advertised to provide four to six servings, when steamed down will only fill a couple of tablespoons.*

ROOTS AND TUBERS

Many plants store energy underground. This can be in the form of an actual root or as a modified stem called a tuber. Carrots, sweet potatoes, beets and parsnips are examples of roots. Other types of potatoes such as red potatoes and baking potatoes are examples of tubers. Tubers tend to be much higher in starch. Smaller potatoes such as the red skin variety have less starch. All are good sources of minerals and nutrients, and the colors are provided by carotenoids, those potent anti-oxidants so important for our health. As long as they do not come fried or in a box or bag, root vegetables and tubers are an important part of a healthy diet.

Almost in a class by themselves, onions and garlic have many health attributes that go beyond flavor. The chemicals that cause the pungent odors of these vegetables have anti-inflammatory, anti-oxidant, and cholesterol-lowering characteristics. Regular consumption may provide protection against heart disease, diabetes, cancer, osteoporosis and possibly even the common cold.

Health Tip *All plants contain trace amounts of natural toxins, but the chief concern is toxins added by agriculture. Most toxins are fat-soluble and are not retained well by the stems and leaves; therefore, they are less of a problem in "true" vegetables. The highest concern for pesticide retention is in thin-skinned fruits and vegetables that hold a lot of water. Buying organic, especially when it comes to fruits such as lettuces, tomatoes, apples, and berries, and getting to know the habits of your local farmers are wise food practices.*

Down the road, we have a vegetable and fruit stand set up by a local farmer. As often as I can, I buy fresh produce there. Usually the owner is around, but sometimes I pick out what I want, weigh it myself, and place money into a slot on the top of a little metal box. Some of the produce is grown on-site, but this fellow also drives up to the state farmer's market each week to obtain more variety. He can always tell me where each item came from and when it was picked. Now and then I have the opportunity to engage him in discussions about pesticide use, living soil, global warming and the like. We do not always agree on every topic, but somehow this dirt-floored, open-air fruit stand feels more comfortable than the cold and seemingly sterile aisles of the grocery store.

SEEDS

The category of seeds includes grains, beans and nuts. A single seed is the origin of new life and thus is truly a powerhouse of nutrition. Seeds are almost (but not quite) complete packages of nutrition, containing fiber, protein, fat, carbohydrates, and other nutrients. Unlike vegetables and fruits, seeds are good sources of fat, and even more importantly, are good sources of amino acids, the building blocks of proteins. Because they are such complete foods and can be easily cultivated and stored, grains and beans now make up the majority of food for the world.

GRAINS

Grains are the seeds of grasses or similar plants. The most commonly grown grains in the world are corn, wheat, rice, and distantly behind, oats. More corn is grown than any other grain, but much of it is used for livestock production. Wheat is the most widely consumed grain by humans overall, but rice is the most common grain in the Far East. All three of these grains have significant health value, but this value rapidly declines with over-consumption and excessive refinement, ever-prevalent in the commercial food industry.

> **Health Tip** *From a health point of view, whole grains are everything that their overly-refined cousins are not. Refined grains increase the risk of many, if not most, diseases—especially diabetes, heart disease and cancer. Whole grains (with the bran and germ still intact) slow the absorption of glucose, such that "sugar surges" are less of a concern. Fiber provided by the whole grain increases the motility of the GI tract and provides food for some types favorable bacteria in the gut, thus protecting against colon cancer. Regular consumption of whole grain fiber decreases cholesterol and lowers the risk of gallstones. The fiber in whole grains assists in removal of toxins from the body. Consumption of whole grains is also associated with a decreased risk of hormonally related cancers such as breast or prostate cancer.*

Wheat

The stuff bread is made of. The reason bread is made of wheat instead of other grains is because of a special protein called gluten that allows it to rise when mixed with yeast. The amount of gluten in the flour has a lot to do with how the final product turns out. Most people do not realize how much wheat flour can vary depending on the climate and soil where it is grown. Wheat flours with high levels of gluten are termed *hard* wheat. Typically, hard wheat comes from dry, cool climates and is used to make better quality bread and pasta. Flour with very low gluten content is termed *soft* wheat and is used to make cake flour. Pastries and cakes are made from cake flour. All-purpose flour is often a mix of the two.

> **Health Tip** *This simple lesson about wheat is very important for those trying to be mindful of glucose intake.* **The higher the gluten content of the flour, the slower glucose is absorbed from products made from it.** *Bread and pasta made from hard wheat can be an acceptable part of a healthy diet. Whole grain wheat, especially when from hard wheat, is even better from a nutritional point of view. Fiber found in the bran as well as minerals and oil contained within the wheat germ provide added nutritional value and slow the absorption of glucose even further.*

Be aware of the latest strategy by the commercial food industry to appeal to health-conscious consumers seeking a taste and feel that they are used to. Whole grains, most probably from softer wheat, are ground to a fine powder similar to plain white flour. The resulting product does have a similar feel and taste to white bread, but releases glucose almost as rapidly. If your "whole grain bread" is as fluffy as a pillow, pass it by. Look for "stone ground" whole grain products with a firmer feel.

Health Tip *While the majority of people tolerate gluten just fine, some people are sensitive to it. Gluten allergies can cause a host of symptoms ranging from gastrointestinal to neurological. Gluten intolerance can cause vitamin deficiencies, can mimic other medical conditions and can aggravate established medical conditions. Often gastrointestinal conditions, allergy symptoms, arthritis, and other chronic medical conditions will respond favorably to a gluten-free diet. Other gluten grains include oats, barley, rye and spelt, but wheat has the highest concentration of gluten and is the least well tolerated by gluten-sensitive individuals.*

Following a diet completely free of gluten grains for several weeks or specific sensitivity testing can tell you if you have this problem. For "gluten sensitive" individuals, there are many gluten alternatives and many recipe books allowing normal life without wheat or other gluten grains.

Rice

Rice is a daily staple for all of Asia and is popular worldwide. Rice comes in even more varieties than wheat, and again the amount of processing and the protein content are key to their nutritional value. Everyday white rice is the most processed, with high amounts of starch and low amounts of protein. The more "sticky" the rice is, the higher the starch and the lower the protein. Sushi rice is the stickiest. From a dietary point of view, this trait is undesirable (but I confess to love sushi). *Basmati rice* has the highest protein content and lowest starch. *Brown rice* is less processed and contains more fiber.

In my house, brown basmati is the staple. It has a wonderful "nutty" flavor. Also look for other varieties such as mahogany rice. These flavorful rices are both high in fiber and protein.

Wild rice, native to North America, is actually related to cattails and not to typical rice, which originated in Asia. It is very high in fiber, protein and nutrients, and has a flavor all its own. For variety, it is definitely a candidate for addition to a healthy diet.

Corn

Because it is inexpensive to produce and has a high sugar content, corn is the most widely produced grain in the world. High fructose corn syrup and hydrogenated corn oil are some of the most over-used products in the commercial food industry. Corn oil, especially when commercially refined, offers no significant health benefits. Aside from these factors, whole grain corn is a good source of vitamins, especially B vitamins, and is a good source of minerals. Sweet corn on the cob, whole kernels of corn in a stew, whole grain organic corn chips, and popcorn can all be included within the confines of a healthy diet.

The "big three" need to share space with all the other important grains. Grains such as barley, oats, buckwheat, rye, millet, quinoa and amaranth are becoming more available and should frequently be incorporated into a healthy diet. Each of them has its own individual health characteristics. Look for these very healthful grains in cereals, bread, and other products. They can also be bought in bulk and used in cooking for variety and taste. Below I have featured several that should definitely be given consideration.

Barley

Most Americans know barley mainly for its connection with one of our most popular beverages. Barley provides the sugar maltose or "malt" for fermentation of beer. Barley is the fourth most widely produced grain in the world with the majority being used for livestock feed. Aside from use in brewing beer, barley is not as flavorful as the "big three" and therefore very little of it makes its way to the dinner table. This is unfortunate, as barley is truly a wonder grain in many ways. Because of the types of fiber and carbohydrates found in barley, absorption of glucose in the intestine is drastically slowed for up to ten hours after consumption. This is especially good news for diabetics, as blood glucose levels can actually be lowered with regular consumption of barley.

Barley provides the highest concentration of fiber of any of the grains (13 grams per cup). The fiber in barley lowers cholesterol and raises HDL levels. Though this fiber is considered indigestible, it does provide food for favorable bacteria in the gut, not only reducing intestinal disease, but also reducing the risk of colon cancer. Beyond fiber, barley is a good source of B-vitamins and minerals. Chemicals in barley may also decrease arthritis.

For consumption, the inedible outer hull of the barley grain must be removed. "De-hulled" barley is considered a whole grain, since the germ and bran are still present. "Pearled" barley is further processed to remove the bran, thus lowering some of the nutritional value. Barley can be eaten as a hot breakfast cereal similar to oatmeal, used a side dish or incorporated into a wide variety of other dishes.

See *www.barleyfoods.org* for recipes and more information about barley as an edible grain.

Oats

Oats can claim similar health attributes to barley but have better taste. The fiber content is not as high, but it shares similar characteristics. There is nothing better on a cold winter morning than oatmeal with a little brown sugar, raisins, and a pat of butter.

Quinoa *(pronounced "keen-wa")*

Cultivated by natives of South American for thousands of years, quinoa is just becoming known to the rest of the world. Quinoa is a complete source of protein, containing all of the essential amino acids necessary for life. Animal food sources provide a complete complement of essential amino acids, but few vegetable food sources can make this claim. Quinoa, with a taste all its own, is one of those few. It is also high in fiber, low in starch, low in fat, and high in minerals.

The taste and texture of quinoa is slightly similar to corn grits. It cooks quickly and stores well in the refrigerator after being cooked. Quinoa can be eaten it for breakfast as a substitute for grits. "Shrimp and grits" with quinoa instead of grits is quite tasty.

See *www.quinoa.net* for recipes and more information about quinoa.

NUTS

Nuts are nature's storehouse of energy and nutrition. Though there are over 300 varieties, we are generally aware of only a handful. Most commonly we think of almonds, Brazil nuts, cashews, pecans, walnuts, hazelnuts, pistachios, and macadamia nuts. Peanuts are actually a type of pea (legume), but they usually get thrown into the mix. Coconuts are of course a nut but seem to stand in a class by themselves.

Though we tend to think of nuts as a group, they originate from different climates, soil types, and plant types and have origins from diverse places. This allows each nut variety to contribute its own array of nutrients, including valuable minerals. For example, because the soil in Venezuela (where most Brazil nuts are grown) is high in selenium, a single Brazil nut will provide an entire day's allotment of that mineral. A handful of different types of nuts may provide all of the different minerals that you need for an entire day.

Nutrition Nuts as a group are very low in glucose, moderately high in protein, and high in favorable unsaturated fat. The fats in nuts are favorable for decreasing inflammation and are especially "heart healthy." Coconuts are the only nuts that are high in saturated fat, but the unique type of saturated fat found in coconuts is considered healthful to consume.

Health Tip *The polyunsaturated fats in nuts easily become oxidized when exposed to air. We call such foods "stale." If nuts have a stale smell, do not eat them: oxidized fats are very unhealthy. Many packaged snack foods and snack bars (even the ones labeled as health food) are stale before you open the wrapper. I generally buy nuts fresh from a reputable source and store them in the freezer. The canned varieties are fresh, but may be loaded with salt. If you purchase nuts from open bins, make sure that they are in a cool place and that turnover is high. There are several reputable mail-order vendors found on the Internet. I often order from www.sunnylandfarms.com.*

BEANS

"Beans, beans, they're good for your heart...." Actually, it's all true: they *are* good for your heart. High in complex carbohydrates and fiber, frijoles help remove toxins and cholesterol from the body. Beans contain chemicals called flavonoids, potent anti-oxidants that prevent plaque formation in the vessels of the heart. These same chemicals moderate the effects of reproductive hormones in disarray, thus minimizing symptoms of menopause in women and decreasing the risk of prostate cancer in men. Beans are a good source of protein. Added to brown rice or millet, beans become a "complete" source of protein providing all of the essential amino acids that we need to survive.

The list of different kinds of beans is long and includes black beans, kidney beans, pole beans, peas (many varieties), navy beans, peanuts, garbanzo beans, aduki beans, lentils, lima beans, and mung beans, just to name a few. Beans are good sources of B vitamins and some minerals, iron, calcium, potassium, and phosphorus. As with nuts, different beans provide different varieties of nutrients.

It is true that some people get increased gas with consumption of beans, but this effect tends to be more pronounced in individuals who are not regular consumers of these vegetables. To minimize flatulence, try rinsing canned beans before use; if using dried beans that have been soaked overnight and then drained, pour off the cooking water after it reaches a full boil, refill with water, and then cook as usual. In general, black beans, lentils, and mung beans produce less gas. An enzyme supplement can also help ease the discomfort.

The problem usually improves over time with consumption of a better diet. Until then, only invite your closest friends and relatives over for dinner.

The omnipresent soybean is so versatile that Henry Ford once made interior car parts out of them. Almost anything can be made out of soy. Considered a health food by some, use and especially overuse of soy does have some concerning aspects. Soybeans are heavily used in the commercial processed food industry as inexpensive sources of oil and protein. They are also heavily used in the livestock industry. The polyunsaturated oils are very susceptible to oxidation caused by heat. The oil is extracted using high heat and/or chemicals, making its ubiquitous use in food products somewhat concerning. The oils found in soy are "pro-inflammatory" when consumed in processed food products and contribute to increased risks of disease. Like many foods, the health potential of soy is related to whether it is whole or processed.

Soybeans contain chemicals called "isoflavones" that act like estrogen in the body. Whether this is good or bad is a matter of opinion. Products containing soy are well known to reduce menopausal symptoms in women, but this estrogenic effect has some experts concerned that isoflavones found in soy could increase risks of breast cancer. The estrogenic effect of soy, however, is extremely weak. These chemicals actually block the activity of estrogens that are already circulating inside the body; hence, they appear to offer protection against estrogen-induced cancers. The very low incidence of breast cancer in Japan, where consumption of soy is very high, supports this theory. Likewise, consumption of soy by men is associated with decreased risks of prostate cancer.

The anti-cancer potential of soy is related to the isoflavone content. Steamed green soy beans, dried soy beans and tofu contain the highest levels of these important chemicals found in food sources. Soy milk contains low to moderate amounts of isoflavones. Soy sauce is low in isoflavones and processed soy oil has none. Interestingly, isoflavones only seem to be concerning when they are highly concentrated within dietary supplements. For this reason, isoflavones should only be acquired from natural dietary sources. Women who have had breast cancer should best avoid soy altogether.

Soy does have a reputation of being a "goitrogen," a substance that blocks the formation of thyroid hormones, but very likely this is a concern only with excessive consumption of soy. The incidence of thyroid dysfunction is not reported to be higher in cultures that consume large amounts of soy. Reasonable consumption of soy products should not pose a threat.

The answer to soy is the same as to any other dietary dilemma: avoid excessive use and avoid processed forms or additives. Stick with whole foods and whole food products. Steamed soybeans, which go by their Japanese name edamame, are being discovered by the rest of the world as tasty and nutritious, with a flavor somewhere between a pea and a butterbean. Tofu and tempeh, fermented soy products, have not made a big hit in the U.S. but are consumed daily in Asian countries. Whole soy products are rich in essential amino acids and stand by themselves as a source of protein. They are low in glucose and low in fat but high in other nutrients. I use soy milk in cooking and on my cereal fairly regularly. Though high in sodium, soy sauce is one of my favorites, and when used to season vegetables, is balanced by the potassium therein.

OTHER NOTABLE SEEDS

A partial list of other seeds with the right kind of nutrition includes flax, sesame, sunflower, and pumpkin. These seeds contain all-important essential fatty acids that moderate inflammation in the body. As with other seeds, the oils are very susceptible to oxidation and should only be consumed when fresh.

Though much attention is given to flaxseed oil, whole flax seeds contain beneficial fiber and chemicals called *lignans*. *Lignans* present in whole flax seeds not only reduce cholesterol but also have anti-estrogenic effects felt to have value in reducing risk of both breast and prostate cancer. Consider adding 2 tablespoons of ground flax seed to cereal, salad or a cup of yogurt each day.

Health Tip If you use flax seeds as a source of essential fatty acids, store them in the freezer. When ready for use, grind them in a portable coffee grinder and add to food. When consumed whole, flax seeds go "straight through" and add little nutritional benefit. Sometimes an easier route is buying unrefined flax seed oil or ground flax seeds in the refrigerated section of a health food store. Sometimes you pay for convenience.

SEED SPROUTS

Young bean sprouts and newly sprouted grasses such as wheat and barley retain all of the nutrition of the seed with the added benefit of nutrition added by the sun. They are high in nutrient value and high in beneficial essential fatty acids. Many people consider juices made from sprouted grass seeds to be very healthy for regular consumption. Those not enthralled with consuming a daily ration of sprouts may choose to obtain these healthy benefits from "super-green" supplements. (Whether freeze-dried supplements carry the same benefit as fresh food is unknown.)

Health Tip One small downside to whole grain consumption is the presence of proteins called "lectins" which have been implicated as inciting factors in many diseases including food sensitivities, inflammatory bowel disease, and arthritis. Lectins are destroyed in the sprouting process and products such as bread and pastas made from sprouted grains are free of this problem.

SEAWEED

Seaweed is dense in anti-oxidants, nutrients, and minerals, but it is, admittedly, an acquired taste. Quality is highly dependent on the water from which it comes. Seaweed is a good source of iodine, an element often lacking in land-based diets that is important for thyroid hormone synthesis. Try a seaweed salad the next time you happen by a sushi bar. Shellfish is another excellent source of iodine in the diet.

FUNGI

The only fungi that most humans consistently consume are mushrooms and some others that make our cheese taste sharp and turn blue. Thirty years ago, mushrooms were shriveled-up, tasteless food items that only came in a jar. Now, not only are fresh mushrooms widely available but many different varieties of them are on the produce shelves. Each of them has a little different flavor, adding a signature touch to dishes. Mushrooms can impart a "meaty" flavor to certain recipes.

> *Nutrition* The little white variety most people are familiar with offers the least nutrition of any of the mushrooms and is colonized by a fungus that produces a toxin called aflatoxin. The fungus and toxin are destroyed by cooking; these mushrooms (and all mushrooms) should not be eaten raw. Many other varieties are becoming commercially available. Mushrooms as a group are low in glucose and fat energy, moderate in protein, moderate in fiber and high in nutrition. Several edible mushroom species have been found to contain potential cancer-preventing chemicals.

FOODS FROM ANIMAL SOURCES

Animals survive by consuming plants, other animals, or both, thus repeating the cycle of life. The nutritional value of food derived from an animal source is very dependent on the nutritional value of the food that sustained that animal. For terrestrial animals, it all goes back to *living soil*. For aquatic animals, the key factor is *clean water*.

TERRESTRIAL MEAT

The two concerns associated with meat consumption are toxin concentration and the complement of fatty acids present. Large animals such as cows and hogs tend to have the highest concentration of toxins and the most saturated fat. Poultry has a higher concentration of polyunsaturated fats and retains fewer toxins. Of course, all meat is much more favorable for consumption if the animal is allowed free range to forage on grasses and other natural foods. Going even further back to our roots, meat from hunted wild animals may be the healthiest of all.

The topic of bird flu certainly makes a case for vegetarianism. Bird flu likely originated as a virus found endemically in ducks. Recent years have seen the emergence of more lethal strains of the virus that have rapidly spread into chicken and other domestic bird populations. Some people, mainly in the Far East, have apparently contracted the virus from handling birds; to date, the virus has not adapted to spreading well within human populations. The rapid spread of these lethal viruses within bird populations has been almost exclusively limited to birds confined to overcrowded, industrial-scale production facilities. The spread of disease in any animal population raised for food is always higher when overcrowding is standard procedure.

Free-range meat is always the best choice. Some groceries are starting to carry these meats, and free-range meats of many varieties can be ordered through the Internet. The ultimate source for finding healthy meat in your region is www.eatwild.com.

Nutrition Depending on the source, meat is low to high in fat, high in quality protein, and has no sugar. Beef and pork are high in saturated fat. Poultry has a higher ratio of polyunsaturated to saturated fat and is lower in fat in general, especially with the skin removed. Though meat does not provide the wealth of nutrients available in vegetables, some important minerals such as iron and selenium are present along with the important nutrients B-12, carnitine, and conjugated linoleic acid that are difficult to obtain from other sources.

Health Tip *When it comes to meat I generally stick with the real thing. Knowing what goes into processed meat foods such as hot dogs, bologna, and souse keeps them off my menu. Oxidized fat content present in these meat products contributes to diseases such as heart disease and cancer. Even hamburger has some pretty scary things ground into it and except for an occasional summer picnic, I tend to steer clear of it...and call me a weenie if you like, but when it comes to sausage, I generally save it only for special occasions or use the soy variety.*

SEAFOOD

The nutritional value of seafood tends to reflect the quality of the water from which it was harvested. A polluted body of water will definitely affect the level of toxins in the animals that come out of it. For up-to-date information about this topic in fish and shellfish, check out *www.oceansalive.org.*

Fish Fish would be the ideal source of quality protein if it were not for the mercury problem. Fortunately, many species of fish are less susceptible to this problem than others. It is an up-the-food-chain phenomenon, and, in general, large predators that feed on other larger-sized fish tend to have significantly higher mercury concentration in their flesh than fish that feed on smaller fish and crustaceans.

> *Nutrition* Fish are high in quality protein and of course have no sugar.
> They are low in fat, but high in those all-important essential fatty acids.
> Seafood in general is high in minerals, especially less common dietary
> minerals such as selenium, iodine, and zinc.

Fish to avoid Shark, swordfish, king mackerel, tilefish, tuna, sea bass, Atlantic halibut.

Fish to choose Wild salmon, Alaskan halibut, flounder, Spanish mackerel, bluefish, grouper, light canned tuna, mahi-mahi, catfish, trout (fresh and saltwater), anchovies and—my personal favorite—sardines. (My wife makes me eat them outdoors.)

> *Health Tip* *Though farm-raised fish may be healthier than terrestrial sources*
> *of meat, aquaculture has some issues that can affect product quality. Because*
> *of the type of meal used as feed, farm-raised salmon do not have the same*
> *complement of essential fatty acids for which wild salmon are so well known. In*
> *addition, farm-raised salmon often have 6-10 times higher concentrations of*
> *toxins than those found in the wild. Avoid farm-raised crustaceans for the same*
> *reason.*

Shellfish
Crustaceans Once maligned for the cholesterol they contain, crabs, shrimp, and lobster are back on the menu as healthy food items. Crustaceans are high in protein, nutrient dense, and low in glucose. Though consumption of crustaceans such as shrimp may increase LDL levels a small amount, favorable HDL levels are increased even more. Consumption of shellfish is only a problem for individuals who have inherited a cholesterol metabolism problem (but consumption of pork or beef would be even more of a problem in these individuals). On a positive note, shrimp and their relatives tend to have high levels of favorable essential fatty acids; also, mercury contamination is not an issue here.

Bivalves Clams, mussels, and oysters are filter feeders. They actually make the surrounding water cleaner, but they tend to concentrate any toxins and microbes in their own bodies. Mollusks should only be consumed when extracted from very clean waters.

> **Health Tip** Interestingly, this is an area where aquaculture really shines. Because feeding is not necessary, mollusks contained in special cages can be placed in pristine waters and end up being some of the healthiest seafood you can buy. Again, make an effort to know where your seafood comes from.

Our shellfish are only as clean and healthy as the water that surrounds them. Even if you do not live near the coast, your local supplier should be able to provide information about the origins of the seafood in the market. Support your local commercial fishermen. Seafood items found in many restaurants and grocery stores are sourced from foreign markets where water quality may be alarmingly poor. You can also let your voice be heard about the quality of the seafood that ends up on your plate simply by joining grassroots organizations and supporting politicians who work for better water quality and air quality.

DAIRY

Milk is not quite the health food that commercial milk producers would have you think. Milk and milk products are high in saturated fat and fat-free varieties are just not as palatable. Also, the dairy industry is known to use hormones to increase production and antibiotics to maintain animals in unhealthy environments. Another reason to reduce dairy consumption is the fact that many of us, as adults, lack the enzyme necessary to break down lactose (milk sugar); we call this condition "lactose intolerance." Symptoms of lactose intolerance are primarily gastrointestinal. Allergies to milk proteins are yet another common problem.

Calcium and the Great Milk Myth: Milk is high in calcium, but whether it has a positive long-term effect on bone density is still widely open for debate. For years the dairy industry has held that the calcium content alone defines milk as being good for your bones, but there is little firm evidence to back up these claims. Skeptics suggest that the large dose of calcium associated with consuming a glass of milk raise blood calcium levels too rapidly. To summarize one hypothesis: In order to prevent toxic blood levels of calcium, it must be removed from the bloodstream as rapidly as possible. Bone is the only place for it to go, but the excess calcium is, in effect, "dumped" into the bone, instead of being structurally placed in a stable, organized fashion. This unstable calcium gradually leaches out of the bone, leaving holes in the bone matrix. This may explain the typical "Swiss cheese" appearance of osteoporosis.

Though arguments on both sides offer valid lines of reasoning, population studies are hard to ignore. The United States and Europe have the highest rates of milk consumption in the world—and the highest rates of osteoporosis in the world. Inversely, lower consumption of milk is associated with lower rates of osteoporosis. China has the lowest consumption of milk and milk products of any country on Earth and concomitantly has the lowest rates of osteoporosis of any culture. Interestingly, in Hong Kong, where milk consumption is now at European levels among the Chinese people there, the incidence of osteoporosis is equal to that of European countries.

Conflicting opinions leave the rest of us caught in the middle. The fact that calcium is necessary for strong bones is a given, but how calcium is delivered to the bones seems to be significant. As with many things, moderation is probably the best option.

Calcium—whether from milk, natural sources or supplementation—is best when consumed in intermittent, small amounts, not enough to raise blood calcium levels too rapidly. Nondairy calcium sources are the best sources, but dairy in certain forms may be acceptable. Cheese (combined with other foods), small amounts of milk with cereal, or small amounts of yogurt with fruit or nuts would not raise blood calcium levels nearly as rapidly as gulping a glass of milk. The same guidelines go for calcium supplements which should be taken in small doses several times daily.

One dairy product that appears to offer health attributes is cultured low-fat yogurt. Yogurt is a good source of protein, live bacteria and other important nutrients. The bacteria break down milk sugars, making the milk more digestible. These bacterial cultures also contribute to a favorable bacterial balance in the large colon and vagina. Yogurt contains a substance called conjugated linoleic acid (CLA), which may inhibit cancers and decrease serum cholesterol and triglyceride. All of this, and you get some calcium, too!

If you enjoy and tolerate milk and milk products, be willing to pay a little extra for organic products, free of the hormones and antibiotics used in standard milk production. For a milk substitute consider soymilk. Newer brands are more palatable than ever. Cooking with soymilk works quite well.

Cheese is an acceptable addition to a healthy diet, especially if excessively processed versions are avoided. (You know what I'm talking about, the kind that pours or comes wrapped in plastic and looks like plastic.) Stay with "hard" cheeses such as parmesan, Romano, sharp cheddar or Swiss because they have less fat. Cheese (limited to small amounts) is almost essential for certain types of cooking.

For a change in taste, clarified butter works well for cooking. Called "ghee" in India, clarified butter is butter with the milk solids removed. It is almost pure saturated fat and therefore must be used sparingly and only occasionally.

EGGS

Like seeds, eggs have everything necessary to nurture new life, and therefore are packed with nutrition. Eggs are important sources of certain vitamins and minerals and are an excellent source of quality protein. Eggs have high levels of lecithin, a very important ingredient for healthy cell membranes. Although they have been maligned in recent years because they are high in cholesterol, eggs also tend to be high in favorable essential fatty acids. Increased risk of cardiovascular disease and stroke need not be of concern unless you have inherited a cholesterol metabolism problem or you tend to gorge on eggs. Never forget the story of the man who won an egg-eating contest by a wide margin on one day and promptly had a stroke on the next.

At one point I was thinking that it might be nice to have a couple of hens around to provide a ready supply of our own free-range eggs. I made the mistake of sharing this thought with friends who owned a farm. Within a week a cage arrived containing one over-protective hen and five biddies. A hutch that had been constructed for a series of pet rabbits sufficed quite nicely for a chicken coop. We quickly developed a routine of letting the chickens out in the morning to forage for food and putting them back into the hutch at night. By the end of fall it was apparent that we had three new roosters and only two new hens; still, the two new hens in addition to the mother would be enough to fill our egg needs.

All went well until the mother hen began to usher her little band into the adjacent woods regularly to forage. With each visit she returned in the evening minus one chicken. Finally the mother hen did not return at all and we were down to only two roosters and zero potential for fresh eggs.

The roosters did have some aesthetic value and ate garden pests, so initially we decided to keep them around. They seemed to have gotten the idea about the woods and stayed exclusively in our yard. Within a couple of months, however, they were crowing continuously from 4 am to 4 pm and becoming a real nuisance. At first we started rooting for the local fox and hawk populations, but when they began destroying my wife's garden we began plotting their demise in earnest. We considered the hatchet; this was, after all, an ideal opportunity to obtain valuable free-range chicken meat at no cost, but the mess that would be associated with cleaning made the whole process seem unpalatable. I guess we have become too far removed from our carnivorous origins. At last a local "4-H'er" agreed to take them off our hands and we were out of the chicken business. The thought of fresh eggs from my own hens still intrigues me and this adventure may be attempted again, but for now I'll settle for eggs from a local market.

The best bet for finding healthy eggs is buying from local farmers, preferably those who have a reputation of allowing their hens to forage for food naturally and supplement with processed food only minimally. I was somewhat taken aback the first time I opened a box of true "free-range" eggs. Having been accustomed to the commercial variety— uniformly bright white, evenly sized and shaped eggs—anything else seemed a little odd. Inside a box of free-range eggs will be found a wonderful assortment of sizes, ranging from seemingly very small to large enough to have wonders about the capabilities of the hen to have produced it. Shell pigmentation varies from light gray to mottled brown. Egg differences do not stop at the shell. When cracked into a frying pan, the yolks are of varying colors, all much more intensely orange than the commercially-produced equivalent.

Although the taste may not be significantly different, the nutritional value very much is. Hens that are allowed to forage for natural foods produce eggs that are generally about one-third lower in cholesterol and have a much more favorable complement of essential fatty acids. The mineral content is higher and the probability of the egg harboring unwanted toxins is much lower. All in all, they are better for us and better for the chickens that produced them. A "second best" option is buying commercial eggs that are from chickens fed with organic feed that is high in omega-3 fatty acids. These eggs can be found in almost all grocery stores.

Do not make the mistake of buying eggs that are simply labeled "cage free." The "cage free" label only implies that the chickens are allowed to stay outside of cages. Generally it means that they live on a concrete floor and eat the same foods fed to other commercially-raised poultry. Eggs from chickens raised on organic feed are a step better, but they may not be true free-range eggs.

If it's not scratching in the yard for worms, it's not a true free-range chicken!

MISCELLANEOUS FOOD SOURCES

OILS AND FATS

Vegetable oils are liquid at room temperature and are predominantly composed of unsaturated fats. Saturated fat and hydrogenated oils that we know of as butter, lard, and margarine are solid at room temperature.

The health potential of all types of fat depends on several variables. The enemies of oils and fat are oxygen, bacteria, heat, and chemicals used in processing. Saturated fats easily become rancid from bacterial growth, even if pasteurized. Saturated fat from animals raised under unhealthy conditions may contain toxins, hormones, and other contaminants. Vegetable oils processed with heat and chemicals are very unhealthy, especially if hydrogenated. To the contrary, both saturated and unsaturated fats from fresh, unprocessed, organic sources can be extremely healthy for regular consumption.

For the healthiest diet, a combination of different sources of fat is important, with the ideal ratio favoring unsaturated fats over saturated fats. The best sources of polyunsaturated fats are found within fresh vegetables, beans, nuts, and grains. Saturated fats are best consumed in smaller amounts such as in lean meats and occasional butter on toast or in cooking.

For cooking and oils added to food, monounsaturated oils are preferred because of their resistance to oxidation. Monounsaturated oils are excellent for cooking, dipping bread, and adding to dishes for flavor. The first on the list is *olive oil* with a wonderful flavor and the highest concentration of mono-unsaturated fat. *Macadamia nut oil* is also very high in monounsaturated fat and, of course, has a characteristic nutty flavor. *Sesame oil*, another oil high in monounsaturated fat, is stable enough for cooking and has its own unique flavor. *Peanut oil* is stable enough to be used for cooking, but has a higher concentration of saturated fat. Oleic versions (high in monosaturated fat) of *sunflower*, *safflower*, and *canola oils* are stable for cooking, but tend to be more processed. *Grapeseed oil* is becoming more available and is stable for cooking. Use only moderate heat, not high heat, when cooking with any of these oils. *Walnut oil*, higher in polyunsaturated fat, is best reserved for salads and not for cooking. *Flaxseed oil* is very prone to oxidation; it should never be used in cooking and should always be stored in the refrigerator.

Picking a good oil is like picking a good wine. The label tells all. Most commercially-processed oils are exposed to high heat or damaging chemicals during the extraction process. Oxidized fat and fat damaged by heat are very unhealthy for the human body. Better quality oils will have the terms "expeller pressed" or "cold pressed" on the label. This implies that the oils have been extracted using only pressure and low heat. The very best oils will have the terms "unrefined" and "unfiltered" implying that they are even less processed and retain all of their natural nutrition. You will pay more, but the cost is worth it.

A unique oil that seems to be gaining favor these days is *coconut oil*. Once condemned because of a 90% concentration of saturated fat, coconut oil is now being raised to the level of health food in some circles. The saturated fat in coconut is composed of "medium chain triglycerides" (MCT's for short).

These fatty acids are much shorter chains than the long ones found in animal fats. Experts are suggesting that MCT's are absorbed more rapidly than other saturated fats and are much more apt to be burned immediately for energy than stored. In theory, a person could actually raise his or her metabolic energy level (and therefore lose weight) by regularly consuming MCT's. I am still of the school of thought that too much of any one thing is not a good thing, but using coconut milk in cooking every now and then certainly is a nice way to add flavor and variety.

Another high-fat food that has gained status in recent years is the avocado. Avocados contain very high amounts of monounsaturated fats and are excellent by themselves or made into guacamole. A satisfactory substitute for a BLT is an ALT—avocado, deep green lettuce, and tomato on whole-grain bread. The taste is surprisingly similar.

Life is full of compromises, and cooking with oil is one of mine. My favorite form of cooking is stir-fry, though I recognize that some damage occurs to the oil during the cooking process. I try to minimize this effect as much as possible by using only a small amount of oil and taking steps to prevent the oil from burning. Usually I use olive oil, but macadamia nut oil, with a natural buttery flavor, has also become a favorite. When compared to deep-fat frying, the level of health concern with stir-frying or sautéing is miniscule. Occasionally, for flavor variation, I use clarified butter (butter with the milk solids removed) for cooking. The saturated fat found in butter is very stable for cooking, but of course the caveat is not to use too much.

FERMENTED FOODS

More by necessity than choice, fermented foods have always been a normal part of human diets. Edible fermented foods contribute to the normal complement of bacteria in the human GI tract, helping to insure normal gastrointestinal function. Americans consume a lower proportion of fermented foods than any culture on Earth and have higher rates of gastrointestinal problems than any culture. In Japan, about a third of the foods that make up an average diet are fermented, and, correspondingly, the incidence of gastrointestinal disturbances is very low in the Japanese population.

Cultured yogurt is about the only fermented food that most Americans will consider eating. Yogurt is considered a "functional food" in that regular consumption of certain cultured yogurt products can be used as an adjunct for prevention and treatment of gastrointestinal disorders. Less commonly known, but also beneficial for GI function, is a cultured dairy product called kefir.

In Asia fermented foods are much more common. Examples include tempeh, a fermented soybean product common in Japan, and kimchi, a fermented cabbage product relished in Korea. Another fermented cabbage product that is a little more familiar to our European-based palate is sauerkraut. Wine, beer, and vinegar are, of course, fermented products, but they do not retain live bacteria.

> **Health Tip** *Especially for individuals who have any type of gastrointestinal disturbance, foods fermented with favorable bacteria should be a frequent dietary addition. For those who find the taste of fermented food products to be unpleasant, a daily probiotic supplement should be considered. This dietary supplement can provide the daily equivalent of bacteria found in common fermented foods.*

It should be noted that not all fermentation is healthful. Many processed foods and certain uncooked foods are colonized with unfavorable bacterial and fungal species that produce harmful toxins associated with increased risk of cancer and immune suppression.

Examples of fermented foods to avoid include these:
- *Sausage, bacon, salami, ham and all processed meats are often colonized with harmful types of fungi and bacteria. If they are consumed at all, they should be very well cooked.*

- *Uncooked mushrooms are colonized with fungal species and should be thoroughly cooked before consumption. One of the most common toxins often associated with raw white mushrooms is called aflatoxin. Avoid raw mushrooms from a salad bar.*

- *Raw peanuts and cashews can also be colonized by fungal species, including those that produce aflatoxin.*

- *Meat from terrestrial animal sources of any kind may be colonized with undesirable strains of fungal species and should only be consumed when fresh and thoroughly cooked.*

- *Milk products including milk, cheese, ice cream, butter and especially cottage cheese are colonized with fungal species. Cottage cheese is by far the worst offender and should probably be avoided. Milk products, such as yogurt or kefir, cultured with favorable bacteria, are not colonized with fungal species.*

- *Raw eggs are colonized with fungi (and bacteria), but these are destroyed by cooking.*

There is good and bad in everything. You can't avoid all the bad, but you can minimize your risk by being judicious about your consumption of food. Eating a wide variety of fresh foods is a wise choice.

SPICES

Spices and herbs are an excellent way to add flavor without adding extra sugar and fat. The art of cooking is truly defined by the combination of herbs and spices. They can turn an everyday dish into something special. Beyond flavor, most herbs and spices have medicinal value. Turmeric, found in most curries, is one of the most potent natural anti-inflammatory substances known and regular consumption is likely to lower your risk of cancer. Cinnamon can help you control your blood sugar, and ginger can settle your stomach when you are sick. Capsaicin, found in cayenne pepper, is another potent anti-inflammatory that is an effective topical treatment for arthritis. Garlic is an anti-microbial, anti-hypertensive, anti-coagulation, anti-cholesterol wonder food that also keeps vampires away. We could go on with enough information to fill a book, but you do not have to know everything about spices to enjoy their flavor and health benefits; just toss them in.

SALT

Though Americans do tend to vigorously overuse the saltshaker, the story on salt again appears to be another one of refined versus unrefined. Sodium and chloride ions found in shaker salt are vital for all functions within the body; sea salt includes these as well as the wide variety of trace minerals found in seawater, most of which are necessary to human health in modest amounts.

The health issue behind salt has to more with the ratio of sodium to potassium than the amount of sodium by itself. The average American diet is very low in potassium, with abundant sodium from our salty diets only compounding the problem. A diet high in vegetables is very high in potassium, with a favorable average ratio of about 5 parts potassium to 1 part sodium.

When using a salt shaker, moderate use of unrefined sea salt appears to be the healthiest option. The minerals in sea salt help maintain an alkaline pH in the blood and tissues. "Lite salt" with half sodium and half potassium is another option for those transitioning to a healthier diet.

CONDIMENTS AND SAUCES

- Mayonnaise generally contains soybean oil, eggs, vinegar, some type of sweetener, and preservatives; it is okay if only used in moderation. Better quality spreads contain unrefined monounsaturated oils, have sugar instead of corn syrup, and use natural preservatives. Olive oil is becoming an available ingredient in mayonnaise. Better products are now becoming standard in average grocery stores.

- Salad dressings with something a bit healthier than soybean oil and high fructose corn syrup are fine. Look for salad dressings with unrefined oil instead of processed soybean oil. Avoid the low-fat varieties, which tend to substitute cheap carbohydrates for oil. The best salad dressings are those that you make yourself.

- Soy sauce adds flavor to many types of dishes and is the base for many types of sauces. Look for low salt varieties or better quality brands with sea salt.

- Bottled sauces are an easy way to enhance cooking, as long as they are not used in excess. Scrutinize labels for high amounts of sugar, refined oils and undesirable preservatives—remember, you can always make your own and put in exactly what you want.

- Ketchup, my son's favorite vegetable, has been found to contain a potent antioxidant called *lycopene*. The biggest problem with catsup is sugar, but if you are avoiding sugar otherwise, the amount in catsup does not add up too much.

- Mustard is fine as long as you can give up the hotdogs.

- Don't forget hummus—it makes a superb condiment.

- Vinegar is an excellent way to add flavor to food. Some tout it as a health food and others strongly argue the opposite. I cannot find very much firm evidence either way. Experiment with vinegars from different sources, which have interesting flavor variations.

BEVERAGES

Soft drinks are a natural complement to all the unnatural foods well known to a generation raised on processed food. Beyond being saturated with high fructose corn syrup or artificial sweeteners and often loaded with caffeine, these products shift the blood pH toward acidity and have a concerning link to early bone loss. There are better options for quenching your thirst.

Now an all-day beverage instead of just a morning pick-me-up, coffee has become wildly popular the Americas and Europe. Though it has a reputation for being a gastric irritant and containing significant levels of caffeine, coffee does have some chemicals that are beneficial for human consumption. The problem with coffee drinks is not the coffee itself, but the large amounts of sugar and milk fat that usually accompany them.

Most of the rest of the world drinks tea. The Asian world drinks "green tea" because the plants grow fresh there. When Europeans discovered the beverage, they fermented the tea and dried the leaves in the sun for the long trip home. This became the "black tea" beverage to which our taste buds are more accustomed. Both forms contain anti-oxidants and other beneficial chemicals, but green tea retains a higher concentration of the original chemicals that have not been altered by the drying process. Milder and lower in caffeine than green tea, "white tea" comes from tender newly picked leaves from the tea plant. Green tea, white and to a lesser extent, black tea contain some of the most potent anticancer chemicals known to man and should be a regular inclusion in a healthy diet.

Tea can be made from other ingredients than the leaves of the tea plant. Herbal teas are becoming very popular and many have medicinal attributes. Chamomile and passion flower are known for relaxing qualities and ginger tea soothes the stomach. Holy basil tea has potent anti-inflammatory properties.

Fruit drinks provide another alternative for staying hydrated. The number of different types of fruit drinks out there is expansive, with the spectrum extending from healthy to very unhealthy. The most healthy fruit drinks are those with no added sweeteners, *not even natural fruit sweeteners*. Some examples include natural cherry juice, blueberry juice, and pomegranate juice, all which are high in anti-oxidants. Citrus juices are a good source of vitamin C, but are high in sugar.

For something lighter and less expensive, try a glass of ice water with a fresh lemon squeezed in and a teaspoon of sugar, Stevia or Xylitol as a sweetener.

Do not forget that the basic ingredient of any beverage is plain H_2O. When you are really parched, water in its purified form quenches thirst better than anything on the planet. Of all beverage possibilities, pure water is nature's original beverage and should be consumed in greater amounts than anything else.

ALCOHOLIC BEVERAGES

Anything containing sugar can be fermented into an alcoholic beverage. The metabolites of alcohol (ethanol) are definitely classified as toxins, but alcohol does seem to have some value in small doses as an anti-anxiety agent. Red wine (and, to a lesser extent, white wine) contains potent anti-oxidants and anti-inflammatory chemicals found in skins and seeds of the grapes. Beer contains beneficial anti-oxidants as well as the vitamins folate and B6. Beer and wine both increase favorable HDL levels and decrease unfavorable LDL cholesterol levels. Numerous studies have shown that one to two 6 to 8 oz. glasses of wine daily or the same number of 12 oz. beers daily is associated with a decreased risk of cardiovascular disease and general good health, while *anything more* is associated with the opposite.

Liquor has little or no medicinal value because of higher alcohol content and because it is often mixed with other beverages containing large amounts of sugar.

SWEETENERS
What about table sugar?
Refined sugar (sucrose) is a molecule of glucose bonded to a molecule of fructose. This "double" sugar is referred to as a disaccharide. Surprisingly, table sugar contributes to a slower blood sugar rise that does pure starch. This is because the enzyme necessary for breaking the bond between these two sugars is present in the intestine, but not in saliva or in the stomach. Nevertheless, sucrose should be consumed only in minimal amounts because it still contributes to the problems of insulin resistance and diabetes.

Another concern about excessive consumption of disaccharides such as sucrose and lactose (milk sugar) is their effect on intestinal bacteria. Disaccharides can cause alterations in the balance of bacteria in the colon, contributing to disorders such as irritable bowel syndrome and overgrowth of yeast in some individuals. Though more common with disaccharides, any sugars (including high fructose corn syrup) can cause overgrowth of unfavorable bacteria in the gut. Imbalances in intestinal flora (gut bacteria) can have wide-ranging, adverse affects.

Refined sugar, in the amounts consumed by most Americans, is a major contributor to America's health problems, but like many things, sugar is only a problem if used excessively.

Natural sweeteners such as honey, maple syrup, and agave nectar add pleasure and flavor to food. The types of sugars within these sweeteners vary, but the potential for harm is limited unless they are used excessively. A small amount of any of these sweeteners in your tea, bread dough, cereal or anywhere else you might want to add just a little bit of sweet is perfectly acceptable.

Honey provides glucose and fructose derived from sucrose found in the nectar of flowers. The sucrose is broken down by enzymes inside bees. Honey offers much more than sugar. A wealth of nutrients derived from flower pollen including vitamins, minerals, enzymes, anti-microbial substances, and other essential nutrients are found within honey. Honeys with the most health benefits are not cooked and come from mixed varieties of wildflowers, as opposed to the more common monoculture varieties such as clover.

Maple syrup is another natural sweetener not to be overlooked. Beyond sugar, maple syrup also offers B vitamins and minerals, especially zinc.

Agave nectar is sweeter than sugar, but low in glucose, such that it can be enjoyed by diabetics without concern. It has a milder taste than honey and maple syrup, providing an ideal way to sweeten beverages or cereal.

And artificial sweeteners?

Saccharin has been around the longest. It has an aftertaste and carries that lingering concern associated with cancer studies in laboratory animals. It is probably one best to be avoided.

Aspartame (**NutraSweet**) consists of two amino acids, aspartic acid and phenylalanine, joined in a way that touches our taste buds for sweet. Many diet soft drinks and a host of other products contain aspartame. Aspartame is not heat tolerant and therefore cannot be used in cooking. Individuals who cannot metabolize phenylalanine must avoid the product completely. There seem to be some concerns surfacing regarding symptoms related to chronic intake of aspartame. Excessive aspartic acid and phenylalanine could cause imbalances in serotonin and other neurotransmitters, which may contribute to depression and other neurological symptoms. Aspartame is approved by the FDA as a safe substance but excessive use should be avoided.

Sucralose (**Splenda**) is the newest arrival on the artificial sweetener scene. This product is 600 times sweeter than table sugar (sucrose). Sucralose is derived from cane sugar, but three of the oxygen atoms in the sucrose molecule are then replaced with chlorine atoms. This creates stronger chemical bond that is not broken down by enzymes in the human body. According to the company, sucralose is non-toxic, is eliminated unchanged in the feces, does not affect insulin levels, and can be used anywhere that regular sugar would be—even by diabetics.

While the safety statistics presented by the company look good, it's still too early in the game to tell for sure. In my opinion, any substance that isn't natural to the human body has at least some potential for harm. Strong chlorinated chemicals are used in manufacturing and I wonder how much residual chemical is left behind. I also wonder about how efficiently sucralose is completely removed from the body.

Stevia is a natural alternative that is functionally similar to Sucralose. Stevia is an extract of leaves of a plant native to South America. It has been used by humans there for over a thousand years. The sweetening capability of the plant comes from several molecules of glucose fused together in a way that cannot by broken down by the human body.

Presently the FDA has not approved Stevia as a food additive and it is still relegated to the supplement aisles. This is mainly because no one has taken the time or had the funding to prove that it is safe, though no significant adverse effects have been reported. The only "side effects" noted so far are that it lowers blood sugar and also lowers blood pressure. Stevia has been used in Japan for over thirty years. There are several cookbooks available for cooking with Stevia. Look for *Stevia Sweet Recipes* by Jeffrey Goettemoeller.

Xylitol is not yet well known, but may be the best option for a sugar substitute. Xylitol is a sugar-alcohol found naturally in berries, plums, mushrooms, and corn husks. It is as sweet as sucrose, but only carries 1/3 the calories. There is no aftertaste. Xylitol is absorbed more slowly than glucose and has less impact on insulin levels, thus it is safe for diabetics. An interesting feature of xylitol is that it appears to prevent tooth decay and reduce plaque. There is some evidence that regular consumption may have a favorable effect on bone density. At present there is no known toxicity.

My greatest concern about sweeteners such as sucralose, Stevia, Splenda and even Xylitol is the possibility of tissue damage from adherence to proteins or unknown effects on chemical messengers in the immune system. Theoretically, Stevia and Splenda pass through the system unchanged with little or no absorption through the GI tract, but I'm not completely convinced. Xylitol and sucralose are broken down completely, but are not regulated by insulin.

The best overall strategy is using small amounts of a variety of sweeteners, with sugar sometimes included. Stevia does appear to have some health benefits and I recommend it, just not excessively. Xylitol, agave nectar, honey and maple syrup are the best options for everyday use, because the body has the ability to break these substances down completely. Xylitol and agave nectar do not affect insulin levels, making them ideal for use by diabetics.

CHOCOLATE

What can I say? For some of us, chocolate is an essential ingredient for life. I could not start my day without a lump of dark chocolate. Other than being pleasant to eat, chocolate contains anti-oxidants and other chemicals that are beneficial from a health point of view. Chocolate seems to be a natural mood elevator. There is also good evidence that a small amount of chocolate, consumed on a daily basis, is associated with lower blood pressure in individuals with hypertension. The recommended daily dosage is 1-2 oz. (about 1/5 of a bar) of dark chocolate with at least 60% cocoa content.

For more extensive information on food and food sources, spend some time at the following websites:
www.localharvest.org
www.organicconsumer.org
www.whfoods.com   Extensive resource for information about healthy food.

CHAPTER 8

Healthier Food, Healthier Eating

Changing to a healthier way of eating is a real challenge, especially if it means going against the established norm. Often, it's like paddling upstream against the current, while everyone else is happily floating downstream, seemingly oblivious to the rapids just around the bend. Overcoming personal cravings is one thing, but doing something different than everyone else around you is truly difficult, all while the commercial food industry is constantly trying to lull you into a comfort zone of being happy with what they provide.

In the last chapter and in this one, I have provided solid information and guidelines for individuals interested in making a real change. These guidelines are drawn not only from present day knowledge about nutrition, but also from what our past dictates a healthy diet should be. For those willing to paddle upstream, the rewards are great.

GUIDELINES FOR CHOOSING HEALTHY FOOD

1. **Choose unrefined whole foods, avoiding processed foods.** The health potential of food is defined by how close it is to its natural origins. Any food loses nutritional value with processing. Commercially processed foods are low in nutrition and are the chief source of excessive dietary glucose, abnormal fats, and toxins that define an average American diet. *The first and most important step in changing to a healthier diet is getting rid of them.*

We could stop right here and make this our one and only rule of healthy food, but life is not so straightforward. Can you imagine if you had to make everything from scratch, right down to the bottle of ketchup on the table? Even then, some processing would be inevitable, as cooking is a form of processing. The question becomes: how much and what types of processing are we willing to accept?

Time is the issue. If we each had an abundance of free time and a flare for creative cooking, healthy foods would grace every meal. Few of us have this luxury. The pace of life today makes the goal of cooking every meal very challenging.

The solution is finding creative ways to fit whole foods into a busy American lifestyle and being very selective about which commercially available products we buy. The FDA has helped us out in this respect by requiring the commercial food industry to tell us what is in our food. Information about fiber content, carbohydrates, fat and protein, vitamins and minerals are listed along with a list of specific ingredients for all packaged foods. Most importantly, the ingredients contained within the product are listed in decreasing order by quantity.

When using packaged or bottled products, get into the habit of reading labels, but remember that the majority of the daily diet should be made up of foods <u>without</u> labels.

Below are some "red flags" to look out for when scrutinizing package labels.
- **Any food items that contain any of the threatening three:** *white flour, high fructose corn syrup,* or any *partially hydrogenated oil* should be avoided completely. This of course means that cookies, pastries, doughnuts, white bread, potato chips, and the like all have to go.

- **Any food product that contains chemical additives that you do not recognize should be avoided.**

- **In general, any food product with more than six ingredients on the label should be scrutinized carefully.**

- **My advice for counting carbohydrate and fat calories is specifically not to.** Whole foods have the correct amount of what you need, in the correct ratios. Whole foods have healthy carbohydrates and healthy fats that do not need to be counted. Put away the calculator and the notebook and start eating right! The same goes for using "glycemic indices" to determine "glucose potency." These values are determined by measuring how quickly glucose is absorbed from a certain food when it is consumed. Because most foods are rarely consumed in an isolated fashion, these values have little real meaning. Adding foods together dramatically affects the overall glycemic index of the foods combined. For example, vegetables, beans, barley, or oats slows the absorption of high glycemic foods such as carrots or red potatoes when they are eaten together. Following a healthy whole foods diet obviates the need for any type of calculations.

- **Avoid processed meats of *any* variety.** Yup, the hotdogs and bologna have to go. For so many reasons, they are just downright unhealthy.

- **Avoid refined oils and products that contain refined oils.** Refined oils are liquid at room temperature and have not been hydrogenated, but the high heat and/or chemicals used in the extraction process create oxidized fats. Finding them in food is not always straightforward, since refined oils are hidden in everything from mayonnaise to salad dressings. At better quality groceries and health food stores look for "unrefined" oil on product labels.

- **Do not eliminate food groups.** Eating a wide variety of foods containing a mix of nutrients is important. Avoid strict low-carbohydrate or low-fat diets. Eating fats and carbohydrates that are healthy is more important, and eating whole foods helps ensure that you get the correct balance. Avoid products labeled as "low-fat" such as salad dressings and mayonnaise; these products substitute poor-quality carbohydrates for fat and generally have more of a detrimental effect on blood lipids and blood glucose. Try using smaller amounts of the regular variety.

- **It's a matter of time.** Commercially-prepared or processed food is nothing more than a time-saving device. The acceptable standard for processed food should equal the same product made at home using whole food ingredients. Even so, anything made fresh from scratch is going to be healthier.

- **Be aware of the new wave of "healthy" processed foods.** New items with sensational labeling are showing up in both regular groceries and health food stores. From olive oil potato chips and natural health food bars to vegetarian lasagna and organic breakfast cereals, healthy is in style. To their credit, these products use organic flour, organic sugar, and non-hydrogenated oils, but still have the problem of excessive glucose and low nutrition. A sniff of that "healthy" granola bar will reveal a slightly stale smell that is indicative of oxidized fat. Granted, some of these foods are probably better than their alter egos, but they should not make up the lion's share of what you eat each day. They still fit into the commercially processed food category that generally should be restricted.

- **Be aware that the commercial food industry is more interested in your money than your health.** They are in the business of selling what sells. If health happens to sell, the better for everyone, but be particular about what you buy. The chief concern of any business selling food is the bottom line. Even "health" foods often contain fillers to bring down the total cost. For example, packaged organic vegetable lasagna contains mostly noodles, sauce, and cheese with a meager amount of vegetables. It is twice the price of typical frozen lasagna and is probably not much healthier.

2. **Eat your vegetables!** This is a "must" for healthy eating. The health of your diet is absolutely proportional to the amount of vegetables it contains, and the more variety, the better.

So many individuals feel they need to eat less to lose weight. Our evolutionary history would actually suggest that we should be eating <u>more</u>! The "more," of course, should be fresh vegetables. You could eat vegetables all day long and not gain weight. What you would gain is abundant nutrients and minerals, fiber to remove toxins, and potent anti-oxidants, all in just the right proportions. No vitamin pill on Earth can come close!

Strive to eat a higher proportion of vegetables by volume than anything else. *Vegetables and fruits should account for 50% or more of your total daily diet.* For individuals who have not learned to enjoy the flavor of vegetables, this is a tall order. Spices, seasonings, and creative dishes can help you accomplish this goal. Start with vegetables you know and like. Regularly incorporate them into meals.

As an exercise in eating healthily, each week pick a new vegetable that is unfamiliar. Do an Internet search for recipes that contain that vegetable. Look for recipes which incorporate the new vegetable with other foods, such that the flavor is not overwhelming. After a while, new flavors and new foods will become enticing instead of threatening.

3. **An apple a day...** Try to eat an apple, a peach, a plum, or a handful of some type of berries every day. Red grapes, blueberries, cherries, blackberries, and other types of berries contain potent ant-oxidants. Add them to cereal or yogurt, or just eat them plain. Follow the seasons when different types of temperate fruits are available, but frozen or dried will do in the colder months when nothing fresh is at hand. Daily variety is a key principle for all food sources. Fruits can be part of the 50% daily target for vegetables and fruit, but should not make up the majority of the total.

Berry juices such as blueberry, cherry and cranberry are brimming with anti-oxidants and can be consumed regularly as long as there is no added sugar. Pomegranate juice is another fruit juice packed with anti-oxidants. Other juices with more exotic names such mangosteen, acai and gogi are purported to offer significant health benefits, but are probably not any healthier than our native berries. (Read labels to be sure the main ingredient is the desired juice and not other, high sugar fruit juice concentrates.)

4. **Whole grains are whole foods.** Completely avoiding grain as a food source is difficult. Whole grains offer considerable nutritional value and can be considered as part of a healthy diet. Whole grains offer a healthy source of carbohydrates, vitamins and minerals, and are typically high in fiber. Having said this, however, grains should be consumed in moderation; they should not replace vegetables as the primary source of food. Whole grains are high in calories and inflammatory conditions are associated with high consumption of wheat and corn, especially in processed forms. Whole grains should not make up more than 25-35% of the daily food total.

From a food sensitivity standpoint, it is a good idea to incorporate a variety of grains into your daily diet and rotate grains as you would any other foods. Breads and pastas can be made from other grains besides wheat. Many dishes go well with brown basmati rice and quinoa is becoming very available. Barley and oats, which can stand alone as side dishes, function to actually slow the absorption of glucose for hours after they are consumed.

Be aware of gluten allergies. Individuals with any type of health condition should consider following a gluten-free diet for several weeks. The gluten grains include wheat, oats, barley, spelt and rye. (See detoxification diet at the end of chapter 11.)

Some individuals do not tolerate any type of grain product. Many sufferers of irritable bowel syndrome and inflammatory bowel disease harbor abnormal bacteria within their gastrointestinal tract that thrive on complex carbohydrates found in grains. The only way to get rid of the bacteria and the symptoms is to exclude grain products completely (at least for a while) until abnormal bacteria are eradicated.

5. **EAT MORE BEANS!** Beans contain high quality protein, are generally low in fat, and provide complex carbohydrates that do not adversely affect blood glucose; in fact, beans slow the absorption of glucose from other foods. They are also high in fiber and contain antioxidants and other chemicals that may prevent cancer and atherosclerosis. Beans come in a wide variety of flavors, shapes, colors, sizes, and can be incorporated into a wide assortment of dishes or eaten alone. Hummus is excellent as a mayonnaise substitute on sandwiches, as a thickener in dishes, and as a dip for crackers or raw vegetables.

6. **Don't be afraid to snack on NUTS.** Nuts contain favorable types of fats and are a good source of protein and important minerals. They satisfy hunger without raising blood sugar. Look for raw or low salt varieties. Nut butters are a good snack food and make excellent thickeners in dishes. Try some varieties other than peanut butter. Nuts and nut products are high-

calorie foods, though—a factor that should be taken into consideration if trying to lose weight. A variety of nuts should be a regular part of your diet.

7. **Humans are omnivores and meat has always been on the menu.** Fresh lean meat including seafood and terrestrial sources obtained wild or raised "grass-fed" can certainly be included as part of a healthy diet. Even with healthier meat, however, consumption should probably be appropriately limited. It is time for meat to step out of the spotlight for a change. Use meat within a dish or as a side-dish, rather than as the main course. Small amounts of meat can be used to add flavor to dishes that are predominantly vegetable. Poultry is preferred over beef and pork. As a general rule of thumb, meat should make up 15-20% <u>or less</u> of your total food.

8. **Compromise as needed with the use of dairy products.** Lactose intolerance and milk-protein allergies are common. Though milk does provide calcium and other valuable nutrients, high consumption of milk is actually associated with increased risk of osteoporosis. People with any kind of gastrointestinal problems, allergy problems, or chronic inflammatory disorders should probably avoid milk products altogether. Yogurt is an exception to the rule, as most people can tolerate cultured yogurt. Those who tolerate milk and milk products can include low-fat organic milk and cheese in moderation. Cottage cheese should be avoided due to possible fungal contamination.

Plain, low-fat yogurt is a good snack food, especially when lightly sweetened and combined with fresh berries and nuts. Plain yogurt is also excellent for adding a creamy taste to recipes, in place of cream or sour cream. Other fermented foods are acceptable on a daily basis. If you do not have a taste for any fermented foods, a daily probiotic supplement is recommended, especially if gastrointestinal disturbances are present.

9. **Strong bones.** While the verdict is still out as to whether milk consumption is a wise way to obtain your daily calcium, there are other excellent dietary sources of calcium worth mentioning. Excellent sources of dietary calcium include calcium-set tofu, nuts (especially almonds), beans (especially soy, chick peas and mung beans), figs, kelp, collards, broccoli, kale, okra, chocolate! and fish (especially sardines, salmon and scallops). Only about 30% of calcium from dietary sources is absorbed.

Maintaining a slightly alkaline pH in the blood and tissues is the best way to keep calcium and other minerals in bones. The natural way to maintain alkaline pH is by adhering to a high vegetable & fruit diet, free of processed and refined foods. The minerals in sea salt may also help maintain alkaline pH.

10. **A fish a day?** Centuries ago, we would have all done well to eat some type of oily fish every day. In these times, however, with mercury contamination of large fish and water pollution being ever-present concerns, we need to carefully consider our seafood choices. Follow the suggestions in the "food classification" section for safe consumption of fish and seafood. Eating seafood at least twice a week under these circumstances is a reasonable practice.

    The evidence in favor of a daily fish oil or essential fatty acid supplement is quite strong, especially in individuals over age 40. Choose a quality supplement that is free of any contaminants or oxidation. A high quality supplement should not have a fishy taste or odor. Better supplements blend a variety of essential fatty acids from both vegetable and marine sources.

11. **Eggs can be a dietary staple.** For individuals with normal cholesterol metabolism, consumption of somewhere between two to six eggs per week is reasonable. Eggs from organic "free range" chickens have a better complement of omega-3 essential fatty acids and are worth the extra money. As always, moderation and variety are the key words.

12. **Salt.** When adding salt to food, choose unrefined sea salt. Most probably life originated in the sea and the trace minerals present in sea water are important for all living things.

13. **Spice up your food!** Spices not only make food more interesting and add flavor without adding extra sugar and fat, they also make food healthier. Many of the spices and herbs have anti-inflammatory properties and virtually all of them have some positive medicinal value.

14. **Balance the oils and fat in your body.** Poly-unsaturated fat should come mainly from natural foods and not added oil. Oils used for cooking and added to food should be un-refined and predominantly mono-unsaturated. A smaller amount of saturated fat and cholesterol found in natural food is actually healthy for consumption.

15. **Getting enough protein.** Proteins make up the machinery and structural components of the body. Every day, old proteins are broken down and replaced with new. Proteins are constructed from amino acids. A complete protein source is one that provides all of the essential amino acids. Meat,

eggs, and dairy are complete sources. Soybeans are also complete sources of protein. Combinations of foods that do not by themselves provide all of the essential amino acids can be complete sources of protein. An example would be combining brown rice with beans.

Americans seem to be obsessed with getting enough protein. It is true that we need to consume enough protein to account for the daily turnover of amino acids in the body, but this amount is easy to acquire. We really do not need more than this amount. In fact, consuming large amounts of protein is hard on the kidneys and can be toxic. High protein diets push the pH of the body toward acidity which must be balanced by leaching minerals from bones (increasing risk of osteoporosis). The dietary recommendations in this chapter more than allow for an adequate amount of quality protein.

16. **Drink plenty of water.** Clean, pure water should be your primary beverage. Strive for a couple of liters every day. Green or white teas with minimal sweetening are the best options for flavored beverages.

17. **To cook or not to cook.** Some individuals advocate strict raw food diets, but light cooking helps break down food, releasing vitamins and nutrients. Also, cooking destroys toxins produced by fungal species and unfavorable bacteria that colonize many food sources. Heated food, especially in winter, encourages the enzymatic processes of digestion and warms the body.

Raw foods in the form of salads, cut vegetables, and occasionally sushi are perfectly acceptable, but do not necessarily need to form the majority of your diet. The normal practice of consuming salads at the beginning of the meal actually makes sense. Raw foods very likely provide natural enzymes that aid in digestion of other foods.

Juicing is a healthful way to obtain all the benefits of fruits and vegetables without having to consume a large volume of fruits and vegetables. Health benefits, however, are very much dependent on what goes into the juicer. Organic and fresh are the by-words for juicing. Fruits and vegetables have the potential to contain both natural and synthetic toxins. Some fruits are very high in sugar. Fresh frozen is acceptable if not freezer-burned. Vegetables and temperate fruits such as berries should be the main source of the juice.

When it comes to cooking, steaming is by far the healthiest. Steam breaks down fiber, renders food more digestible and seals in nutrients. Steaming does not destroy natural enzymes found in food. Baking is healthy, but takes time and energy. Stir-frying and sautéing are tasty ways to seal in nutrients, but have the disadvantage of adding heated oil. Grilling seals in nutrients and removes some fat, but adds toxins in the form of smoke and char. Avoid charring as much as possible when food is on the grill. Boiling is not an ideal form of cooking because nutrients are leached from food. The verdict is not yet final on microwave cooking. It would seem to be similar to steaming, but there are suggestions that microwaves may adversely change the structure of chemical nutrients within the food. Overcooking should always be avoided, with the exception of meat which should be cooked through and through.

Deep-fat frying is the only method of cooking that I discourage completely. It is true that deep-fat frying is the ultimate marriage of glucose and fat and that anything, even shoe leather, coated in flour and dropped into a deep fat fryer for several minutes tastes good; nevertheless, deep-fat frying is a true health hazard.

Before about 1900 acquiring enough fat to totally immerse something was very expensive. The abundance of grain has brought with it a cheap source of vegetable oil, such that deep-fat frying has now become a staple in fast-food restaurants. This method of cooking may hit all the right taste buds, but fried foods are major contributors to the obesity problem, cardiovascular disease, and cancer. In my opinion, the only good thing that comes out of frying food is the leftover oil, which can be converted into biodiesel to fill the tank of your car and help conserve our precious petroleum supplies.

18. **Fresh is best.** Excessive cooking and excessive processing quickly decrease the nutritional value of food. Age and spoilage allow the growth of toxin-producing fungal and bacterial species. For most foods, fresh is best. Fresh frozen is almost as good. Avoid excessive use of foods containing preservatives. Fish, canned beans and tomatoes retain most of their beneficial nutrients, but most canned vegetables do not. We live in a time when fresh food and refrigeration are readily available. Take advantage of it.

19. **Select food that has origins in living soil.** Industrial-scale production of food depletes minerals in the soil and therefore decreases the nutritional value of the harvest. Foods produced using chemical pesticides, hormones, and antibiotics also have obvious health concerns. We all pay the costs in the long run—in our health and in damage to the environment.

Choose organic whenever possible, but when choosing vegetables, fresh trumps organic. If the organic vegetables in the produce aisle are covered in plastic and appear to be past their prime, pass them by.

20. **Support your local farmer and the local vegetable stand down the road.**
Produce purchased from a familiar face is pleasant and comforting. It may
not be organic, but many small farmers are using better farming practices
and fewer chemicals than mega-agriculture. All you have to do is ask!

One step further is growing your own. Having a small garden is pleasing in
many ways and may be the way to have the healthiest food around.

See *www.localharvest.org* for information about finding local food sources.

21. **The high cost of food?** Cost is always relative. Americans like their food
quick and cheap, with little concern for quality, but the cost of cheap food
goes well beyond what you pay at the grocery store. Presently America
spends only about 7% of the gross national product (GNP) on food. We
spend 15% of the GNP on healthcare. The math behind the real cost of
better food is simple. If we were to spend twice as much on healthier food,
very likely we would spend only half as much on healthcare costs, thus
breaking even. And this estimation does not even include the
environmental costs of producing cheap food that we all pay for in the long
run. When all variables are added in, better quality food is not only cost-
effective but also offers a better life for everyone. *Loosen up your pocketbook:
you deserve better food!*

The high cost of food is often more about the high cost of convenience
than the actual cost of food. Even the priciest grocery stores have a good
supply of raw food products (rice, beans and such) at very reasonable prices.
Whole vegetables, in season, are generally not expensive. Meat is generally
the most expensive item in the grocery cart, but cutting back on meat
consumption is a good practice anyway. Organic, free-range meat costs
twice as much as the grocery store variety, but if you eat half as much, the
cost is the same. Organic whole grain stone-ground flour is a fraction of the
cost of fresh-baked bread. The cost of flour comes down even more and the
quality goes up even further if you grind the kernels yourself.

*A container of fancy organic hummus costs as much as $6.00. Enough garbanzo
bean flour, tahini, and other ingredients to make about 10 containers of hummus
costs about $16.00, or $1.60 a container. It's all a matter of time. A batch of
quality hummus only takes about 30 minutes to prepare.*

*Remember, the closer you get to the source, the more you control the quality and
flavor of the end product.*

22. **Variety is the spice of life**. There are many reasons why variety is important, but, first and foremost, it is essential for providing adequate nutrition. No single food source is complete. Consuming a wide variety of foods increases the probability of obtaining all of the vitamins, minerals, fiber and other nutrients necessary for good health.

    Other reasons to avoid monotony are less obvious, but even foods we consider "healthy" can be problematic on occasion. Some people just do not tolerate some foods. There may be a small amount of hidden toxin, the potential to cause an allergic reaction, or an adverse affect on a certain hormone in the body. For example, soy is a wholesome food, but excessive soy in the diet can inhibit thyroid function. The same is true of cruciferous vegetables. The point is that eating the same things repetitively is *un*healthy, even if they are healthy foods. Make a habit of varying foods from season to season, week to week, and even day to day.

23. **The pH debate:** Many people seem to be concerned that certain foods make the blood acidic. While the actual acidity of food has no bearing on the acid/base balance of the human body, certain foods may affect the ability of the body to maintain a normal pH.

    Enzymes in the body function optimally when the blood and tissues are at a slightly alkaline pH of 7.4. The body has complex buffering systems that guarantee maintenance of this specific pH, and only in states of severe disease does the pH of blood and tissues waiver toward being too acidic or too alkaline.

    Mechanisms for balancing pH include removing acid via the kidneys and lungs, as well as neutralizing acid by adding alkaline minerals. Forces within the body are continually generating acid. The body must constantly counterbalance this effect to maintain stable pH. Metabolism of certain amino acids (found in the so-called "acidic foods") creates additional acid. Certain other foods provide a neutralizing effect in the body by providing alkaline minerals that neutralize acidity. If alkalinizing foods are not present, the body must pull minerals such as calcium phosphate from bones to ensure a stable pH.

    Continually leaching calcium from bones to neutralize acid may be a contributing factor to osteoporosis. Regularly consuming foods that push the pH toward acidity may also be a factor in the formation of stones in the kidneys and gallbladder, bone spurs, and calcium deposits at other locations in the body. Deposits of these minerals form when excessive acid is neutralized. The deposition of uric acid crystals in joints associated with gout could be driven by this same process.

While the above is simplification of a complex process, it may be a plausible explanation for the origins of osteoporosis. If you have spent your life leaching minerals from your bones, putting them back is not going to be easy. Medical therapy may be a necessity, but you can start slowing the loss right now by changing your dietary and lifestyle habits.

Common foods that are considered to have a positive, alkaline effect include fruits and vegetables, pumpkin seeds, flax seeds, coconut oil, olive oil, sesame seeds, almonds, avocado, lima beans, white beans, lentils, tofu, Stevia, sea salt and alkalinized water. Alkaline grains include buckwheat, quinoa and spelt. Just another reason to eat your fruits and vegetables every day!

The main foods considered to have an acidic effect include soft drinks, refined sugar, corn, wheat, rice, dairy products, meat, refined oils, artificial sweeteners (especially aspartame) and alcohol drinks.

THE GREAT REFRIGERATOR AND PANTRY MAKEOVER

An exercise for learning about food starts in your own home. After thoroughly digesting the information and guidelines on food and eating, remove all food items from the refrigerator, cabinets, and pantry. (No, it doesn't have to be done all at one time and yes, it was high time for it anyway!) Create two separate areas in each of the places you store food. Items that would be classified as "acceptable" according to the food guidelines are placed in one area and everything else in the other area. In most homes the "acceptable" pile is going to be rather small at first (but hopefully not non-existent). Gradually change the ratio until the "un-acceptable" items are an insignificant part of the pantry and 'fridge. Every couple of weeks, re-read the guidelines to monitor progress. You are on your way to having a healthier diet and living a healthier life!

TIPS FOR BETTER EATING HABITS

1. **CHEW YOUR FOOD THOROUGHLY AND COMPLETELY.** The digestive system works better if it has time to digest and if food is well chewed before it is presented to the stomach. Chewing food thoroughly causes you to eat slower. Eating slower allows time for the normal physiological signals that gradually reduce hunger and allow a feeling of satiety. Chewing food thoroughly is also a first step in alleviating any sort of gastrointestinal problem.

   For most of us, chewing takes practice. We live in a world where gulping down food on the run is the norm. Eating slowly and chewing thoroughly takes practice. As a general rule of thumb, chew food thirty times before swallowing. Of course, this is a general guideline and varies depending on the food. With time, it should become an unconscious effort.

   Following a rapidly consumed meal with a large cold drink also is not a good idea from a digestion point of view. Liquid consumed in large amounts during or immediately after a meal dilutes enzymes necessary for proper digestion. Cold liquid slows enzymatic processes even further.

   This one was really tough for me. I have always eaten very rapidly and for most of my life I consumed large quantities of iced tea or soft drinks with every meal. I am just starting to be able to slow down enough to savor meals and often have hot tea or just a glass of water without ice. Sipped wine or beer is also a natural accompaniment to food.

   Make an attempt to sip a beverage that accompanies a meal, rather than gulping several drinks. If you are thirsty, drink your beverages well before beginning the meal. Room temperature liquids are more ideal than iced beverages.

2. **Portion sizes.** Statistically, long life is much more associated with eating less and being hungry than staying satiated. Even so, living life with chronic hunger pangs is not a necessity to be healthy. Most people have trained themselves to chronically eat more food than they actually need. So often we eat food, not because we're hungry, but because it's there. Before putting food in your mouth, get in the habit of asking yourself...*do I really need those calories...am I really hungry?* Eating more slowly and chewing food thoroughly is an automatic way to learn to eat less food. Filling up on vegetables instead of starches and sugar is a good practice. *Another helpful tip is using smaller plates and bowls.* The perception of a full plate goes a long way towards relieving hunger...but a smaller plate doesn't mean refilling it repeatedly.

At age fifty I eat about half the amount of food I ate at age twenty-five. My appetite is very comfortable. I do not want for more food. After purging processed carbohydrates and fat from my diet, hunger is not a problem. With better quality food as the norm, I actually derive more pleasure and relaxation from eating than ever before.

3. **How often should you eat?** It probably does not matter—whatever feels comfortable is the right answer. Most experts are now recommending five to six small meals a day. Contrary to that opinion, I have met plenty of folks in their nineties who owe their longevity solely to the fact that they typically eat only one meal a day. *The type of food seems to be more of an issue than the frequency of eating. High intake of vegetables is directly associated with improved longevity and better health.* Insulin-resistant individuals (most of the people reading this) tend to best tolerate small, frequent meals until insulin levels gradually return to normal.

   Personally, I like to start my day with breakfast. It gets me going in the morning. Through the day I will generally have several snacks and one other full meal. Whenever it comes during the day, a full meal should be a relaxed event.

4. **A word of caution about changing to a healthier diet.** Let's face it: by the time they get around to changing to a healthier diet, many people are not very healthy. This includes the gastrointestinal tract. Gastrointestinal dysfunction is caused by poor dietary and eating habits. Normal gastrointestinal function is essential for digestion of the complex foods found in a healthy diet. When they first change their diets, people who are not used to healthy food will often initially notice that symptoms of bloating and gastric discomfort actually increase. Do not worry—these symptoms should gradually resolve. A healthy diet encourages healing and generally, with time, gastrointestinal function improves.

   Consider supplementation with probiotics and digestive enzymes to aid in digestion of newer and more complex foods when you are making an abrupt diet change.

5. **It's only human to cheat every now and then.** Make an "exceptions list" for foods that are decidedly unhealthy but are difficult to leave behind.

   My father makes the best peanut brittle in the world, a perfect crunch made from real butter, raw sugar, and the best peanuts available. Not to be outdone, my mother makes chocolate dipped coconut balls that would rival those of any candy maker. Both are pure decadence, but the few times a year when these treats are available, I refuse to miss out. Though they are the antithesis of health food, eating such treats on an occasional basis produces a significant amount of pleasure.

Exceptions can be an important part of health and well-being, just as long as they are kept in proper perspective.

My "exceptions list" includes items such as ice cream, soft drinks, and cake, but I do not have them very often. As time goes on, it seems the list is getting shorter and shorter, and I "need" these things less often. I also feel much better if I stay away from them. Keep an "exceptions list" for yourself and use it wisely.

When first changing to a healthy diet, you may find that many of your everyday foods are on the "exceptions list." In the beginning, at least for several months, it is probably best to "purge" your system completely and avoid them altogether. (The detoxification diet at the end of chapter 11 is a good place to start.) Gradually they can be added back on an occasional basis. When you get around to doing this, consider asking yourself questions such as: Is it something I really need right now? How much do I really want it? How bad will it make me feel if I do eat it? Can I get by with just a bite or two and still be happy?

Every now and then, life demands a special treat. Why waste it on some artificially-sweetened-processed-tofu thing, when what you really want is an ice cream sandwich? Go ahead, get the real thing. Just make it an exceptional treat to be savored on an occasional, not a daily, basis.

CHAPTER 9

Daily Bread

The most challenging part of changing to a healthy diet is learning to like it. Children start with a very limited palate and gradually accept new foods as they are continually exposed to them. If, as an adult, you have never been exposed to varieties of vegetables and whole grains, it is unlikely that you will have a taste for them. We could ship you off to an island where only these foods were available, and leave you there until your tastes change, but rarely are such drastic steps necessary.

Anyone can learn to like a wide variety of foods if he or she makes the effort.

Start slowly. Begin to substitute brown rice, whole grain bread, and whole grain pasta for the processed versions in your daily diet. Gradually replace part of your grain consumption with vegetables. Use the Internet and the guidelines below to find ways to adapt your palate to vegetables and other foods. Use recipes that combine different healthy foods in one dish. Add small amounts of unfamiliar foods to a main course that you like very much, such that the taste is not overpowering. This is an especially good strategy for learning to like beans or certain vegetables. Before you know it, your tastes will change—I guarantee it.

When hunger strikes, most people will eat whatever is handy. Keep healthy food around. If only healthy foods are available in your kitchen, then you and your family will transition more rapidly toward eating better foods.

STARTING THE DAY OFF RIGHT

Every day should begin with the most important meal of all, breakfast. This simple and often overlooked meal is the only one that should not be skipped. The energy provided by breakfast gives your body a jump start on the day. This is the time to have your simple carbohydrates and grain products, since they will be burned with activity of the day, but stay with whole grains and steer away from donuts, pastries and the like.

Breakfast does not have to be complex or time-consuming, but also it does not have to be boring. If you are not in the habit of eating breakfast every day, your stomach may need some time to adjust. Start with familiar foods. Beverages are an important part of breakfast. Variety is always important. If you are a strict coffee drinker, try substituting hot tea (regular or green) occasionally. Fresh orange juice is great way to get a boost of Vitamin C and folate in the morning. Breakfast is the time to gain benefits from fruit juices because the sugars will be burned through the day.

Here are some healthy ways to start your day

- **A quick bowl of cereal** in the morning has always been a reliable mainstay. Many choices of low sugar, high fiber cereals are available. If your favorite cereal is still "Lucky Charms," it's time to grow up. Look for cereals that are completely whole grain and are minimally processed. Four to six grams of dietary fiber per serving is a good guideline to follow. Organic is preferred. Avoid cereals with added nuts or flax, as the oils become stale rapidly. Adding your own nuts and fruit is preferred.

  What should I put on my cereal in the morning? *Some health concerns associated with consuming cow's milk appear to be legitimate. I still use some low fat organic milk, but often choose soymilk. Even excessive consumption of soymilk may have some health concerns, and so I have found rice milk, almond milk, and coconut milk to be acceptable alternatives. More than ever before, I am choosing other options than cereal for breakfast and avoiding the milk issue altogether.*

- **Fresh fruit and yogurt.** Opt for the plain, unsweetened variety of yogurt with a spoonful of fruit jam, fresh fruit and/or some type of sweetener such as maple syrup, agave nectar, Stevia or Xylitol. Granola, wheat germ or flax meal can be added to the yogurt for texture. Making your own yogurt saves expense and is easier than you think. Yogurt makers are available at most department stores and online. Yogurt mixed with nuts and berries seems very similar to bowl of cereal, but without the grains.

- **Any type of fresh fruit makes a nice breakfast.** Try to consume some fruit every morning, even if it is only a glass of orange juice. Consider a mix of cantaloupe, pineapple, bananas, blueberries, raspberries, strawberries, grapefruit, oranges, or other fruits. Again, the sugars will be burned as the day goes on.

- **Eggs are fine several times a week** (unless you have a hereditary cholesterol problem). Hard-boiled, poached, fried, or scrambled, eggs take very little time. Whole grain toast with jam is the traditional side dish, but shredded toast and butter mixed with the egg can be a variation.

  I have found several varieties of soy sausage to be satisfactory and generally save the real stuff for rare and special occasions.

- **Poached eggs, toast and quinoa with butter.** Quinoa is very good for breakfast and is reminiscent of corn grits. It can also be served like oatmeal with milk, butter, brown sugar and raisins.

- In a pinch, **whole grain toast with jam and a glass of orange juice** is perfect for an "out-the-door" kind of breakfast.

  What do I put on my toast in the morning? *I don't know about you, but I refuse to eat my toast or my waffles dry. For a spread, use low-fat cream cheese or butter with canola oil. Products combining olive oil or unrefined canola oil with butter may be the best option yet. Plain old butter is a better option than margarine, especially if it is organic. Some newer margarines contain "plant sterols" known to lower cholesterol, but they still contain processed fat. These products are probably reasonable, as long as they are not used excessively.*

- **Whole grain pumpernickel bread with butter and a bowl of baked apples with cinnamon.** A large baking dish can be filled with Macintosh or similar apples and baked the night before for dinner, providing leftovers for breakfast or snacks.

- **Whole grain bagel with low-fat cream cheese and smoked salmon.** Many cultures eat some type of fish everyday for breakfast.

- **Organic oatmeal** with a little brown sugar, raisins, soymilk, and a pat of butter. Do not stop with oatmeal. Most other whole grains can be used in this fashion as a breakfast cereal. Consider quinoa, barley or a mix of several different whole grains. A large pot of barley can be used in various ways for both main meals and breakfasts.

- **Out-of-the-freezer waffles.** The commercial food companies have nothing on me. On weekends, I frequently make whole grain waffles from a high quality mix and then freeze extras for use over the following couple of weeks. Thaw in the microwave for a few seconds, pop them in the toaster, and they taste even better than right out of the waffle iron. A little bit of maple syrup is nice, but fresh fruit with yogurt works well on top also. For variety, waffles or pancakes can be made from mixes with different grains such as buckwheat. Consider substituting cooked, mashed sweet potatoes or pumpkin for some of the liquid in the mix. Pecans or walnuts are a tasty addition.

- **Whole grain French toast.** This breakfast can be reserved as an occasional treat using a high quality round loaf of whole grain bread left over from dinner the night before. With a fork, whisk a couple of eggs, a splash of soymilk, nutmeg, and cinnamon together. Soak the slices of bread for several minutes. Spray a little grapeseed oil on a cast iron skillet heated to medium. Brown the slices on each side and serve with a little honey or maple syrup.

- **Healthier hash browns.** Potatoes with less starch, such as the little red ones, are okay for occasional eating. Start with pre-cooked potatoes (a good way to use leftovers). Chop up an onion and a bell pepper. Use an amount equal in volume to that of the potatoes. Cut the potatoes up into cubes or small slices. Sauté the potatoes, onions, peppers in olive oil on medium-high heat until brown. Add salt and red pepper to taste. Serve with a fried egg. This recipe is also quite good using sweet potatoes (avoid overcooking potatoes prior to use in the sauté).

- **Frijoles in the morning.** Beans for breakfast? Absolutely! Scrambled eggs with salsa and seasoned black beans on the side make an excellent breakfast. Add plantains or bananas sautéed in macadamia nut oil with cinnamon and a touch of brown sugar, and you have really gone south of the border!

WEEKEND BREAKFASTS (also make great light evening meals)
- **Whole grain waffles.** Several good quality mixes are available. Of course you need a waffle iron. Top with pure maple syrup or try fruit and yogurt. For variety, add mashed sweet potatoes or pecans in the mix. For a side item, some varieties of soy sausage are surprisingly palatable.

- **Veggie omelet with whole grain toast.** Here's how to make a perfect omelet. By hand, beat 4 to 6 eggs with salt, pepper, and a splash of soymilk. Season a 10-inch, rounded edge sautéed pan with non-stick cooking spray. Pour the egg mixture into the cold pan about a half inch deep. *It is very important that the pan and stove are cold in the beginning.* Place the pan on the stove with medium heat. Sprinkle fresh grated parmesan cheese on top. The omelet is done when there is no liquid on top and the cheese is melted. While the omelet is cooking, sautéed chopped onions, mushrooms, peppers, tomatoes, garlic, and fresh oregano in olive oil. Spread this mixture on top of the omelet and fold with two spatulas. Serve with toast and soy sausage.

- **Salmon patties, boiled egg, and toast.** In many cultures, fish is a breakfast staple. For the patties, mix leftover grilled salmon or canned wild salmon with an egg, chopped onion, chopped bell peppers, garlic, salt, pepper, and some dry oats or shredded bread as a thickener. Form into patties and cook in a frying pan seasoned with non-stick spray. Cook until brown and serve with toast and an egg.

HEALTHY FOOD ON THE GO

Here in America we tend to eat lightly during the day and save our big meal for the end of the day. Many experts would suggest the European plan of eating a main meal in the middle of the day and eating lightly in the evening is healthier. No doubt, this style of eating is better for digestion and probably less conducive to weight gain, but fitting a large meal into the middle of an American day is challenging. Avoiding a big meal altogether may be a possible solution. Eating small amounts throughout the day prevents and suppresses the urge to eat large amounts. On some days, consider having several substantial snacks during the day and then a lighter meal at night. Eating lunch instead of dinner at a nice restaurant is pleasant way to break up the day. Midday meals at better restaurants tend to be lighter and healthier.

For on-the-go days there are many options to choose from without resorting to typical fast-food fare.

SMALL AND EXTRA-QUICK MEALS

Some of the most pleasant meals I can remember in my lifetime have been the simple ones. A favorite pastime for my family has been hiking in various different national parks around the country. Day hikes usually include a simple meal along the way. A quick stop off at a bakery or general store on the way to the day's hike provided pick-up items to toss into my backpack. Standard picks include a loaf of hard bread, Swiss cheese, apples, berries, chocolate bars, oatmeal cookies, and bottles of water. Any preparation is done with my pocket knife and the "table" is usually a rock overlooking some gorgeous valley, waterfall, or equally magnificent scene miles away from civilization. Food cannot taste any better than after you have walked half a day to end up in such a special place. These simple meals have become the most celebrated of our lives.

Simple meals can be some of the best because they do not require much preparation or cleanup. They can be fixed anytime during the day or evening. A wide assortment of simple meals is possible. Though some of the items mentioned below may seem foreign to your taste buds, that will change with time.

My office staff constantly makes fun of my lunches. I think nothing of microwaving a collection of cabbage and mushrooms seasoned with olive oil and ginger and eaten with a hunk of whole grain bread spread with almond-butter. Of course, I give them as much flak about their "supreme" grease-oozing taco. It's all a matter of what you get used to. Sometimes good health is worth a little compromise.

Vegetable bowls. Fresh vegetables, the most important of our food sources, are often left off the menu completely. Even those of us who like vegetables sometimes find it hard to consume our full quota each day. My solution to the problem is a concept I call "vegetable bowls." It is my answer to microwave dinners. At the office, I keep a selection of fresh and frozen vegetables in the refrigerator at all times. It takes about five minutes to fill a bowl with a varying assortment of different chopped vegetables. The only tools necessary are a large (4 cup) glass bowl with a lid, a cutting board, a large knife and a spoon. Five to six minutes in the microwave and you have a bowl of fresh steamed vegetables (I actually prefer steaming and may purchase a portable steamer at some point).

The key to making vegetables palatable is the addition of spices, a little bit of fat and sometimes something sweet. I keep a variety of bottled sauces, pesto and spices on hand and always have a bottle of olive oil in the cabinet. Brown rice, whole grain pasta, chicken or shrimp brought in from home also make flavorful additions. This concept can also be prepared at home the night before and microwaved at lunch the next day. Below are some suggestions for items and possible seasoning combinations:

Vegetables   carrots, cabbage, peppers, celery, edamame (fresh soybeans), broccoli, fresh green beans, zucchini, onion, and peas.

Other items   kidney beans, black beans, black-eyed peas, hummus, brown rice, whole grain pasta, pre-cooked chicken, pre-cooked shrimp.

Seasonings   *Italian:* green pesto or sun-dried tomato pesto, garlic, parmesan cheese. *Oriental:* ginger, garlic, soy sauce. *Indian:* ginger, garlic, curry paste. Olive oil can be added to a dish for more flavor.

Try it. Add a vegetable bowl to your routine at least several times a week. There are almost an infinite number of possible combinations. With a slice of fresh bread, this is a very satisfying meal that could never be rivaled by something out of a bag or package, in quality or taste. When you first start out, stick with items that seem familiar, and then gradually expand your tastes. Do not be afraid to think outside the box.

Other suggestions for quick meals during the day or in the evening

- **Leftovers!** Some of the best and quickest lunches are leftovers. Often I will make a large meal in the evening with intentions of allowing for several lunches. Often extras from one meal can also provide the raw ingredients for subsequent meals. You just have to get into the habit of thinking ahead when cooking a meal. Rarely does food go wasted in my house.

- **Soup.** Some of the best leftovers are homemade soups. Soups are so easy to make and can be frozen for later use. During winter months, a large pot of soup made on the weekend can provide a couple of evening meals and several lunches. Avoid canned soups (except for those containing mainly beans or lentils, which tend to retain their nutritional value when canned). Because of the amount of heat required for canning soups, the nutritional value of most vegetables is lost.

  Recently, a soup company came out with a campaign advertising "0" calories and "0" fat. What they did not advertise was "0" nutrition.

- **Sandwiches.** Sandwiches are the quintessential on-the-go American food, and they can be made into healthy choices. Sandwiches are, by definition, two pieces of bread with something in-between. The "something" can include some type of quality meat with a quality cheese, tomatoes, cucumbers, avocado, shredded carrots with other vegetables, leftover grilled vegetables, banana with peanut butter, and anything else you can think of. The healthy part always starts with good quality whole grain bread. If trying to lose weight, ask for very thin-sliced bread. High quality mayonnaise (not containing processed oils) is fine, but also consider other types of spreads. Hummus is a great spread with vegetables. A little bit of olive oil and vinegar also works wonderfully well.

  At one point when considering vegetarianism, I lamented that sandwiches would have to go because of the meat and cheese, as well as the white bread. This is a perfect example of how tunneled our thinking can become in regard to eating.

- **Mixed greens salad.** With a choice of fresh cut vegetables, boiled egg, crumbled walnuts, avocado, grapes, berries, raisins, chopped red bell peppers, carrots, canned wild salmon, and/or tofu, there are almost unlimited combinations. Learn to think outside of the box. Good quality lettuce is now very available. This is one item I often buy pre-washed and packaged to save time. Organic spinach and several organic lettuce combinations are available. The deeper the green, the more substantial the nutritional value. Iceberg lettuce has virtually no nutritional value and I recommend avoiding it.

- **Beans and rice.** Whenever I cook rice, I always cook a double amount for use in other dishes. This basic dish can made any number of ways. Different types of beans change the flavor of the dish. Spice it up with the addition of stir-fried vegetables, fresh minced herbs and garlic, Mexican spices like cumin and chili powder, seafood, or chicken. You can even throw in vegetables like zucchini or carrots. This same idea can be used with other grains such as barley or quinoa.

- **Whole wheat pasta (gluten-free pasta can be substituted) and sauce.** This is a reliable standby at our house. It takes no time to fix the pasta. There are some outstanding bottled pasta sauces available. Try it with soy-based "meatballs" (some brands are better than you think). With a salad or a side of steamed broccoli, this dish makes a full meal.

- **Leftover quinoa mixed with a spoonful of red-pepper hummus and canned crushed organic tomatoes, microwaved for a minute, is surprisingly tasty.** As a side, add a simple slaw made with shredded cabbage and carrots, diced apples, raisins, a bit of mayonnaise (try the olive oil variety), a little mustard, salt, pepper, paprika, and you have a nutritious meal.

- **Tofu** with ginger dressing, baked for 20 minutes. To most people tofu, by itself, is bland and relatively tasteless, but the neat thing about tofu is that it soaks up any flavor you add to it. It isn't so bad once you learn how to cook with it. Serve with steamed cabbage.

- **PB&J** is my surfing lunch or a quick bite before going on a midday bike ride. Use whole grain bread with peanut or almond butter and a little honey. Quick, easy, and nutritious.

- **Steamed fresh salmon** with ginger sauce along with steamed edamame, mushrooms, and soy sauce. Edamame is the Japanese name for fresh soybeans. The taste is somewhere between a pea and a butterbean.

- **ALT.** Avocado, lettuce and tomato on whole grain bread.

- **Pick-me-up smorgasbord.** A meal does not always have to be well-defined. Sometimes an odd assortment of anything around can make for an adequate meal.

FULL MEALS

Ideally the largest meal of the day should be casually consumed in the company of family and friends. In Europe this meal typically occurs in the middle of the day and is frequently almost a celebration. Though it is a healthy style of eating, it is not practical for most American families. Here we typically eat a light midday meal and follow it with a full meal at the end of the day. With busy lifestyles, cooking seems to be a real inconvenience for working adults. It should not be. Meals prepared from fresh ingredients are always healthier than those prepared in a restaurant or by a food factory.

Where so many health cookbooks offer recipes and menu plans, I would like to offer concepts instead, knowing full well that diet fads fade and most people will gradually return to old habits. I would like to help you grow as a person, to teach you how to rustle up a healthy meal. Following a healthy diet is a lifetime commitment that requires new skills and habits.

In the following section I assume that you know nothing about cooking and need to start from ground zero. It will include suggestions on what to stock in your kitchen and even suggestions on how to shop at the grocery store. This will be followed by a series of meals that even a novice can handle and that anyone should find tasty. Try several different ones each week. From here I hope that you can go "solo" and move on to ideas of your own without being encumbered by a recipe book.

CREATING A WELL-STOCKED KITCHEN

I am often asked to provide shopping lists and menu plans. My response is to suggest having a well-stocked kitchen instead. Extensive planning is exactly what I would like to help you avoid. People who try to live by planning out each meal for each day of each week generally tire of the practice and go back to whatever they were doing before.

Have you ever gone out of your way to plan to cook a specific recipe on a specific night, only to find out that key ingredients are missing, necessitating yet another trip to the grocery store?

Simple cooking means learning how to improvise. One of the most important concepts of simple cooking is that, without any significant planning, you can go to the pantry and refrigerator, pull out several items, and create a healthy and tasty meal within a short amount of time, with minimal stress. The key to success is having a reasonable selection of items on hand all of the time.

While many individuals will find their pantry and refrigerator to be complete, others will need some basic suggestions. The idea is to save planning and shopping time so that only essential items need to be purchased from week to week. My shopping list is more like a re-stocking list. Though I will occasionally shop for a specific recipe, most of the time I cook with items that are already at home.

Basic condiments and spices

Seasonings

Spices, herbs, oils, and vinegars are a very important part of simple cooking. These ingredients allow the addition of flavor without added salt, sugar, and fat. Different combinations can completely change the style or taste of food. I try to keep a basic assortment on hand all of the time.

Oils

There are many varieties of oils, each adding their own particular taste to food. Of all of them, olive oil is probably my personal favorite. Here are some I keep in the cabinet. Oils should be minimally refined and cold-pressed. Notice that corn oil is not on the list. I cook with butter only occasionally.

Olive oil	walnut oil	sesame oil
Canola oil	grapeseed oil (a spray can is handy)	
Macadamia nut oil		

Vinegar

Vinegar has a way of bringing out the flavor of food and can be used in many types of dishes. Different vinegars, of course, have different flavors.

Apple cider vinegar – an all-purpose vinegar.

Rice vinegar – a light vinegar for light cooking. Often used in Oriental dishes.

Malt vinegar – a tasty vinegar great for seafood and potato dishes.

Balsamic vinegar – a robust vinegar made from red wine. Excellent for Italian dishes.

Fresh herbs

I try to keep fresh herbs growing in a garden out back from spring until fall. I do not claim to have a green thumb. Herbs are basically weeds and are easy to grow in any pot or sunny corner of the yard. Also grocery stores are beginning to regularly stock fresh herbs in the produce section. Though I keep some jars of dried herbs on hand for emergencies, they truly pale by comparison. If forced to use dried herbs, remember to use a much smaller amount since the intensity of flavor is concentrated.

My favorite fresh herbs include basil, oregano, thyme, rosemary, marjoram, and cilantro. Other popular fresh herbs include lavender, dill, tarragon, fennel, and lemon grass.

Dry spices

Cinnamon, nutmeg, curry powder, cumin, chili powder, turmeric, Mexican oregano, saffron, allspice, garam masala, paprika, mustard powder, and cayenne pepper are all found in my spice rack. I also keep dried thyme, oregano, basil, and bay leaves in case fresh varieties are not available.

In the refrigerator Keep on hand some low-sodium soy sauce, Worcestershire sauce, mild curry paste, a large jar of minced garlic, fresh ginger root or a jar of minced ginger, and hot chili sauce. There are various other bottled sauces that I keep around to make life easier, but lately, I seem to be making my own more and more often.

Salad dressings and mayonnaise are now readily available with unrefined oil and better quality ingredients, but those that you make yourself are probably tastier and healthier. Making salad dressing is not very difficult, and recipes for every variety you can imagine can be found on the Internet.

Yogurt is a great snack food, but is also a healthy way to make a dish creamy. I generally keep a large container of organic plain (unsweetened) yogurt for use in both purposes. Strained or Greek yogurt (sometimes called yogurt cheese) is excellent for cooking. Look for low-fat favorites.

Hummus is another multi-purpose item handy to have around. Hummus is a tasty dip for vegetables and crackers, an alternative to mayonnaise as a spread for sandwiches, and a thickener for use in cooking. Though readily found in grocery stores, I often make my own from garbanzo bean flour, tahini (sesame paste), and other fresh ingredients. It really has a better flavor than anything I have found in the grocery. By the way, garbanzo bean flour is a healthy alternative to corn starch or white flour for use as a thickener.

My refrigerator always contains an assortment of fresh fruits and vegetables which vary by season and availability. Follow the seasons and let the availability of local food dictate what's for dinner. Other staples include organic milk, soy milk, several varieties of fruit juice, several blocks of hard cheese such as sharp cheddar, Swiss, and parmesan, free-range eggs, a container of butter/canola oil blend, and a couple of jars of pickles that have been back there as long as I can remember. Occasionally tofu or tempeh will also find its way to the shelf. Several jars of fruit jams are a necessity. I also generally keep whole grain pancake mix in the refrigerator instead of the pantry.

In the freezer The primary staples found in my freezer are nuts. My nut supply includes almonds, walnuts, cashews, Brazil nuts, macadamia nuts, pecans, and hazel nuts, all kept in tight containers where they will not spoil or become freezer burned. Usually there will also be a piece of wild red Alaskan salmon (often available for an amazingly good price), a small amount of free-range beef and chicken, and occasionally a piece of wild elk meat from a friend in Colorado. Sometimes there will be frozen shrimp (which freeze very well if covered in water), but I buy most seafood fresh from local markets. In the winter there are a variety of fresh-frozen organic berries and vegetables.

In the pantry I always keep certain items on hand, such as bottled pasta sauces (always organic), several types of whole grain or high quality pasta, a large container of brown basmati rice, several other kinds of rice, wild rice, barley, quinoa and canned items. A couple of cans of crushed organic tomatoes and a can of tomato paste are handy to have around. A small can of coconut milk is a necessity for Thai cooking. A jar of peanut or some other nut butter (almond is my favorite, but expensive) and a jar of salsa are always present. I usually keep several kinds of canned beans on the shelf including dark red kidney, black beans, cannoli beans, navy beans and pinto beans. I generally do not buy other canned vegetables, as they are low in nutrition. The only dried beans that I keep regularly are red and green lentils. Other dry goods include items such as whole grain cereals, whole grain crackers, and whole grain corn chips.

TIPS ON SHOPPING

My trips to the grocery would be best described as restocking trips. Sometimes I carry a list, but most of the time I have a fairly good idea of what I need. The first stop is the produce section, where I buy a general selection of fruits and vegetables that my family and I can consume within a week. Seasonal fruits and berries are always on the list. Greens and vegetables such as summer squash, broccoli, cauliflower, and cabbage are more perishable and are generally purchased in smaller amounts with plans to use them over the upcoming several days. Vegetables such as carrots, winter squash, onions, and sweet potatoes will keep for a while and can be kept on hand all of the time. Occasionally a seasonal vegetable will spark an idea for a specific meal.

Next on my route is the bakery for a fresh loaf of organic stone-ground whole grain bread. Fresh meat and cheese are sometimes on the list. The remainder of my shopping trip is usually just replacing staples such as pomegranate juice, 2% organic milk, soymilk, organic plain yogurt, free range eggs, organic peanut butter, bottled sauces and salsas of different varieties, whole grain cereal, tea bags, dog food, etc. (Lately I have been trying to feed my dog more fresh food or a can of wild salmon instead of just the processed stuff). In winter I purchase frozen berries and vegetables, when fresh items are not available for a reasonable price. Dried berries also keep well in the off season. They are kept in the refrigerator.

As a physician with a keen interest in nutrition, it's hard not to notice what people have in their carts at the grocery store. As they are placing their items on the conveyor in line in front of me, I'm ticking off in my head that person's health potential. Sometimes I think I could do a better job assessing someone's health status by following them around in the grocery store than doing a screening exam at the office. Maybe I could offer it as a way to save money in the new healthcare system. Instead of going to the office I could be paid to hang around the grocery store and give nutritional advice.

It often surprises me that my cart full of fresh items is usually about the same price as the same amount of packaged goods that other people are willing to pay for. Packaging adds cost, and meat especially adds cost. People who buy packaged food often tend to buy a lot of meat. I like the flavor of meat as much as anyone else, but a little bit of it should go a long way. Our healthcare expenditure would immediately go down if everyone in the country started buying half as much meat and packaged foods as they are right now.

During the warmer months shopping trips are more frequent, with many destinations. In addition to regular visits to local seafood markets, I frequent fruit and vegetable stands for locally-grown produce. Buying from local markets and growers whenever you can is an important way to support your community. Trips to the state farmer's market with a large cooler are a special treat.

Mail order can be a practical way to obtain quality food at reasonable prices. Free-range meats of different varieties are available online. My freezer always contains a large package of mixed nuts obtained from a reputable source.

Remember to bring your own cloth bags on shopping trips!

SIMPLE COOKING FOR ONE, A COUPLE, OR A WHOLE FAMILY

With the aim of simple cooking in mind, anyone should be able to go to the refrigerator, open the door, remove several items already on hand, and construct a tasty healthy meal with a minimal investment of time. This is a very achievable goal, whether for a single individual or a whole family. Most of the meal guidelines and recipes that follow work for one person or a whole crowd. Leftovers and leftover ingredients can be saved or used with other ingredients to make a different type of meal.

It is possible to make tasty meals without becoming a slave to sugar and fat. These preferential tastes must be respected, but should not be allowed to become dominant. Herbs, spices and combinations of food can enliven a dish without it becoming laden with starch, fat and sugar.

When you do go to the refrigerator, start with the most perishable vegetables. This is often my guide to meal planning. I regularly check the vegetable bin and try to use items while they are fresh, so as to avoid allowing the vegetable bin to become a compost pile!

Next add other items to make a whole dish. Take advantage of "batch" items. Whenever I cook rice, I cook enough to make several different dishes during the week. The same goes for steamed vegetables. I can make a week's worth of different meals using these basic ingredients with different spices, sauces, and added meats.

BASIC STIR-FRY

Have you ever been to a Chinese restaurant that features a Mongolian barbeque, the kind that has about twenty different varieties of fresh raw vegetables presented in a salad-bar-like fashion? Customers individually fill bowls with their favorite ingredients and present them to a cook, who runs them around a large flat grill and hands back a plate of piping-hot, fresh food of the customer's own creation. This is the essence of simple cooking: fast, easy, and with endless variations.

Simple cooking is not difficult, does not take a lot of time, does not require lots of expensive cookware, and offers an almost unlimited amount of variety. New tastes can be gradually incorporated along with familiar ones. In fact, just the concept of cooking fresh food is a step in the right direction.

Following the lead of the Mongolian barbeque, let's start with a simple stir-fry. Any frying type pan will do, but a wok is preferred. A good steel wok is not expensive and can be purchased almost anywhere. I could survive just fine with a large steel wok, a large rounded knife, a slotted spoon, and pan to cook rice in. Throw in a large soup pot, a vegetable steamer, and an outdoor grill and I have all the cooking utensils I need! For pots and pans I generally use steel and stay away from aluminum and non-stick coated cookware.

Now for the ingredients. The neat thing about a stir-fry is the variety of stuff that can go into it. Almost an unlimited number of flavors to suit any tastes are possible. Even the pickiest individuals should be able to mix up a list of ingredients that they can enjoy.

Most any of the following items could be included on your shopping list:

Vegetables

broccoli	cabbage	cauliflower	firm tofu	green peas
carrots	onions	bell pepper—red, green or yellow		snow peas
zucchini	eggplant	spinach	green beans	spring onions
celery	bok choy	yellow squash	mushrooms	
edamame (soy beans)				

Pick your favorites first and then add smaller amounts of others that are less familiar. The foreign flavors will blend and will be hardly noticed.

Meats

chicken	shrimp	scallops	squid
fish	pork	beef	crab

Basic seasonings for a Chinese style stir fry

canola oil (heat tolerant)
(olive or macadamia nut oil is fine if care is taken not to overheat the oil)

soy sauce (low salt)	vegetable or chicken broth
minced garlic	fresh grated ginger
fresh minced cilantro	fresh minced basil

Generally this dish is accompanied by rice, but grain is not essential. Brown basmati rice has much more fiber and protein than regular rice and has less starch. It also has more flavor.

What goes into this meal depends on your personal tastes. Start with things that you genuinely like. Cooking two versions is easy. When my kids were younger, I would stir-fry the meat first with seasonings and put it aside. Then I would stir-fry vegetables for my wife and me and add some of the meat mixture in for flavor. Adapting to the taste of vegetables takes time for some individuals. We would usually have some type of stir-fry every week. As time went on I would mince small amounts of vegetables into the kids' version until only one version was necessary for all of us.

The meal we are about to cook blends flavors to come up with a unique taste. Different vegetables, oils, meats, and seasonings all affect the flavor of a dish. The amount of variety possible is almost infinite. Healthy foods can be added gradually as tastes adapt. Broccoli may not be your favorite, but instead of being pushed aside or ignored altogether, it becomes incorporated into a blend with other flavors.

Before we get started, study some basic cooking skills:

How to chop vegetables

Obtain a good quality wide blade knife with a rounded bottom across the edge. Good does not necessarily mean expensive. A reasonable quality knife of this description can be found at most large chain stores. On a wooden cutting board (use plastic for meat) lay out a vegetable such as a zucchini. Place the tip of the knife on the board. Using a downward rotating motion, slice through the vegetable with the middle of the blade. Gradually advance the vegetable forward between continuous slicing motions with the knife. The knife stays stationary, with the tip on the board. Keep a steady rhythm. (Watch out for your fingers!) Who needs a food processor?

How to mince herbs

Fresh herbs are widely available and have much more flavor than their dried counterparts. Lay a handful of herbs out on a wooden cutting board. Grasp the top of the blade of a wide rounded knife with both hands. Chop across the pile of herbs with fine rapid chopping motions. After one pass use the edge of the blade to pull the pile into a row. Chop across the row. Repeat until the herbs are finely minced.

How to stir-fry

A good quality steel wok is preferred, but not essential. Look for one with a flattened bottom if you are using an electric stove. A cover for the top is an important accessory. Place the wok on medium-high to high heat. After the wok is hot, add the oil and then immediately add the ingredients to be stir-fried. This is important to keep the oil from burning. Smoking oil is a sign that the oil is being damaged. ***Never let your oil get hot enough to smoke.*** Special "wok" oils can be purchased that have been selected to have a very high "smoke-point," but any oil can be used if you are careful. Olive oil and macadamia nut oil are my personal favorites. Sesame oil is also very stable and imparts a unique flavor.

Once the food goes in, use a rounded metal spatula or large spoon to stir the food away from the bottom to prevent burning. The motion is a scoop, moving food off the bottom of the pan followed by a flip of your wrist to spread the food along the cooler upper parts of the pan. The idea is to constantly keep the food moving away from the hot spot in the middle so food will not burn. This is done repetitively to circulate the food around the pan. It takes a little practice but is not difficult to learn. Start with a small amount at first so that food does not end up flying all over the kitchen. With time you will be able to cook a whole meal easily in one round.

Stir-frying is healthy because only a small amount of oil is required and flavor and nutrition are sealed in by the brief exposure to high heat. I generally stir-fry for only 3 to 5 minutes, usually just enough to brown the onions. After a brief stir-fry, add liquid ingredients and lower heat to simmer. Cover the pan and continue cooking on simmer until the vegetables are tender. This gives the food the taste of a stir-fry, but most of the cooking is actually by steaming. Avoiding overcooking, with the idea being to release nutrients, not destroy them. I like my vegetables to stay crunchy.

Sauté versus stir-fry

Stir-frying generally involves higher heat and only a small amount of oil–just enough to prevent food from sticking to the pan. The food is constantly and vigorously moved in order to prevent burning. Sautéing uses a flat bottom pan with the entire surface of bottom heated equally (i.e., your basic frying pan). Only low to medium heat is used. The food is continually but gently stirred in the pan. Slightly more oil or other liquid is used to prevent sticking and burning. Because less heat is used, most unrefined cooking oils works well. Again, olive oil is a favorite. Some recipes will work better with one than the other, but for most dishes the two methods are interchangeable.

How to make perfect brown rice

Start with good quality rice. I recommend basmati brown rice. For most rice, add about 2-2 ½ cups of water per cup of rice. Place rice and water in a pot over high heat. Add a teaspoon of olive oil and a dash of salt. Bring to a boil. Turn the heat down to low. *Allow several minutes for the water to return to a low simmer before covering.* This will prevent the mixture from boiling over. Cook covered on low for 45 minutes or per the instructions on the package. White basmati rice will take less time. Remove from the heat and allow to stand (covered) for 5 to 10 minutes before serving. Rice keeps well in the refrigerator, and I always make extra for use in other meals during the week.

Home made Teriyaki Sauce

Mix ¼-½ cup of low salt soy sauce with a cup of organic chicken or vegetable broth. Add a teaspoon of rice wine vinegar. Grate in a tbsp. of fresh ginger. Add a tsp. of fresh garlic and a tbsp. of brown sugar. This a great sauce for many dishes and as a marinade for grilling.

Finally we can move on to the kitchen. Rice takes the longest amount of time and needs to be started first. Meat should be thin-sliced about 1/3-inch thick and free of as much fat as possible. I usually leave it sitting on a small cutting board until ready to cook. Next I chop the vegetables. Zucchini squash seem to take longer than anything else to cook, so I usually slice them fairly thin. Which vegetables and how much of each really depends on your tastes. I would expect that some people will start with mainly meat, and that's okay as long as more vegetables are added in each time this dish is made. Don't be afraid to try new things; the tastes become blended more than you would think.

For four people I generally chop enough vegetables to almost fill a two quart pitcher. Don't worry about cooking too much. Plan on a little extra to take for lunch the next day. The first time around, do not try to cook everything at once. Plan on cooking in several batches. With experience it will become a one pot meal.

Place the wok on a burner and turn on high heat. Let the pan heat for a minute or so. *After* the pan is hot, add enough oil to cover the bottom, about 1-2 tablespoons. With experience you will need less oil. Just as soon as the oil is hot, add food. *Do not let the oil get too hot before adding the food.* Cook any meat first until no raw areas are noted. Add a little of the teriyaki sauce if the meat alone is going to be served to some individuals. Place the meat in a separate bowl. Add more oil to the wok.

Next, stir-fry onions, mushrooms and peppers. When the onions are brown, add other vegetables, herbs and seasonings. Continue the stir-fry for only a couple of minutes until they are seared. Add the meat back in. Remember to keep the food moving. Add the liquid ingredients, lower the heat, cover and simmer for about 5 minutes. The whole idea is not to overcook. Vegetables sometimes need more oil than meat; don't be bashful when you are first starting out.

Serve the mixture over a bed of rice with hot green tea as a beverage.

If you have never done this type of cooking before, the first time can be a bit of an adventure. If things get too fast, you can slow it down by taking the wok off the burner, turning down the heat, or using a little more oil. Be careful not to slosh hot oil on yourself or a burner. Again, with experience you will be able to cook all of this meal at one time. I usually give meat such as beef or chicken a head start before adding the vegetables. Seafood, such as shrimp, is added toward the end of cooking the vegetables. Often somewhere in the middle I will add in a small handful of minced fresh cilantro or basil for added flavor.

The really cool thing about this style of cooking is that it can be adapted to an almost unlimited variety of dishes. Change the ratio of meat or vegetables and have a different flavor. Change the seasonings and have a different dish altogether. Below I offer a series of dishes that follow the same format and use many of the same ingredients, but taste very different from the basic Chinese stir-fry.

Southeast Asian Stir-fry

The choice of vegetables will influence the flavor. I usually use milder flavored vegetables such as snow peas or spring onions, but any from the list will work. The best choices of meat include chicken or shrimp. Minced herbs can include either basil or cilantro. Lemon grass is also excellent for this dish. This is a good dish in which to introduce tofu instead of meat. At first glance tofu appears to be a tasteless, gelatinous mass, but it has the ability to pick up and concentrate all the flavors in the dish. In a very flavorful dish such as this one, it makes a nice addition. This dish can be served over brown rice, brown rice pasta, or udon (a Japanese thick whole grain noodle similar to spaghetti).

There are many sauce possibilities; here is just one, but its many flavors combine to give this dish a savory flavor: Combine 1 cup vegetable or chicken broth, ¼ cup low sodium soy sauce, 2 tablespoons minced fresh ginger, ½-1 cup light coconut milk, 1 teaspoon brown sugar, ½ teaspoon red chili sauce, ½-1 teaspoon mild curry paste, 1 lime halved and squeezed into the sauce, 1-2 teaspoons of rice wine vinegar, and 1 teaspoon minced garlic. Peanut butter is also often found in Thai cooking.

Cook and serve this dish in exactly the same manner as the previous one.

Middle-eastern Stir-fry

This dish can use the same vegetables as the one before, but again the sauce gives it a totally different twist. It can be centered on chicken, shrimp, or tofu; most often I prepare this as a totally vegetarian meal. It can be served over rice, but it seems to go best with good quality brown rice pasta or lentils.

A little prep work is required for the sauce. Start with a small to medium onion and a red bell pepper, chopped and sautéed in olive oil. Add 1-2 teaspoons of minced garlic. Stir in one can of crushed tomatoes or tomato sauce (preferably organic).

Now for the spices: 1 tablespoon of chili powder, 1 teaspoon of ginger powder, 1 teaspoon of ground cumin, 1 teaspoon of ground turmeric, 1 tablespoon of mild curry paste, a half teaspoon of red chili sauce or minced red chili (cayenne), a pinch or two of sugar, and salt to taste.

Cook this dish in the same fashion as the previous ones. Mix in enough sauce to cover the vegetables. Serve over the pasta. Save the unused sauce. This spicy tomato sauce can be used in a variety of dishes. I usually make a double amount and save half in the refrigerator.

Pasta Primavera

Next we move over the Mediterranean for an Italian-style pasta dish. Vegetables that work well include zucchini, onion, mushrooms, bell pepper, and carrots. Shrimp are especially good in this one. The "sauce" is not made separately, but is added as you go along. I usually prepare this dish in a sauté pan (basic steel frying pan) over medium-high heat with olive oil.

Sauté the vegetables in olive oil until tender. Along the way add in 1 teaspoon of minced garlic (though it does lose some potency, I usually buy minced garlic in jars to save time). Add in a handful of minced fresh basil and oregano. When I say a handful, I mean just that. It is hard to overdo-it with fresh herbs. The dried variety in jars will do in a pinch, but the flavor will not be quite the same. Use a much smaller quantity of dried herbs, as the flavor is concentrated. Other seasoning additions can include pine nuts and chili powder.

Next add in 2 cups of fresh cherry tomatoes or 1 can of crushed tomatoes. For extra flavor stir in a teaspoon of balsamic vinegar. Bring down the heat and simmer until the tomatoes are broken apart and mixed in (you can help them with the back of a spoon if you like). Add salt to taste. Add in 2 tablespoons of low fat sour cream or strained yogurt and sprinkle freshly shredded parmesan cheese on top. Serve over good quality pasta. I usually use whole grain wheat pasta, but any type of pasta will work.

How to make perfect pasta

Pour one to two quarts of water (depending on the amount of pasta) into a pot and bring to a boil. Add salt to taste. Add one tsp. of olive oil to prevent sticking. Add the pasta. Stir often, checking frequently to see if it is ready (remove a piece or two to taste). When the pasta has just lost its crunchiness, pour into a strainer in the sink. This is referred to as *al dente* or "to the tooth."

Fish fajitas

This quick and simple stir-fry includes fish, but it is another opportunity to introduce more vegetables into your daily diet. Use any firm-textured fish such as triggerfish, grouper or Mahi-Mahi. Any of the vegetables from the previous list will work, but I typically use onions, bell peppers, shredded cabbage, and sometimes zucchini or mushrooms. How much of each ingredient depends on your taste. Again, the spices make the dish.

Stir-fry the vegetables in your choice of oil with as much garlic as you like and a handful of minced cilantro. Add heat with minced hot red pepper. I usually use one small pepper with the seeds removed. The seeds account for much of the "hot" of the pepper (hot red chili sauce will do in a hurry). Mince very finely. Be careful about touching your face or eyes if you handle the pepper with your fingers. When the vegetables begin to soften, add the fish (cut into chunks). Stir in about 2 tablespoons of chili powder. I like to also add in ½ to 1 can of organic black beans.

This mixture can be served over shredded deep green lettuce or shredded cabbage and tomatoes as a salad, or wrapped inside a whole grain tortilla. Toppings can include fresh salsa, shredded cheese, sour cream, guacamole, or avocado. Chicken works as well if fish is not available. If chicken is used, cook it thoroughly before adding the vegetables.

Easy Shrimp Creole

The vegetables and spices are the real treat in this dish. Traditionally the vegetables include tomatoes, onions, bell peppers, and celery, but virtually any of the other vegetables can be added. I often add zucchini. Depending on the crowd, plan on about ¼ pound of peeled shrimp per person. Usually about one onion, one bell pepper (green, red, or yellow), 2 stalks or celery, and a large can of crushed tomatoes along with 1-2 lbs. of shrimp will do it for four people. You can stretch this recipe with extra vegetables.

The spices include 1-2 teaspoons of cumin, 1-2 teaspoons of minced garlic, one minced cayenne pepper without the seeds (unless you want it hot), and 2 bay leaves.

Sauté the vegetables in 1-2 tbsp. of olive oil. Add the spices and the shrimp. Simmer until the shrimp are completely pink, stirring as needed. The tomatoes will generally add enough liquid. Serve over a bed of brown basmati rice.

Beef Stroganoff

For those who want a traditionally meat version, use a good cut of lean beef (free-range, if available) cut into thin strips. The meat in this recipe can easily be replaced by either a medley of mushrooms or tempeh. The vegetables include onion, mushrooms (any kind), and tomatoes but many other vegetables such as eggplant can complement the flavor of this dish.

Stir-fry the meat first in oil of your choice. When the meat browns, drain the fat and add the vegetables. I often cook the meat and vegetables separately to compensate for differing tastes in the final meal. When the vegetables are tender, add a large can of crushed tomatoes or a couple of chopped tomatoes. This usually provides enough liquid, but water can be added if needed.

The seasonings for this dish include a handful of minced fresh oregano, a tablespoon of Worcestershire sauce, a small can of tomato paste, a teaspoon of garlic and a splash of balsamic vinegar. Stir in the seasonings at the same time as the tomatoes, lower the heat, and simmer covered for about 10 minutes. Remove from heat and stir in a couple of spoonfuls of low fat sour cream or yogurt. If you add these too early, they will curdle. Serve immediately over whole grain egg noodles.

Wild rice and mushrooms

This next selection uses many of the same ingredients and spices as the other dishes, but the flavor is completely altered by the presence of wild rice. Wild rice is prepared in the same way as brown rice and takes about the same amount of time. Start the rice ahead so that it can be cooking while preparing the main part of the dish.

Generally I use several different types of fresh, chopped mushrooms. Other vegetables can include chopped onion, red bell pepper, and zucchini. If you desire meat, the selection could include chicken, shrimp, or crab. Sauté or stir-fry the vegetables and meat in olive oil with seasonings including garlic, freshly minced thyme, freshly minced cilantro, and salt to taste. Rosemary is also a nice spice for this dish.

Once this part is cooked, add in 2-3 tablespoons of low fat sour cream, 1-2 tablespoons of freshly grated Parmesan cheese, and 3-4 tablespoons of garbanzo bean paste. I know this is a new ingredient that you probably have not used before, but garbanzo bean flour is an excellent substitute for cornstarch for use as a thickener. Garbanzo bean flour can be found at most health food stores and some grocery stores. Look for the "Bob's Red Mill" brand (www.bobsredmill). Follow the instructions for the garbanzo bean mixture on the back. I usually make enough to also make the hummus recipe (the best hummus I have ever had). If you want a short cut for this recipe or cannot find the flour, simply substitute plain hummus for the paste.

After all of these ingredients are mixed together, mix in several large spoonfuls of wild rice. The taste will be completely different from any of the dishes above.

When following the concepts of simple cooking, do not get uptight about a missing ingredient left off the shopping list or not being able to find a particular ingredient. The whole idea is being able to improvise. These dishes will all taste just fine with one or two of the recommended ingredients missing. Also, there may be a spice or some other ingredient that you just do not care for. Leave it out! It will not hurt a thing.

Now that you have the basic concept, try making up your own stir-fry. For inspiration pick up a cooking magazine that follows the lighter side of cooking. Instead of following a specific recipe, try adapting one to a simple stir-fry. It can also be a creative way to clean out the vegetable bins.

Special cases Make note that any of the above dishes can be made without using *any* added oil. If you are trying to lose weight, you may want to get by with as little added fat as possible. Also individuals who are healing from illness or recovering from a heart attack may want to completely avoid *any* abnormal fats created by heat. Though the level of concern with stir-fry compared to deep-fat frying is miniscule, you may want to avoid it completely in these cases.

To avoid using oil, simply place the ingredients in a steamer instead. Steam just until tender and then move the vegetables into a sauté pan, add with the spices and simmer for about 10-15 minutes. Seafood does very well steamed, chicken does okay, but beef tends to lose flavor.

All of the dishes can be modified to accommodate a gluten-free diet by using rice or by serving the dish over gluten-free pasta. Any of the recipes can be prepared without using grain products.

SOUPS AND CHOWDERS

You remember the old story of "stone soup" where three hungry soldiers wandered into a small town, commandeered a large pot, filled it with water, placed it in the center of town over a fire, and added a stone. Curious onlookers strolled by and each added an ingredient. Before long there was a rich, hearty soup, enough to feed the entire community plus the three soldiers.

Soup is the ultimate one pot meal and an excellent way to add nutritious foods to your diet. Homemade soups and stews are generally more tasty and substantial than those found in restaurants or out of a can, which are often mostly broth. An excellent way to use leftover vegetables, soup is just as good on the next day and it tends to freeze well.

Creating most soups is simple. Place the ingredients into a large pot, cover with liquid, bring to a boil, and simmer for about 20-30 minutes. The list of ingredients can include almost any vegetables, meat, whole grains such as brown rice or barley, and herbs and other seasonings. For thicker and creamier soup, stir garbanzo bean flour into whole milk or soy milk over medium heat until smooth and then stir this into the soup.

STANDARD AMERICAN FARE

I grew up with the standard plate of a meat, a vegetable, and a starch at many evening meals. Meat usually was the centerpiece with the other items relegated to the side. I can still envision a T-bone steak hanging over the edges of the plate with a large baked potato at the edge. A separate bowl of iceberg lettuce salad would offer a token vegetable. At one time I considered this a healthy meal. Times have changed. If you still consider these options healthy, we have some work to do.

These days meat needs to give up its place in the center and move to the sidelines. Meat can be a tasty addition to a meal, but just a small amount of it will do. Vegetables need a more prominent place; in fact, an assortment of several vegetables can make an adequate meal. Better quality starches such as whole grain pasta and brown rice need to replace white rice, macaroni & cheese from a box, and potatoes from a box. Fresh potatoes cooked in various ways are okay from time to time, especially the smaller ones such as the red skin variety.

Think of a restaurant that serves only side dishes. For a meal, pick any two to three items from the list.

grilled wild salmon	steamed shrimp	chicken breasts
lean steak	baked sweet potatoes	baked red potatoes
tofu or tempeh	mashed cauliflower	rice and beets
rice and beans	slaw	

steamed vegetables (*any kind and any combination*)
baked beans (*homemade, not out of a can*)
scrambled eggs *with sautéed onions, peppers and tomatoes*
butternut/acorn squash
whole grains *such as barley or quinoa*
fresh potato salad with red potatoes
green peas with sautéed mushrooms
black eyed peas (without the fatback)
steamed or sautéed greens such as collards, kale or Swiss chard
sautéed mushrooms of different varieties

Try to avoid using a starch with every meal. A meat with two or three different types of vegetables, such as butternut squash and steamed cabbage can make a perfectly acceptable meal. Eat fish and seafood more often. Plan some meals without using a meat at all.

For more suggestions and some additional recipe ideas, turn to the appendix of this book. Thousands of recipes are also available on the Internet.

SNACKS AND HUNGER BUSTERS

Snacking during the day, as long as you don't over-do-it, is important. Snacking provides a break from the everyday grind and helps stop hunger in its tracks. Hunger, built up to a ravenous level, can lead to eating too fast and over-eating at mealtimes. The types of snack foods, however, are extremely important.

For many individuals, being overweight is directly related to eating the wrong types of snack foods.

Typical American snack foods are a processed-food nightmare. You know the kinds I'm talking about – cakes, cookies, donuts, potato chips, etc. They all have all three of most concerning ingredients of processed food – the cheapest variety of refined flour, lots of fructose, and hydrogenated oils.

I have noticed that as I have purged sources of excessive glucose from my diet, the drive to snack during the day has decreased substantially. Those old temptations no longer have a hold on me, but to prevent being enticed, it is important to have healthy alternatives on hand. Here are a few suggestions:

- Apples, oranges, cherries, pears, bananas, plums, melons, and fruit in general are a great way to fill the hunger void. (fresh, frozen or dried)

  Bananas never go bad around my house. As soon as they ripen, whole bananas are peeled, wrapped in aluminum foil and placed in the freezer for a treat that is nearly equal to ice cream. Shave on dark chocolate for an extra special indulgence.

- Dried fruit such as prunes, raisins, apricots, and dates are great snack foods.

- If you have a juicer, fruit and vegetable juices make refreshing, healthy treats. Try carrots, fresh ginger and celery. Fresh berries and citrus are a tasty combination. The possibilities are unlimited.

- Sliced vegetables are healthy snacks, but often don't do an adequate job of breaking hunger. Dips such as salsa, hummus (there are many different types available), bean dip and guacamole can make this a satisfying snack. Celery spread with nut butter is a personal favorite. Avocados make great snacks by themselves. High in monounsaturated fatty acids, minerals, and vitamins, and low in carbohydrates, they can be consumed regularly as part of a healthy diet.

  Celery contains important cancer-fighting chemicals, can lower blood pressure in hypertensive individuals and is natural way to help normalize low testosterone levels in men. Several stalks a day are recommended.

- Whole grain corn chips (in moderation) with some of the above dips.

- Brown rice cakes drizzled with wild honey and tahini (sesame seed paste) is surprisingly tasty.

- Whole grain crackers or whole grain bread with nut butters. Organic peanut butter with no additives is very healthy. Stir in the oil, which separates naturally from the ground nuts. Try other nut butters such as almond butter and cashew butter.

- Nuts in general make great snacks. A snack mix can be made with almonds, pecans, Brazil nuts, cashews, walnuts, sunflower seeds, raisins, and carob or chocolate chips. This keeps very well in the freezer. Nuts are high in fat, but the fats are very favorable. You could gain weight if you ate enough of them, but a handful or two a day should not be a problem with regular exercise.

- Whole grain cereals are good for occasional snack foods. Bite-sized shredded wheat baked with canola oil and garlic or cinnamon is a satisfying healthy snack.

- Yogurt with wheat germ or ground flax seed mixed in. Try the organic varieties of yogurt. Organic varieties of yogurt use sugar for sweetener instead of high-fructose corn syrup. Often I will add berries and walnuts to plain unsweetened yogurt and use agave nectar as a sweetener.

  The very best yogurt is homemade. Yogurt makers are inexpensive and the process is very simple. Homemade yogurt costs a fraction of the store-bought version.

- A "smoothie" takes no time at all. Toss several different types of frozen berries or fruit into a blender. Add a scoop of low-fat yogurt along with a squirt of fresh flaxseed oil and a package of Stevia or a little honey as a sweetener. Pour in enough soymilk to cover everything. Turn on the blender until the contents are smooth and pour an extremely refreshing and healthy snack. I make smoothies several times a week.

- Organic popcorn is a satisfactory snack, especially if you stay away from the processed and packaged varieties. As long as I can remember we have had used a device called a "Whirley Pop" (www.popcornpopper.com) popcorn popper that agitates the kernels of corn as they are being heated on the stove. One teaspoon of macadamia nut oil, a pat of butter, a little salt and you will have the best tasting popcorn on earth.

- Don't forget snack foods that aren't typical snack foods. There is nothing wrong with eating leftovers at times other than a formal meal. Most of these items are much lower in calories than average snack foods.

- I generally avoid processed snack foods. Even the ones labeled as "health foods" contain sugar (sugar is sugar, organic or not) and fats that are always a bit spoiled. I do have to admit to a weakness for whole grain fig bars.

- A cup of hot tea with a little sugar can, by itself, be an adequate appetite suppressant.

Style of snacking is dependent on the activity level of the day. At the office, low energy snacks are preferred, whereas a five mile hike in the mountains would dictate the need for high energy snacks such as chocolate or peanut butter. Thru-hikers on the Appalachian Trail actually eat large amounts of peanut butter just to maintain weight.

COPING IN THE WORKPLACE

If your workplace is anything like the average, there is a constant stream of cakes, cookies, and pastries coming through the break area. The snack machines are full of honey buns, candy bars, soft drinks, and assorted other processed food items. They are hard to resist. Trying to avoid snacks completely is probably not a good idea, especially while trying to lose weight. Snacks provide an energy boost and a moment of relaxation, both of which are helpful in getting you through the day.

Going for snack foods that are healthy and nutritious generally means bringing your own. It also means getting used to snack foods that aren't traditional. See the previous section for some ideas. Make a habit of always bringing something to work or having something on hand. Your body will reward you for your discipline. *Most people could be healthier and lose weight by simply avoiding typical snack foods alone.*

EATING OUT

The best way to deal with most of the typical fast-food restaurants is to avoid them completely. Even though they generally carry token "healthy" items on the menu, most of those have low nutritional value. Also, it is really hard to sit and eat a salad while everyone else around you is chowing down on cheeseburgers. Local delis and similar restaurants are often good bets for fast food that fits the guidelines. This is especially true if you can find a deli that makes everything from scratch.

Health food stores and many grocery stores can be a good source for fast food. Many now have salad bars, delis, and quality food to go. In a pinch, a handful of fruit, a whole-grain baguette and carrots with hummus make an adequate meal or snack. Cafeterias and steakhouses with food bars are also a good avenue for meals within the guidelines. Sushi bars also offer healthy choices.

In restaurants, be aware that most chefs rely on sugar and fat to make food appealing. This is true even in the best of restaurants. Expensive is not necessarily synonymous with healthy. Some of the healthiest meals out are often found in midrange restaurants, usually with an ethnic flair such as Thai, Indian, Japanese, or Mexican. Restaurants that make legitimate boasts of healthy menus are gradually becoming more common.

For a night out on the town don't save up your hunger. Go ahead and eat a normal midday meal. That evening, consider ordering just a salad and an appetizer for your whole meal. Often these are the healthiest and lowest calorie items on the menu. The wine and the company will be just as good, I promise. Don't forget, you can always ask for an item to be prepared in lighter fashion. Ask for double vegetables instead of rice or potatoes. I have never been turned down with this request. Maybe if enough people ask, restaurants will get the message. Consider sharing an entrée with another person or taking half home for another meal.

For something different, occasionally plan an extended lunch out with family or friends. Most restaurants serve lighter and healthier meals at lunch.

TRAVEL

Travel offers a wonderful opportunity to enjoy food. We traveled as much as possible when my kids were growing up. I always insisted that chain restaurants were to be avoided unless there were no other alternatives. This opened up a wide variety of fresh foods that were not available at home. Fresh salmon and blackberries in Oregon, cherries and apples in Washington state, artichokes and apricots in California, oranges and grapefruit in Florida, lobster in Maine; we sampled wherever we went. With tips from guidebooks, local fare can, of course, be found at restaurants, but meals need not be confined to the indoors: items picked up at local markets, bakeries and roadside stands can make great picnics along the way.

Food is often the centerpiece of experiencing new places and cultures. Add this pleasurable dimension to travel wherever you go.

SPECIAL OCCASIONS

The act of sharing a celebratory meal with friends and family can be a health experience in itself. Holiday meals can be made to be healthy. Just the fact that people tend to cook fresh food is a step in the right direction. Holidays tend to be centered on times when there are plenty of healthy foods available, such as citrus fruit, apples, pears, cranberries, and fresh nuts of many varieties. Try to keep the cookies and cakes to a minimum and be mindful of portion control and eating more slowly, but certainly do not let any of it get in the way of enjoying the food and the company. As long as celebratory feasting is reserved for a seasonal treat and is not a weekly indulgence, you should not get into trouble.

PILLAR II

Body Purification

Toxins are the most prevalent and insidious of all causes of disease. Removing toxins from the body is an essential step for achieving optimal health.

CHAPTER 10
Toxins, Microbes, and the Common Social Good

Carrot Island is a beautiful protected coastal area near my home. The marshes and bays are favorites for kayakers. Along with the beauty, there are mosquitoes. On any given day between May and December, there is a good chance of being bitten by one. A century ago the threat of malaria was very real. Because of the efforts of a Swiss chemist in the 1940's, I can regularly paddle these waters with no concern for contracting malaria. His discovery was a chemical pesticide that was inexpensive to produce, lethal to mosquito populations, easy to disseminate, and purportedly harmless to humans. Thousands upon thousands of lives were saved as malaria carrying mosquitoes were eradicated from much of the planet. In 1948, chemist Paul Müller was distinguished with a Nobel Prize for his discovery of the chemical pesticide DDT.

A scant fourteen years later, Rachel Carson alerted the world to the adverse impact that DDT and other chemicals were having on the environment in her book, Silent Spring. As it turns out, DDT was not only lethal to mosquitoes but was lethal to all insects, even those vital to a balanced environment. It was later discovered that DDT also affected reproductive hormones in birds, such that the shells of their eggs were too thin and easily cracked, leading to an alarming plummet in certain bird populations worldwide. The potential for harm to humans was much greater than originally thought.

While she was writing Silent Spring, Rachel Carson spent her summers doing research on Carrot Island. At that time, the site of a brown pelican was probably rare. Because of her efforts, my excursions around Carrot Island are complimented by flocks of brown pelicans skimming across the water and the sharp call of ospreys overhead.

THE COMMON SOCIAL GOOD

As a society we make decisions that affect our collective health and wellbeing. As individuals we can let our voices be heard to influence those decisions. Eliminating malaria was a decision our society made to do away with a microbial threat. In doing so, we created another type of threat. The second threat was recognized and dealt with because of the voice of a single individual. Life is a give and take of which we all share a role. We all want the best of life and must work together to achieve that goal. This concept can be referred to as "the common social good."

The common social good has done much to change the standard of living in this country over the past hundred years. Epidemics of microbial infections, childhood illnesses, and secondary bacterial infections are much less of a threat than in the past. Modern antibiotics can be given some credit for this change, but the most influential factors have been improved standards of sanitation and the distribution of vaccines, both being decisions administered by our society as a whole. Seemingly simple concepts such as garbage collection, city sewers, and government bureaucracies that ensure that our cars, appliances, tools, etc. are safer are all aspects of the social infrastructure that have positive influence on our personal health.

Though the common social good has set a high standard of living in this country, all that we enjoy is still threatened. Some threats are invisible and hard to define. Who knows how much fallout from nuclear testing over the past 50 years has influenced our risk of cancer and chronic disease. And some threats seem to never completely go away: microbes will be around long after we are gone. One particular area where we could do a better job is reducing the hidden threat of toxins, but even that task is not straightforward.

The dichotomy of DDT as both friend and foe illustrates why eliminating certain threats to our wellbeing is so challenging. Toxic chemicals do not just appear. Their creation is associated with a purpose that generally enhances our lives in some way. Toxins may be the intended product, as with the manufacture of chemical pesticides or cleaning agents, or they may be a byproduct of a process, such as chemicals that leach into the environment with the manufacture and use of plastics or in the exhaust from the tailpipe of your car.

A common link that many toxins share is an association with petroleum or other hydrocarbon fuel sources. Nonrenewable hydrocarbon energy sources, mainly consisting of petroleum and coal, are the ultimate source of the high living standards to which we have all become accustomed. Petroleum not only powers the planet but also provides for all of our needs and wants. Everything you see around you and everything you touch is associated with petroleum in some way. The carpet on the floor, the paint on the walls, the pen you write with, the dashboard in your car and the plastic bottle holding your beverage are all derived from petroleum. All of our food production is associated with petroleum-driven machines and petroleum-derived pesticides are used heavily in the industry. Even the shirt on your back is made from cotton grown, harvested, spun, and sewn with the help of petroleum.

If petroleum were used more conservatively, it could be used to provide a high standard of living for hundreds of years into the future, without adversely affecting the environment. We would have to learn to live differently, but not necessarily less comfortably.

Because petroleum, natural gas, and coal provide for so much good in our lives, it is easy to overlook the fact that they are also the source of most toxins. As the rest of the world seeks the same standard of living that we enjoy in the industrialized world, the atmosphere is becoming increasingly saturated with toxins, and at the same time cancer and other chronic diseases of immune dysfunction are becoming alarmingly more common.

Just as a gas leak in a coal mine is not obvious to coal miners until it is too late, an increase in human disease from the insidious buildup of toxins in the environment can be difficult to recognize. Traditionally, coal miners used a canary to call alert to the possibility of impending disaster. In Rachel Carson's day, large birds were the "indicator species" for the adverse changes DDT was inducing in the environment. Today, two other groups of animals—amphibians and bees—may suggest that something equally sinister is happening in the earth's environment.

For many years scientists have been tracking a worldwide decline in all amphibian species (frogs and salamanders). This decline has not been limited to industrialized countries. It also has been occurring in amphibian populations deep in the rain forests of the world, suggesting that something is affecting our atmosphere. Though cause and effect has not been established, the decline parallels the increase in petroleum and coal usage worldwide.

Another alarming indicator of widespread environmental change is the worldwide decline in honeybee populations. Without these bees we lose the Garden of Eden: these proficient pollinators are a necessity for production of many of our fruits and vegetables. A recent Nature documentary on public television related the efforts of researchers to find the cause of the global decline in bees. Not surprisingly, they found not just one potential cause but multiple ones, culminating in a "perfect storm" of adverse conditions that may be contributing to a precipitous decline in hive populations. Pesticide use was very high on the list. Microbe infestation was common; this may be related to malnutrition and to the stress of being trucked frequently from farm to farm, following the needs of crop-growers.

Interestingly, as worldwide bee populations remain in decline, the hives of small organic beekeepers are stable and healthy. This observation suggests that if we are wise, we can have our cake and eat it too.

INDIVIDUALS CAN MAKE A DIFFERENCE

Walking or riding a bike is an obvious way to decrease pollution and is good for your personal health at the same time. Carpooling, driving a fuel-efficient car, or using mass transit make a positive statement. Conservation of electricity at home with thermostat adjustments and compact fluorescent bulbs is not only practical but also cost-effective. Tax incentives make a solar hot water heater a better deal than ever before.

Being energy conscious and toxin aware does not necessarily mean giving up creature comforts. In 2005 my wife and I designed and had constructed a passive solar home. The overall cost was no more than any other conventional home of the same size. It is bright and warm, even on the coldest winter day. Our solar room is filled with plants most of the year. I even grow fresh herbs in the winter. The ventilation is such that only in the heat of middle summer do we turn on the air-conditioner. So far, our energy costs have been about half that of a conventional home of the same size. We made a decision to use non-toxic paints, even though they cost a bit more. We are careful about cleaners, and pesticides. We installed a central vacuum to more effectively remove allergens. Our home is truly a refuge from the outside world and a most pleasant place to live.

Another way to use less petroleum is by recycling. Recycling is not a new concept. Before 1950 and especially during World War II, everything that could be recycled was recycled. Liquids were contained in glass or tin and most other items were kept in paper or cardboard. Paper bags were the only option at the grocery store; most shoppers carried their own baskets. Milk was delivered to your doorstep in recycled glass bottles. Soft drinks, the newest drink craze, were available in recycled bottles.

In the 60's and 70's America was just learning to be a throw-away society. Paper trash and bottles littered our highways and byways. Many a young entrepreneur, including myself, earned pocket change by collecting discarded roadside bottles for the five-cent deposit. Those nickels added up. No matter where you happened to be, a ready supply of cash was always lying in the ditches, waiting to be harvested. Because of the simple five-cent incentive, a substantial percentage of those bottles ended up back at the bottler to be perpetually refilled. Though I seldom drink soft drinks any longer, I, for one, am sorry to see that bottle-deposits are no longer mandated in most states.

As our dependence on petroleum deepened, we became more and more of a throw-away society. Plastic containers of all varieties lie buried in our landfills and litter our public places. Unlike glass, which is inert, and paper, which is biodegradable, plastics will be shedding toxins to the environment for hundreds of years—not just on land but also in our oceans, lakes and rivers. Who knows what kind of toxic stew we are creating.

Part of the solution to the plastic problem is using less of it. Every time you wash your dishes instead of just throwing them away, you are recycling. Get back into the habit of drinking out of a glass instead of a plastic bottle. Store your water in glass whenever possible. When you need disposable cups, use paper ones (if you can find them) instead of plastic. At the grocery store, buy fresh food not wrapped in plastic whenever possible. Bring your own shopping bags. When you cannot reuse something yourself, recycle it through a waste management service. Recycling plastic not only conserves petroleum but also conserves energy.

Beyond decreasing our exposure to toxins, there are more pressing reasons to conserve petroleum. Our time in the Garden of Eden is running out. At present usage, petroleum flow will peak soon—perhaps this decade—and the remaining petroleum will be increasing difficult to extract. Natural gas will peak out at about the same time. Coal is much more plentiful, but is very dirty to use.

Many people seem confident that after petroleum and gas are gone, some other energy source will be "discovered," but make no mistake—there is no substitute. Petroleum is raw energy, made by ancient microbes and then encapsulated within the earth for millions of years. Alternative sources of energy, including wind, water, nuclear energy and biofuels, may help us prolong the blessing of petroleum but cannot replace it. Ironically, even alternatives depend on petroleum to some extent—for example, plastics are used in the construction of photovoltaic cells.

If petroleum sources were to suddenly dry up tomorrow, we would quickly plunge into the Dark Ages.

If we could learn to be better stewards of our Garden of Eden, it could be enjoyed by many generations to come. Simply by conservation, the blessings of petroleum could balance the problems associated with petroleum usage. For example, trains, instead of trucks, could be used to transport food and goods across the country with a fraction of the current energy expenditure. Using alternative sources of energy to reduce our dependence on oil and decreasing our total reliance on plastic would not only prolong the availability of our finite reserves of petroleum but would also slow global warming and significantly decrease the burden of toxins in the environment.

SELF PRESERVATION IN A WORLD OF HIDDEN THREATS

Certainly no one would ever think of intentionally drinking or eating pesticides, chemical cleaners, or industrial by-products, and yet we readily allow these substances to enter our homes, our food, and our water supplies. We are not aware because the quantities are too small to see or taste. Measured *independently*, small doses of chemical toxins may not produce immediately visible negative effects on our health, but *cumulatively* the story may be quite different.

The normal level of any toxin in the human body is <u>zero</u>!

Recent science studying concentrations of various toxins in human populations around the country suggests that toxins accumulate within the human body (http://pollutioninpeople.org). The human body seems to be a sponge for chemical toxins and tends to store many of them in our body fat. Common sense would suggest that chemical toxins do have potential for harm and probably do play a significant role in disease, but the question of "how much" is hard to answer because there are so many different toxins and the total load and interactions are hard to quantify.

Waiting around until someone defines the exact amounts of specific toxins the average person can tolerate is not practical, but becoming "toxin aware" is. Avoiding toxins in a toxin-filled world is not as difficult as it sounds. Toxic chemicals, allergens (substances that cause allergic reactions), and microbes can only enter the body in a limited number of ways. For instance, we can breathe them in, consume them via food and drink, or absorb them through our skin. Becoming aware of common sources of toxic substances and how they enter the body is the first step in decreasing their impact.

"GOOD" WATER

It is a sad fact that much of world's water supply is contaminated with chemical toxins, heavy metals, and microbes. In this country sanitation standards are currently quite high, but safe water is not guaranteed everywhere in the world. Water, however, is the easiest entity to fix. Particulate and carbon filters (in-line or hooked up to the tap) remove the majority of contaminants, leaving water safe and drinkable. Any water can be filtered.

Beyond filtration, the question of what constitutes healthy water is a matter of opinion. Minerals-out or minerals-in is central to the debate. All water from ground sources, either well or natural spring, contains dissolved minerals and is considered mineral water. Mineral content varies widely with geographic location. Traditionally, mineral water has been considered healthy, but health potential is highly dependent on the types of minerals dissolved in the water—not all minerals are considered beneficial. There is also the matter of taste: certain minerals improve the taste of water and certain others do the opposite.

Calcium, the most abundant mineral found in groundwater, is considered desirable for healthy bones. Magnesium, common in water supplies but often deficient in food sources, is important for bone formation and normal cardiac function. Iron and copper, on the other hand, are probably best obtained from food sources, since the inorganic forms of iron and copper found in mineral water are not readily absorbed through the intestines. Sulfur compounds present in many groundwater sources give water an undesirable "rotten-egg" smell but are not necessarily harmful for consumption.

The presence of minerals defines water as being "hard." Removing minerals from water appears to be more about aesthetics than health. Since the 1930's, mineral residues (bathtub rings, etc.) have been considered unsightly and many households found in hard-water areas opt for a water softener. Water softeners use salts that substitute sodium for minerals found in the water. While soft water is less likely to leave stains on the tub and sink, health benefits of soft water are questionable. Such water can add significant sodium to the diet.

In 2004, a World Health Organization expert consensus on water suggested that the healthiest water is hard water, filtered of any microbial and organic chemical contaminants, but still containing essential minerals, especially magnesium and calcium. Evidence cited in the consensus strongly suggests that incidences of heart attacks, cancer and other diseases are decreased with increased magnesium and calcium content in water supplies.

The composition of the water spilling from the tap in your home is highly dependent on the source. Well-water varies with location and depth of the well. Municipal water sources can be derived from wells drilled into underground aquifers or from surface waters, such as rain-fed reservoirs and rivers. Mineral content is highly variable and chemicals such as chlorine and fluoride are commonly added to municipal water. Some public water is highly suspect and some is quite good, with all gradations in-between.

For your home, whether the water source is municipal or well, having the water checked for mineral content, pH and contaminants is a worthwhile endeavor. This can be done through any local health department. "Good water" would be defined as having moderate to high levels of calcium and especially magnesium with a slightly alkaline pH of 7.4. Excess iron and sulfur can be removed by special filtration systems. To decrease bathroom stains and scale, having a water-softener for the main house and a separate hard-water line for drinking water may be worthwhile. Drinking water can be filtered with simple carbon and particulate filters to remove any contaminants. Reverse-osmosis systems provide very "safe" water but also removes all minerals—an option that is necessary only if water is highly questionable.

The latest trend in water treatment is ionization. When mineral-containing water is exposed to an electrical current, the minerals within the water form negative ions and shift the pH toward alkaline. Alkaline mineral water is desirable, but before going out and spending a thousand dollars on one of these devices, have your water checked. If the magnesium and calcium levels are high and the pH is near 7.4, a water ionizer is not a necessity. If calcium and magnesium are not present or you have a water-softener, then the ionizer will not do you any good anyway. Distilled water or water run through a reverse-osmosis system has the minerals removed and will not ionize. If you want alkalized water and are averse to spending that amount of money, a poor-man's water ionizer is a teakettle. Water can be ionized by simply bringing it to a boil, as you would do for making tea.

Mineral water that has been alkalized by ionization or boiling is the tastiest water you can drink and possibly the healthiest. Alkalized water may be beneficial for decreasing the risk of osteoporosis, kidney stones and possibly gallstones.

If your best source of drinking water ends up being bottled water, take the time to research its origins (www.mineralwaters.org). The mineral content of commercially-sold bottled water is highly variable and dependent on where the water was acquired. Some bottled waters come from documented spring-fed sources, but many are simply municipal water that has been filtered, with minerals added. Though often criticized as not being "the real thing," the latter option may be the best because the water is highly filtered, with specific minerals added back in specific ratios. Groundwater may or may not contain the most desirable types and ratios of minerals, and, if not filtered, may contain contaminants.

Remember that chemicals from plastic bottles can gradually leach into the liquid stored in them. This is especially true if the container is heated. Whenever possible, store your water in a glass container. When plastic is the only option, keep your water bottle out of the sun and in a cool place. Aside from potential toxicity, the sheer load of plastic waste generated by this industry may be the biggest deterrent to bottled water. Hopefully the future will bring a return to recyclable glass containers for bottled retail beverages.

Beyond filtration, do your part to keep our water supplies clean and our landfills lighter. Using fewer disposable products and plastic products, eating organic and eating lower on the food chain translates into less pollution contaminating our streams, rivers, lakes and estuaries. Paper products are a significant source of water contamination. Toilet paper, napkins and paper towels are usually bleached with dioxins. Non-bleached and recycled paper products are becoming more widely available. The extra cost of these products is balanced by better health and a cleaner environment.

www.realgoods.com One of the oldest retailers of environmentally-sound products.

www.seventhgeneration.com Resource for safe cleaning products and non-bleached paper products.

When traveling to other countries, remember that water-borne microbial threats are common in many parts of the world. They are tied to different standards of sanitation and personal hygiene than we enjoy here. Local residents may have adapted to the microbes, but those germs are foreign to you. If you travel outside of this country consider purchasing a portable water filtration system. These can be found at any outdoor or camping supply store. You may look a little odd filtering your glass of water at the dinner table, but it may save you from a severe case of dysentery.

TOXIC CHEMICALS IN OUR FOOD

The steady rise in the types and concentrations of toxins in our food over the past fifty years is concerning. The primary culprits are large-scale commercial agriculture and commercial food processing. Industrial residues and by-products of plastics and petroleum also contribute to soil and water contamination. Fortunately, we are beginning to have some better choices. Organic produce and chemical-free products are becoming more readily available everywhere.

The overall cost of organic food is less than you would think. Though the retail cost of such food steers many away, it is a matter of supply and demand: As more individuals demand organic food, the cost will gradually come down—and our total healthcare bills will also likely substantially decrease. In addition, a switch to organic eating means that our water supplies and the environment in general would be safer and cleaner, an added benefit for every living thing on the planet.

The sheer numbers of potentially toxic molecules to which we are exposed on a daily basis is problematic. Even organically-produced food contains some natural toxins, and other toxins are difficult to eliminate from our soil and water. Many foods, even organically-produced ones, have the potential to cause food sensitivities. A wide variety of medical conditions can be caused or aggravated by sensitivities to certain foods. So, beyond organic, the keyword in healthy eating is diversity.

Eating a varied diet and rotating foods with the seasons is a naturally healthy practice. Make a habit of buying local produce whenever it is available. This helps small farms and decreases transportation costs and associated pollution. Get to know local farmers, many of whom are making efforts to decrease pesticide usage, even though they have not been officially "certified" as organic. It also makes sense to rotate food sources so as to reduce the cumulative impact of any one particular toxin that might be in a product.

One way to reduce your toxin load from food is to avoid products that are directly encased in plastic. Sometimes even organic foods come packaged in plastic. This may sound like paranoia, but the evidence linking chemicals leached from plastic to chronic disease and cancer is too great to ignore. Foods that contain fats are especially vulnerable. Many chemicals associated with plastics and pesticides are hormonally active. Nicknamed "xeno-estrogens," these chemicals mimic estrogen in the body or affect the metabolism of estrogens, increasing the risk of hormonally-active cancers including breast, uterine and prostate cancer. Reducing exposure to plastic is one of the primary ways to reduce the risk of cancer. Importantly, cruciferous vegetables, essential fatty acids, ground sesame seeds and ground flax seeds are several important foods for augmenting the ability of the liver to metabolize estrogens and xeno-estrogens in our "estrogen-dominated" environment.

Local markets and farmers markets where fresh vegetables and fruit are displayed in open bins are often the best places to buy your food. This may be your best opportunity to find the safest, freshest foods possible. When you go, bring your own cloth bags and a cooler for free-range meat. When shopping at a conventional supermarket, choose liquid food products in glass whenever possible and avoid (to the extent practical) food products wrapped in plastic.

CHEMICALS FROM THE MEDICINE CABINET

People readily and voluntarily take pharmaceuticals every day but are unaware that most drugs could actually be classified as forms of toxins. Though they are sometimes lifesaving and useful in many ways, all drugs all have the potential for side effects and are metabolized within the body in the same way as any other toxins. In medical therapy we try to select beneficial effects of drugs over the toxic effects, but for most drugs eliminating the toxic effects altogether is impossible.

The fact is that the majority of synthetic drugs have been in use for less than fifty years—not even one human lifespan. Some of the more commonly used drugs have been approved for use within the past two decades, which is hardly enough time to determine the long-term potential for toxicity.

Gaining the most from pharmaceutical therapy while minimizing side effects is a matter of choosing the lowest dose possible and supporting therapy with appropriate lifestyle and dietary changes. Multiple drug therapy should be avoided whenever possible. Supplementation with high quality multivitamins is indicated because many drugs have the potential to induce vitamin and mineral deficiencies. Coenzyme Q-10, an important component in energy production, should be used in conjunction with any medications for cardiovascular or diabetic therapy.

Not infrequently I see patients with chronic disease who bring with them a long list of medications used to control their symptoms. In some cases I wonder whether their illness is more related to side effects of medications than to the actual disease process.

Most "natural" therapies have been around for a while, but they cannot be completely excluded from concern. Though herbal therapies usually contain beneficial chemicals that promote healing, these chemicals circulate through the liver and kidneys in the same way any other toxin would. It should be noted that many plants naturally contain toxic substances. Tobacco would be a good example. Commonly-used, over-the-counter remedies such as kava, hops, and valerian have been found to cause liver damage in certain individuals. Caffeine, found widely in nature, causes discomfort in some people. *Any* herbal remedy has the *potential* to cause side effects. *Choose supplement therapies wisely under the guidance of a qualified specialist.*

Most people would not argue that illicit street drugs would fall in the category of being toxins. Many of them were originally used for medicinal purposes and some are available by prescription, but recreational use dictates higher (sometimes near-lethal) doses. The most commonly used recreational drug, voluntarily consumed by millions of people worldwide, is alcohol. Like most chemicals, toxicity of alcohol is determined by dose. At a lower dosage— say, a glass of red wine or a bottle of beer daily—alcohol actually has significant health benefits, probably because of its mild anti-anxiety properties and the antioxidants in the wine or beer. Anything more and it is definitely a toxin.

Another obvious source of self-inflected toxins is cigarette smoking. Approximately a third of Americans smoke, and a large proportion of them are young people. Many experts argue that smoking is our leading preventable cause of morbidity, but some evidence speaks to the contrary. In Europe, smoking is still popular and an interesting study documents that lean German vegetarians who smoke do not suffer morbidity significantly worse than non-smoking populations (Heidelburg Vegetarian Study). In this country, smokers tend to follow the worst health habits *and* the worst dietary practices—compounding all of their health concerns. Smoking *is* certainly bad for your health, but possibly not nearly as bad as the average American diet.

FOOD ALLERGIES

True food allergies are not as common as most people think. Food allergies can occur to any food and cause classic symptoms of itching, hives and, in severe cases, difficulty breathing. Top food allergies include: milk and milk products, eggs, peanuts, tree nuts, seafood, shellfish, soy, strawberries and wheat (gluten). Food allergies are generally easy to identify.

Sensitivities to foods occur more frequently. Most everyone can claim at least some sensitivity to some foods, with certain individuals plagued by multiple food sensitivities. Food sensitivities typically cause delayed symptoms of joint and muscle pain, fatigue and general achiness. Generally this situation results from a hyper-stimulated immune system and is often associated with gastrointestinal dysfunction. (Solutions will be discussed further in the next chapter.)

MICROBES IN OUR FOOD

Microbes in our food can be either friend or foe. Our gastrointestinal tract depends on regular inoculations of favorable bacteria from fermented foods for normal function. Furthermore, without microbial fermentation we would not enjoy bread, yogurt, sauerkraut, blue cheese, wine, or beer.

Fermentation with the wrong microbes, however, can be quite threatening. A turkey sandwich left out on the counter overnight warrants a toss into the trash. Food spoilage may be obvious, which alerts a potential consumer, but the presence of undesirable microbes may also be subtle.

As mentioned in the food section, many processed foods and certain uncooked foods are often colonized with unfavorable bacterial and fungal species that produce harmful toxins associated with an increased risk of cancer and immune suppression.

HIDDEN TOXINS

There is mounting evidence that many types of pathologic microbes have the ability to take up residence in our tissues and remain hidden for long periods of time, sometimes for a lifetime. The mission of these microbes is simply to make more microbes: the idea is not to kill the host but to disable it, allowing millions of microbial progeny to flourish. They do so by producing chemicals that compromise or control the host's immune and neurological systems. To us, these chemicals are toxins. Lyme disease may be the best known example of chronic disease caused by a hidden microbe, but there are many others. Research is suggesting microbial links to chronic diseases including as arthritis, chronic fatigue, sarcoidosis and possibly most of the autoimmune diseases.

Heavy metals are another group of hidden toxins, with mercury being one of the most common. Mercury can be a factor in any chronic disease process, from hypothyroidism to heart attacks. The chief source of mercury in humans is amalgam dental fillings. Symptoms vary, but even if you just don't feel well, your amalgam fillings may be the problem. Replacing fillings can, however, be an ordeal; being checked for mercury toxicity first is a good idea. If mercury levels are high, dental fillings can be replaced. Replacement should be performed only by a qualified dentist specializing in extraction of amalgam fillings. After the source of mercury is removed, heavy metal detoxification should be carried out under the guidance of a qualified health practitioner.

The possibility of heavy metal toxicity should be considered if there is unexplained chronic disease. Furthermore, when chronic disease is present, toxins of any type (including heavy metals) are an impediment to healing. It is difficult to totally avoid exposure, but some individuals retain heavy metals to a higher degree than others. Body fat is the most important variable. Toxins of all varieties accumulate more readily in fatty tissue, another reason to stay as lean as possible.

Testing for toxin levels may be worthwhile in some cases, but defining toxicity is not straightforward (since the normal level of any toxin in the human body is zero). Reducing the level of any and all toxins in the body is the best choice. The detoxification protocol at the end of chapter 11 is a good place to start.

*The safest, most comfortable and possibly the most effective way to remove common toxins, including heavy metals, from the human body is **far infrared sauna** (FIR sauna). Toxins are gently pushed to the surface and released through sweat. Often referred to as "healing waves," far infrared radiation is at the opposite end of the spectrum from damaging gamma rays and x-rays. FIR saunas are not exorbitantly expensive (about the price of a two-person hot tub) and can be installed in a home. The effectiveness and safety of FIR sauna is well documented in the scientific literature. FIR sauna is beneficial for many types of chronic disease and has been proven safe for cancer patients and patients with congestive heart failure.*

TOXINS IN THE AIR

Most of us spend much of our time inside tightly sealed air capsules. Our homes, workplaces, and automobiles are, for the most part, sealed from the outside environment. Whatever goes into these atmospheres stays and circulates. Toxic chemicals, microbes, and allergens can build up and become concentrated. The list includes numerous chemical toxins from plastics, paints, carpets and chlorinated cleaning products, and pesticides, dust, mites, molds, other microbes of many varieties, and many, many different types of allergens. The air inside an average home may be more toxic than the downtown air of a major city in summer.

AIRBORNE ALLERGENS

Many individuals are absolutely plagued by chronic sinusitis caused by allergies to dust, mold, and pollen of various sorts. When clinically tested, many of these individuals find that they are "allergic to everything." They spend their lives being chronically treated with antihistamines, nose-sprays, and rounds of antibiotics.

The root of the problem is an overactive immune system. Standard treatments often accentuate the problem instead of relieving it. The real solution is toning down the immune response by decreasing exposure to allergens. Taking steps to ensure clean indoor air (i.e., quality air filters, better vacuum cleaner) is part of the solution. Being aware of ozone levels and different pollen seasons is a must. Clean air, both indoor and outdoor, is of the utmost importance.

The concept of an "allergy threshold" is very important. Most people do not become symptomatic until they reach a certain threshold of exposure. At this point, the immune system becomes overwhelmed and symptoms occur—a single trigger can be explosive. The most important way to avoid going over the threshold is by decreasing exposure. Allergy testing for not only airborne allergies, but also food sensitivities, can assist the individual in avoiding exposure.

Washing away allergens is another tactic. During pollen season, frequent nasal saline washes during the day help to flush away allergens. Facial steam baths can help sooth mucous membranes in the nasal cavity. Try adding a drop or two of concentrated eucalyptus oil. Certain supplements taken on a regular basis during allergy season can optimize immune function and decrease the need for antihistamines and other pharmaceuticals. *Vitamin C, quercetin,* and *bromelain* are well known for calming the immune response to allergens.

Be mindful that the air itself can be a factor in healing chronic sinusitis. Low or high humidity can adversely affect healing. Ideal humidity is between

30 and 50%. Instruments to measure humidity are available at any hardware store. Properly functioning air conditioning lowers humidity and inexpensive room humidifiers increase humidity. Many people find that regular use of far-infrared sauna is very helpful in reducing symptoms.

Chronic allergies do not always start in the nose. As with everything else, all of the factors of disease can play a role. *Symptoms associated with airborne allergies are often closely tied with gastrointestinal dysfunction and delayed food sensitivities.* Poor diets and stress affect gastrointestinal function and can lead to multiple food sensitivities and hyperstimulation of the immune system in general. Food sensitivities can tip the balance of the immune system past the allergy threshold.

AIRBORNE MICROBIAL THREATS

A sneeze or a cough is all it takes to send a cold or flu virus toward its ultimate goal of infecting another victim. Contagious viruses and bacteria are spread by riding microscopic droplets of water carried through the air. The droplets can be inhaled directly or spread by contact after landing on countertops and food or sprayed into a telephone receiver. Constant vigilance by both the patient and others in the vicinity is required. Handwashing or use of an antimicrobial gel is essential, especially for those in the healthcare and food industries. Most important of all, however, is maintaining a healthy immune system.

TOXINS VIA THE SKIN

The outer layer of our skin, called the epithelium, provides a waxy coat that waterproofs and holds moisture in at the same time. Many substances, especially fat-soluble toxins, can be absorbed through the skin. Passage goes both ways, however, as sweating is one of the most effective ways to remove toxins and heavy metals from the body.

Modern humans spray on, rub on, and douse themselves in chemicals on a daily basis. The list of products that contain chemicals applied to the skin includes cosmetics, lotions, toothpaste, soap, shampoo, medicinal creams and deodorants, just to get started. The list of synthetically-derived chemicals approved by the FDA for human use is too long to consider. Without a doubt, some of these chemicals have potential for toxicity, but as with chemicals allowed in our food, the level of toxicity is difficult to quantify.

A partial list of commonly-used products recognized as having at least some potential for causing reactions includes aluminum-containing antiperspirants, sodium laurel/laureth sulfate commonly found in soaps and shampoos, diethanolamine (DEA) found in many skincare products, propyl glycol found in many toiletry products, propyl alcohol used in mouthwash, toluene found in nail polish and perfume, and mineral oil made from petroleum.

Anything coming into contact with skin should be used with discretion. Some people are sensitive to chemicals in new clothing, adhesives in band aids and tape, chemicals in laundry detergents, and rarely even chemicals in toilet paper. Latex is found in many products and latex allergies can be severe.

Be aware of hidden chemicals in objects that contact the skin and use skin care products judiciously. Read labels. Natural is often better, but not always. Toxic chemicals occur in nature. Any products can contain substances that are allergens to certain individuals. Know your own body. Find products that work for you. The best way to keep your skin healthy is from the inside out. A healthy diet with balanced oils and sufficient antioxidants does more to keep skin healthy than anything else.

The final word on sunscreen is open for debate. The ionizing rays of the sun are a known contributor to skin aging and certain cancers[*], but many chemicals found in sunscreens can be classified as toxins. Sun exposure may convert these substances into even more toxic compounds. As with many things, moderation and good judgment are essential. Carotenoids from regularly consumed vegetables protect from the inside out. Sleeves and a good hat may be your best sun protection.

When working with chemicals that are known toxins, such as paints, glues, or cleaners, always avoid direct exposure to the skin. Wear protective clothing and gloves. Do make sure that you have adequate ventilation.

I once burned my lungs while cleaning mildew from the inside of an old sailboat with strong bleach. I had on protective gloves and clothing, but did not bother with adequate ventilation. It took several months before my lungs were completely back to normal.

EVERYDAY TOXIN AWARENESS

Exposure to toxins is continuous and cumulative. "Toxin-awareness" is an important step toward decreasing the total toxin burden of the body. The following choices are easy and require minimal change in habits.

---

[*] Squamous and basal cell skin cancers have a definite link to sun exposure, but melanomas may not. As a gynecologist, having found melanomas between toes and other places where the sun doesn't shine, I tend to side with experts who suggest that melanomas may be more related to toxin exposure. Could it be that the rise in the incidence of melanomas is actually related to increased sunscreen use and not to increased exposure to the sun?

Tips for around the kitchen and bath

- Buy unbleached paper products—paper towels, napkins, tissues and toilet paper. Use washable cloth dish towels and cloth napkins whenever possible.

- Pots and pans: stainless steel is best. Aluminum and non-stick should be avoided. The cast-iron frying pan is safe, if old enough to be blackened. Cooking and drinking directly from copper or brass should be avoided.

  Iron and copper from organic sources (i.e., food) are essential for life, but free iron and copper ions in the bloodstream convert oxygen free-radicals into "super" free-radicals—a significant risk factor for atherosclerosis.

- **NEVER MICROWAVE FOODS CONTAINED IN PLASTIC OR WRAPPED IN PLASTIC WRAP, ESPECIALLY FATTY FOODS.** Heated plastics out-gas chemicals which are readily absorbed into fatty foods. Microwave foods in ceramic containers. Do not marinate foods in plastic bags.

- Plastic storage containers for foods are a necessity, it seems, but should be mostly limited to the refrigerator or freezer.

- Disposable plates and cups for parties and picnics should be paper instead of plastic or Styrofoam.

- Nontoxic natural cleaning agents are widely available. Look for them at health food stores. ***Avoid cleaners containing chlorine and chlorinated compounds.*** Many natural and inexpensive cleaning options are available for around the kitchen and bath. Baking soda (mild abrasive), white vinegar, rubbing alcohol, ammonia, lemon juice, lemon or grapefruit peel, soap flakes and water are some examples. A simple, non-toxic household cleaner can be made from a half cup of sudsy ammonia, a pint of isopropyl alcohol, and one teaspoon of dishwashing liquid mixed in a gallon of water. White vinegar is excellent for cleaning windows.

  Other natural cleaners and non-toxic solutions can be found in the Reader's Digest book *Homemade—How to Make Hundreds of Everyday Products You Would Otherwise Buy.*

- Scrutinize all toiletry products for potential toxicity. Avoid antiperspirants with aluminum if possible.

TIPS AT HOME

- Avoid using carpet in your home, especially if you have chronic allergies. If you have carpet, go for less toxic varieties with less "out-gassing" of chemicals. Some manufacturers provide specifications. All you have to do is ask. Carpets made from natural materials are available, but still readily collect hair, dust and dirt. Cork flooring does not collect dirt and is warm and soft on the feet; it may be the least toxic alternative.

- Nontoxic paints, wall, and floor coverings are more expensive, but are worth the cost.

- Choose minimally toxic ways to deal with pests and bugs. ***Never allow someone to spray chemical pesticides inside your home or office. These chemicals are extremely threatening and stay around for a long time.*** Use baits instead of widespread chemicals for eradicating pests. They are just as effective.

- Dust mites can be minimized with regular damp dusting. Many microscopic insect pests live in bedding. Wash linens and clean upholstery regularly. Consider placing a free-standing HEPA air filter in the room where you sleep, to avoid deep-breathing dust and other allergens all night.

- Change A/C filters frequently. Consider installing a whole house air filtering system. High-quality individual room filters can also be purchased. Look for filtering systems containing charcoal, particulate and HEPA filters. These are readily available for reasonable prices at home supply stores.

- Periodically have the duct work in your house completely cleaned by a professional.

- **Negative ion generators.** Negative ions inhibit free radicals derived from the harmful aspects of oxygen and air-borne pollutants. Negative ions exist naturally in air found over and around bodies of water. Possibly this is why a vacation at the beach or beside a lake feels soothing and healthy. Fresh-smelling air occurring just after a thunderstorm is filled with negative ions. Negative ion generators do have the ability to clean the air, but not as thoroughly as a HEPA filtering system; in some incidences, both are necessary. Negative ion generators can be found on the Internet and most home supply stores.

- Central vacuum cleaners do the best job of actually removing dirt and dust completely from the house, but some better quality free-standing vacuums can also do the job.

- One-third of Americans still using tobacco products for relaxation and recreation. Smoking tobacco is a choice that some people make, but smoking inside an enclosed air space affects everyone in that space. Cigarette smoke is a primary source of the toxic heavy metal cadmium.

Because of pesticide use, tobacco products are probably more toxic than they were a hundred years ago.

If you are a smoker, the need to quit goes unsaid; yet, before you do, there is one often unrecognized benefit of smoking that must be addressed. Smoking releases stress. Deep breathing and concentrated focus associated with smoking is extremely relaxing. Many people depend on smoking for stress management. When stopping smoking, other methods of stress reduction must be cultivated. Medications can be helpful, but have significant side effects. Hypnosis is very beneficial for most people who are trying to quit.

COPING IN THE WORKPLACE
(AVOIDING "SICK BUILDING SYNDROME")

Office setting Office buildings often have poorer air quality than homes. Mold and mildew are very common in large buildings. Most air filtering systems in large buildings are not satisfactory. Consider purchasing a high quality room air filter and possibly a negative ion generator to protect your own workspace.

In the South mold in buildings is almost a given. All it takes is a little moisture and warmth to grow a variety of fungi. Mold spores irritate mucous membranes and are notorious for causing immune system compromise.

My present office is about 30 years old. During a complete renovation, the heat pump/AC systems were replaced and special electronic filtering system was installed. Even so, after a weekend in the summer when two air systems have not been running, the air has that "old building" smell, indicative of mold and mildew. Individual room HEPA filters at strategic locations around the office do a good job of eliminating the odor and most likely the threat.

New buildings are not immune to the mold problem. I know of an office that was of new construction; yet, after only one year, the ceiling tiles were removed to reveal that all of the spaces above were covered in mold and the air systems were saturated with mold.

In an industrial setting, you need to be proactive to ensure that ventilation systems and protective clothing meet the mark. Do not assume that you are protected. Voice your concerns tactfully but vigilantly. Remember that the management is interested in the bottom line and any regulations they have to comply with—not your health.

EXERCISES IN "TOXIN AWARENESS"

- Have your water tested. Install some type of water filter for drinking water.

- Spend a Saturday morning going through cabinets and under counters, reading labels of products in your home. Chlorinated products, products with threatening chemical ingredients, or products that just smell toxic should be noted. With a piece of tape and a pen identify these products as toxic. As they are used up, try to replace them with less toxic alternatives.

- On another Saturday evaluate personal products for potential toxic substances, such as aluminum in your deodorant. Try some of the natural brands of toiletry products to see if they work as well for you.

- Set up a calendar to change the filters in your air vents regularly. The same may apply to water filters and free-standing air filters.

- Consider purchasing a free-standing air filtering system for your office or workspace.

- Make a list of ways you could use alternatives to plastics in your everyday life and try to stick to it. Plastic has moved into a position of being nearly essential in our modern world, but recognize that all plastic has a least some potential for toxicity.

Exposure to toxins, microbes, radiation, and other environmental stresses is nearly unavoidable. By making choices and changing our lifestyle, we can decrease our exposure, but the issue goes beyond avoidance strategies alone. Maintaining the body's internal waste removal and detoxification systems is essential for good health. The next chapter will address this important topic.

CHAPTER 11
Detoxification and Elimination

Silent, but deadly, toxins may be the greatest overall contributor to disease. Toxins increase oxidative stress and disable the immune system, allowing microbes to set up shop. Toxins poison biochemical reactions, disturbing essential functions in the body. Though completely avoiding toxins is nearly impossible, we can choose to reduce our exposure. We can also support our bodies' intrinsic strategies for detoxification and elimination, without which toxins accumulate within our tissues.

The last chapter was chiefly devoted to reducing the burden of toxins acquired from external sources, but toxins are also generated internally by normal metabolic processes. This chapter will focus on how all types of toxins are eliminated from the body. Beyond generation of free radicals, metabolism results in the production and accumulation of toxic byproducts. We depend on a healthy vascular system to move these waste products through the blood to the appropriate waste disposal sites. Carbon dioxide is removed via the lungs, wastes associated with the normal turnover of proteins in the body are removed through the kidneys and most other toxins are neutralized by the liver.

Not to marginalize the importance of the lungs or the kidneys, the liver is our chief organ of detoxification. Most external and some internally-derived toxins are fat soluble and are retained in our fatty tissues. We depend on the liver to convert these fat-soluble substances into less toxic water-soluble substances that can be removed more easily. This is a hard job. With age, some permanent damage to liver cells is inevitable and the liver becomes less efficient not only at detoxification, but also at other functions such as regulating cholesterol and glucose. Liver cells that have sustained significant damage are replaced with fat cells. An overly used/abused liver will take on a yellow color and be referred to as "fatty liver."

Protecting liver function as we age is extremely important. The detoxification process produces significant oxidative stress and regular intake of antioxidants helps protect liver cells. Regular consumption of cruciferous vegetables (e.g., broccoli, cabbage, Brussels sprouts, kale, bok choy, and cauliflower) aids in removal of hormones and hormone-like toxins from the body, a significant factor in decreasing the risk of hormonally-active cancers such as breast and prostate. Milk thistle and dandelion are herbs well known for protecting liver function. Supplements containing these ingredients should be considered by anyone with a history of liver damage, individuals who are on numerous medications, and possibly anyone over the age of fifty.

Toxins neutralized by the liver must still be removed from the body. There are three main pathways for removal: the colon, kidneys, and sweat glands. (A minor fourth one includes expiration via the lungs). Different toxins are processed in different ways. The majority of toxins are removed through the colon but others specifically exit via the urine. Some toxins can be removed directly by sweating, even before they pass through the liver. Working up a good sweat by exercising regularly or going to a sauna is a natural and important way to remove toxins.

The necessity of regular sweating has been recognized for ages. For populations around the equatorial regions, sweating throughout the hot day was a normal part of life, but for people in colder regions this was less true. Sweating had to be initiated. Native North Americans regularly participated in rituals that involved sweat houses. Saunas have been popular in Finland since the Middle Ages. Their use has now spread worldwide.

The vast majority of toxins are removed through the gastrointestinal system. After being processed by the liver, partially detoxified substances are carried by bile into the intestines and colon. Bile, consisting mainly of bile salts made from cholesterol, is secreted by the liver to help break down fat. Bile is tightly recycled in the body: 95% of bile is reabsorbed from the small intestine. *Most toxins can also be reabsorbed. This is where dietary fiber is so important.* Dietary fiber, made of indigestible material in our food, surrounds toxins that are in the intestine, thus preventing their reabsorption. How much fiber is necessary? The bulk of our food should be made up of fiber, but for average American, this is rarely the case: most Americans consume only about 5 to 10 grams of fiber daily, only a fraction of the 25 to 35 grams felt to be necessary for optimal health.

There are two types of fiber—soluble and insoluble. Soluble fiber holds water-soluble toxins within the colon until they are removed. Insoluble fiber makes up the bulk of feces; this type of fiber helps to push everything through. An added benefit of dietary fiber is removal of excess cholesterol from the system. (Inhibited flow of bile may even be a contributing factor to increases in blood cholesterol as we age.) Both types of fiber are important for normal gastrointestinal function and toxin elimination. Drinking plenty of water is important for the process to properly take place.

Gastrointestinal function in general is intimately tied to our overall health. Our neurological system is tightly intertwined with our gastrointestinal system and much of our immune system resides within the gastrointestinal system. Not only is the gastrointestinal system responsible for digestion of food and removal of toxins, it encounters microbial invaders and potential allergy producing substances on a continual basis. *When the gastrointestinal system is out of balance or not functioning properly, every system in the body is affected.* The biggest enemies of normal gastrointestinal function are processed foods (with high sugar, starch, and fat content, but low dietary fiber) and emotional stress. These seem to go together all too often.

Emotional stress shifts the resources of the body toward dealing with the stress at hand and away from dealing with everyday matters such as digestion. Chronic emotional stress almost always results in gastrointestinal dysfunction. Poor nutrition adversely affects both the integrity of the lining of the GI tract (called the mucosa) and our ability to produce the enzymes necessary to break down food. Lack of fiber slows motility (the movement of food through the GI tract) even further and allows the buildup of toxins and abnormal bacteria in the intestines.

When our primitive man was escaping from a tiger, digesting food was the least of his concerns. The resources of his body were temporarily shifted away from the gastrointestinal tract and toward the brain and muscles, of higher priority for the moment. Just suppose he happened to gulp down a burger in the middle of the escape— the burger would sit in his stomach undigested for some time. Gas produced by fermentation would be forced into the esophagus, carrying stomach acid along with it. Fullness and discomfort would ensue until he finally relaxed enough to allow normal gastrointestinal function to resume.

Most Americans live this way on a daily basis. They come home from a day of "escaping the tiger" to immediately sit down to the largest meal of the day—at a time when the GI tract is least prepared to deal with it. Consuming food when gastrointestinal function is suppressed leads to disastrous consequences.

STOMACH

For many people the stomach is where all health problems begin. Gastroesophageal reflux and gastric ulcers are some of the most commonly treated disorders today. Chronic gastric dysfunction leads to erosion of the lining (mucosa) of the stomach, allowing ulcers to develop. The damaged tissues become fertile ground for secondary bacterial infections, most commonly *Heliobacter pylori*.

What happens in the stomach can greatly affect the other organs, including the esophagus. Poor eating habits, processed food, and stress delay gastric emptying, allowing food to stagnate and ferment. Gas and belching splash acidic liquid into the esophagus, causing inflammation and irritation of the esophagus. Painful erosions at the lower esophagus are part of *gastroesophageal reflux disease (GERD)*.

Most treatment protocols assume that increased stomach acid is the total cause of the problem and focus therapy on suppressing it completely. In actuality, stomach acid is an essential ingredient of normal digestion and without it, digestion of food is compromised. Without stomach acid, proteins are not properly broken down for digestion. Important minerals and some vitamins are not properly absorbed. Threatening microbes pass through this normally impenetrable barrier unharmed. Food stagnates in the stomach and gastric motility is slowed. This, by itself, contributes to further mucosal damage. Minimally-digested food is eventually allowed to pass into the small intestine, causing problems further down the line.

Erosions within the stomach are called *gastric or peptic ulcers* and present with classic "heartburn" symptoms along the left side of the upper abdomen. Erosions of the duodenum, where the stomach empties into the small bowel, are termed *duodenal ulcers*. "Infections" with the bacterium, H. pylori, are often associated with peptic ulcers. These ulcers present with pain in the middle of the abdomen in an area called the "epigastric region" and can radiate to the back. All of these ulcers have the same origins and respond to the same therapy.

The first step in maintaining a healthy stomach is following a diet made up of a wide diversity of fresh and natural whole foods with sufficient fiber. Regular consumption of fermented foods such as yogurt is an important practice for replenishing normal bacteria of the entire gastrointestinal system. If esophageal or gastric irritation is present, acidic foods such as citrus and tomatoes should be avoided. Spicy foods such as hot peppers can irritate an established problem, but are not causative. Coffee is a gastric irritant. Tea may also be a mild gastric irritant. Alcohol consumption can aggravate an established gastric disease process. Caffeine increases production of stomach acid.

The American habit of sitting down to a large meal at the end of a stress-filled day encourages gastrointestinal dysfunction. We would all do well to mimic our European neighbors with a main midday meal and a light supper, but most Americans find it hard to make the change. At the very least, a regular practice of distributing food throughout the day instead of a large end-of-day meal is better for digestion. Relaxing and stretching before a meal is another good practice. Never eat on the run.

When you sit down to eat with a group of people, are you the first to finish or the last? If the answer is first, not chewing is very likely a large part of any gastrointestinal upset you may be experiencing. Remembering that digestion starts in your mouth, make a conscious effort to eat more slowly and chew your food thoroughly. Chewing is the only part of the digestive process over which we have voluntary control. Completely chewing food may have more bearing on the incidence of digestive problems than anything else. Overeating is also less common in individuals who eat slowly and chew their food adequately, and it makes for a relaxed meal, which is better for digestion all the way around. A relaxed lifestyle in general has a positively influence on gastrointestinal function.

Large amounts of cold liquids consumed with food slow enzymatic function and impede digestion. Small sips of liquid during a meal are preferred. Again the Europeans are one up on us with a habit of drinking water, wine or beer at room temperature. Large iced drinks should be reserved for quenching thirst after exercise. This advice sounds harsh for most Americans, but it will reduce gastrointestinal dysfunction.

Dietary supplements should be considered before resorting to drug therapy. Since activation of digestive enzymes is compromised by a dysfunctional stomach, supplements containing enzymes that break down starches, sugars, proteins, and fat carry little potential for harm and may be of significant benefit. If bloating and stomach gas are prevalent, then reduced acid may be the problem. Try taking a spoonful of apple-cider vinegar in water with the meal—this strategy has helped many people with reflux.

Favorable bacteria, whether acquired from food sources or probiotic supplements, suppress the growth of secondary infections with harmful bacteria and fungal species. Bismuth subsalicylate, the ingredient found in the well-known over-the-counter remedy Pepto-Bismol, offers anti-inflammatory and protective functions, and effectively reduces secondary infections by the bacterium H. pylori. Deglycyrrhizinated licorice (DGL) and slippery elm are natural substances that can offer protection to the mucosal lining. Antacids containing calcium and magnesium have little potential for harm.

SMALL INTESTINE

After being exposed to the acidic environment of the stomach, food enters the small intestine where the acid is neutralized. Partially digested food is now exposed to more digestive enzymes and to bile, secreted by the liver. Partially digested proteins, carbohydrates and fat are further broken down into component parts for absorption through the mucosa of the small intestine. If the digestive processes of the stomach or small intestine are compromised, partially-digested food is at risk of becoming putrefied by bacterial fermentation, rather than being properly digested—with gas and distension as the immediate result. Consumption of processed food, lacking natural enzymes that aid digestion, compromises the digestive process even further. Undigested and contaminated food materials activate the immune system and cause further problems.

Enzymes are an essential part of the digestive process. Specific enzymes are secreted at key points in order to break down carbohydrates, fats and proteins. (Humans lack enzymes to break down certain complex carbohydrates that are collectively known as fiber.) As we age, digestion of proteins is compromised by reduced gastric acid secretion and gradual decline of digestive enzyme secretion. Digestion suffers and the incidence of gastrointestinal disorders increases.

Digestive enzymes are also naturally found within raw fruits, raw vegetables and raw meat. Pineapple and papaya are well known for containing digestive enzymes. These additional enzymes provide, for us, a boost to the digestive process. Processed and overly cooked foods contain no natural enzymes; this is likely another factor that contributes to the high incidence of gastrointestinal disorders seen today.

The enzymes naturally found in foods may have purpose beyond digestion alone. In Japan, a fermented soy product called "natto" is widely consumed. The bacteria in natto produce an enzyme, now called "nattokinase." When consumed by humans there is good evidence that nattokinase actively dissolves fibrin, the fibrous part of an arterial plaque—possibly one reason the Japanese are known for having the lowest rates of stroke and heart disease in the world. Other enzymes found in foods are known to have anti-inflammatory and analgesic properties in human consumers.

Under normal circumstances, foreign molecules such as proteins occasionally pass through the digestive process intact. Undigested proteins could represent a potential microbial threat or a potential allergen. Allowing such substances to cross the intestinal barrier into the bloodstream is very undesirable; thus, the immune system acts as a line of defense, ready and able to neutralize any foreign substance—especially foreign proteins. Because these food-based threats are relatively common, much of the immune system resides within the gastrointestinal system.

When digestion is compromised, intact proteins of all varieties pass into the small intestine. The immune system quickly becomes overwhelmed and hyper-stimulated. The defensive cells of the immune system congregate and inflammation ensues. Inflammation and the undigested proteins directly cause damage to the intestinal mucosa, allowing a flood of abnormal substances to cross the intestinal barrier. A vicious cycle is thus created. The entire process is commonly referred to as *"leaky gut syndrome"* and the resulting inflammation is a contributing factor to *inflammatory bowel disease*.

Proteins that have been neutralized by the immune system form *"inflammatory complexes"* that pass into the bloodstream and are circulated to other parts of the body, causing symptoms well outside of the gastrointestinal tract. This is the basis for food sensitivities. When a hyper-alerted immune system is continually exposed to the same proteins, even those from everyday foods, it becomes "sensitized" to those proteins (some foods are more apt to cause sensitivities than others because of the type of protein). This explains why food sensitivities often occur to commonly consumed foods and why unusual symptoms, such as fatigue, body aches, chronic skin conditions, headaches, muscle pain, joint pain, and even insomnia may result. Symptoms are often delayed up to one or two days from the time an offending food is consumed.

Food sensitivities associated with leaky gut syndrome should be differentiated from classic food allergies. True food allergies are associated with acute symptoms of itchy skin, swelling and watery eyes, and are relatively uncommon. The offending foods are normally easy to recognize and can be avoided. Generally a person will have allergies to one or only a few different types of foods. True food allergies are associated with a different type of immune reaction, last for a lifetime and are not necessarily associated with gastrointestinal dysfunction.

Bowel dysfunction with associated food sensitivities increases the body's total immune burden. Unrecognized food sensitivities, when combined with airborne allergies, push the immune system toward the breaking point referred to as the "allergy threshold." For this reason, nasal allergies and chronic sinusitis are commonly found in association with gastrointestinal dysfunction and food sensitivities.

Food sensitivities can produce symptoms beyond gastrointestinal dysfunction. Vegetables in the "nightshade" family including tomatoes, eggplant, potatoes, and peppers are notorious for aggravating arthritis. Some foods have a reputation for triggering migraines. Classic examples include caffeine-containing foods, red wine with sulfites, preserved meats containing sodium nitrite, dairy, chocolate, and foods containing the flavor-enhancer MSG. Problem foods and types of reactions can vary widely from person to person.

The first step in management of food sensitivities is recognition. An elimination diet is the best way to recognize and avoid offending foods. Testing for acute food allergies and delayed food sensitivities can also be helpful in defining the problem. Once food sensitivities are recognized, avoidance of offending foods is the next step. Variety and rotation of foods is essential. Following good gastrointestinal health habits further inhibits development of sensitivities to other foods. All of the same supplements and strategies for gastric therapy apply to small bowel health. With time, after the bowel has an opportunity to heal and the immune system is calmed, some foods can carefully be reintroduced on a limited basis.

LIVER, GALLBLADDER, AND PANCREAS

These three organs are intimately tied to each other and to the elimination process. Ducts from the liver, gallbladder and pancreas join to form the common duct which connects to the upper part of the small intestine. The liver secretes bile, which is necessary for the breakdown of fat. An extra supply of bile is stored in the gallbladder for use when excess dietary fat is consumed, such as after eating a double chili-cheese burger. The pancreas secretes enzymes necessary for digestion of everything else.

The flow of bile is a key point in the detoxification cycle. Once the liver cells have extracted fat-soluble toxins from the bloodstream and converted them into less toxic substances, they are shuttled into the bile. The rate of toxin removal is therefore dependent on the flow of bile. Stress and consumption of processed foods, which tend to be inflammatory, can significantly inhibit the flow of bile.

Bile is made up predominantly of bile salts derived from cholesterol. Besides carrying toxins from the liver, bile is necessary for digestion of fat. Bile is dumped into the intestine, but then reabsorbed (recycled) later down the line. At that point, any water-soluble toxins that are not surrounded by indigestible fiber are also reabsorbed; thus, high-fiber diets expedite toxin removal from the body.

The brown color of stool represents bile. Light-colored stools suggest sluggish bile flow or excessive reabsorption of bile. Constipation, as you can surmise, is a risk factor for toxin retention. Loose stools, however, do not necessarily represent adequate flushing of the liver. Often bile flow is inhibited in disorders such as irritable bowel syndrome, and undigested fat contributes to diarrhea. "Congestion of the liver," with decreased bile flow, is very likely is a factor in many chronic disease processes, from elevated cholesterol associated with atherosclerosis to cancer.

The most common threat to this three organ complex is gallbladder disease. Extra bile is stored in the gallbladder. Gallstones, consisting predominantly of bile salts, form when the flow of bile is stagnant. Hereditary factors increase the risk of stone formation, but the most significant contributing factors are poor dietary habits and poor health habits in general. The stones themselves are generally not a problem, unless they become lodged in the common duct, completely blocking the flow of bile from the liver and causing painful back-up of enzymes from the pancreas.

LOWER SMALL INTESTINE AND COLON

Finally we get to the lower portion of the GI tract where the final processes of digestion, toxin removal, and elimination of waste material occur. The concentration of bacteria in this region is truly astounding and may easily exceed a trillion bacterial cells in adults with normal GI activity. The large intestine may be home to approximately 400 different varieties of bacteria, yet the species that predominate in one individual may not be those that are most common in another person:

The bacterial makeup of a person's gastrointestinal bacterial flora is almost as individual as his or her genetic code.

The bacteria of the colon (the first part of the large intestine) feed upon any undigested food particles remaining at this point and assist in the further breakdown of any toxins present. Gastrointestinal bacteria are also important because they produce certain vitamins essential for human health. When out of balance, overgrowths of abnormal or harmful bacteria can produce excessive gas and toxins, which cause pain and can actually slow or stop the elimination process—thus producing the miserable state of constipation.

Poorly digested food, low quality food, and slow motility promote overgrowths of abnormal bacteria in the colon, a condition that is commonly referred to as "dysbiosis." This process is aggravated further by a low-fiber diet, which lacks the bulk necessary to push toxic buildup of bacteria on through.

This can become a perpetual problem. Slow intestinal motility often allows abnormal bacteria to backup into the small intestine causing gas and damage to the mucosa of the lower small intestine. I have commonly witnessed this phenomenon in patients who present with pain in the right lower portion of the abdomen, where the small bowel inserts into the large bowel. These patients are sometimes seen in the emergency room with symptoms similar to those with appendicitis. Most often this problem waxes and wanes throughout a person's lifetime and is a hallmark sign of irritable bowel syndrome.

"Dysbiosis" and "leaky bowel syndrome" are the roots of irritable bowel syndrome, inflammatory bowel disease and chronic constipation. When the digestive process is compromised upstream, problems in the large colon are often going to follow. Poorly digested processed foods feed abnormal bacteria. Overgrowths of abnormal bacteria produce gas and toxins that slow intestinal motility. Distension and discomfort result. The initial result is often constipation, but, as toxins build up, episodes of explosive diarrhea occur. The condition is referred to as *irritable bowel syndrome* (IBS). Some suffers have more of a tendency towards constipation and others toward frequent loose stools. Fortunately, however, damage to the mucosa is not usually severe and inspection of the bowel by colonoscopy typically reveals normal tissues.

Inflammatory bowel disease occurs when severe inflammation and ulceration of the mucosa is present. If inflammation and ulceration affect mostly the small bowel, the condition is termed *Crohn's disease*. When the colon is mostly affected, the condition is called *ulcerative colitis*.

Toxins produced by overgrowths of unfavorable bacteria can have far-reaching effects. Symptoms commonly associated with chronic fatigue and fibromyalgia may be related to dysbiosis. Breast cancer and arthritis may have links to dysbiosis.

Chronic constipation can include irritable bowel symptoms or exist by itself. Constipation occurs when the muscular contractions that move material through the colon are slowed or stopped. This process of intestinal motility, referred to as peristalsis, can be compromised by many things, including toxins in the food we eat, toxins produced by abnormal bacteria in the colon, and chronic distension of colon. Many medications also slow intestinal motility.

The good news is that there are many ways to reduce the frequency of bouts with most GI disorders. Following a diet made up of a wide diversity of whole foods with sufficient fiber is important for maintaining a healthy lower gastrointestinal tract. Regular consumption of fermented foods such as yogurt replenishes favorable intestinal bacteria. Management of stress and regular practice of relaxation techniques are also essential for allowing the gastrointestinal tract to perform its job.

Restoration of normal gastrointestinal function is essential for overcoming any type of chronic health problem. Strategies for overcoming intestinal dysfunction should include recognizing and eliminating foods causing food sensitivities, aiding digestion with digestive enzyme supplements, soothing and protecting the intestinal mucosa with selected supplements, increasing dietary fiber to push abnormal bacteria through the tract, and replacing bad bacteria with favorable (normal) bacteria. The elimination diet found within the detoxification protocol at the end of this chapter is a good place to start.

Supplements that may be beneficial include slippery elm, aloe vera juice and ginger tea (all soothe the intestinal mucosa), digestive enzymes, probiotic supplements and fiber supplements. Most natural fiber supplements consist mainly of psyllium, which can be beneficial for controlling both loose stools and constipation. (NOTE: In some individuals, psyllium feeds abnormal bacteria and causes gas. In these cases, synthetic fiber supplements should be considered. Stimulant laxatives should only be used occasionally or under the direction of a health care provider.)

Another complimentary strategy recognizes that certain carbohydrates commonly found in grain products feed abnormal bacteria in the colon. This strategy eliminates all grain products and other food sources that contain related carbohydrates in order to "starve out" undesirable bacteria. A special diet, referred to as the "Specific Carbohydrate Diet," defines the strategy.

Details can be found in the book *Breaking the Vicious Cycle* by Elaine Gottschall, B.A., M.Sc. The diet has a following worldwide and is supported by several websites offering recipes and food suggestions. The diet often works, to which multitudes of sufferers can attest. *www.breakingtheviciouscycle.info*

Gastrointestinal dysfunction is common and mild symptoms often respond to dietary and lifestyle changes. Any out of the ordinary symptoms including vomiting, vomiting blood, passage of blood from the rectum, or any severe symptoms should be immediately reported to a healthcare provider.

DETOXIFICATION DEMYSTIFIED
—a rational detoxification/elimination protocol

Toxin accumulation is intimately associated with all processes of disease. Only by staying ahead of toxin accumulation can we cut disease off at the pass. Optimal detoxification not only helps us stay healthy but also decreases the risk of chronic diseases, reduces symptoms associated with arthritis, chronic fatigue and fibromyalgia, and expedites recovery after chemotherapy. It may also encourage remission of various autoimmune diseases.

The magic behind detoxification lies within the healing systems of the human body. The body will readily detoxify itself when maintained on a diet of fresh whole foods in a low stress environment. The greatest impediments to detoxification are the burdens imposed by the factors that cause disease—reduce these factors and the body will respond appropriately. That being said, the most effective detoxification protocol is one that supports the normal detoxification processes already in place.

The following detoxification protocol is designed to rejuvenate and support normal gastrointestinal and detoxification processes of the body. Note that it is only a beginning, since normal detoxification is really a lifelong process. For anyone suffering from chronic disease, this detoxification protocol is a way to jump-start the healing process and reduce the stress factors associated with disease. In cases of known toxin overload, detoxification should only be carried out under the careful guidance of a knowledgeable healthcare provider.

To optimize detoxification and regain lost health, the cycle of poor health habits must first be broken. To accomplish this task, most people need a point of departure; a place to start, but also a place to return to when old habits inevitably resurface. A period of fasting, followed by a detoxification and elimination protocol provides the ideal vehicle. While a few individuals will completely easily embrace a healthy diet and never turn back, most people gradually return to old habits. A period of fasting followed by a detoxification diet several times a year is a good way to keep the body in tune and keep unhealthy habits in check.

The most important aspect of fasting is allowing the gastrointestinal system to have a period of rest. Digesting food consumes an enormous amount of effort and energy. Taking a break from it allows the body to redirect resources toward long-overdue repair and maintenance functions. Of course, to make best use of fasting, the whole body should be at rest. While fasting, emotional stress and strenuous activity should be avoided as much as possible.

One to two days of fasting is followed by the detoxification diet. This special diet works on several levels. The chosen foods and activities reduce stresses on the digestive and immune systems of the body, allowing toxins to be extracted from tissues. Toxins brought out of the tissues by fasting end up in the gastrointestinal tract, where they can be eliminated; for this reason, fiber (found in fruits and vegetables) is an important part of this strategy, since the fiber helps to bind the toxins and carry them out of the body with the feces. Dietary fiber also rids the colon of toxin-producing bacterial overgrowth. The selected foods are nutrient dense, providing vitamins, minerals, healthy fats and antioxidants important for rejuvenation. Organic is preferred, so as not to add to the burden of toxins.

This special diet offers the opportunity to eliminate any types of food sensitivities. The diet during the first week should include low-protein foods that rarely cause food sensitivity reactions. Dietary protein requirements are initially met with rice or rice protein powder (whey or soy protein can be substituted with observation for any types of reactions). Rice is rarely associated with food allergies or sensitivities and therefore it is the main grain used in the diet. Brown rice is a good source of fiber, protein, minerals and nutrients. After the first week, other categories of foods are added back one at a time, allowing for enough time between food reintroduction to observe for adverse reactions.

NOTE: *Starches and fiber found in* <u>any</u> *grains or grain products, even rice, can be a source of woe in individuals with irritable bowel syndrome or inflammatory bowel disease. Individuals with persistent symptoms of gas, distension and loose stools should consider reviewing guidelines for the "specific carbohydrate diet."*

After a period of fasting and a week on the detoxification diet, most people feel rejuvenated and well. Aches and pains associated with chronic disease are reduced and energy is increased. After the first week, other foods (preferably healthy foods) can be added back, one at a time. Individuals with concerns for food allergies or food sensitivities should keep a diary. If symptoms of fatigue, arthritis, GI dysfunction, etc, return within one to two days of a food being added back, that food should again be eliminated. Admittedly, this approach is tedious, but it is effective.

ESSENTIAL COMPONENTS OF THE PROTOCOL

Reduce toxin intake

- Purified water—all water or liquids consumed should be free of contaminants.

- Choose foods known to be low in toxins (i.e., most organic foods) and be sure to select foods that have low potential to cause allergic reactions. All refined or processed foods should be completely avoided. Food choices should provide adequate fiber.

- Clean air—follow the recommendations in chapter 10 for a clean-air environment. Not smoking cigarettes should go unsaid.

- Vigilance and a "toxin-aware" attitude are essential. Special attention should be paid to avoid toxins derived from plastics.

Balance cell membranes

- Healthy cell membranes, essential for normal communication between cells and for optimal cellular function, require essential fatty acids,

- Certain essential fatty acids also balance the inflammatory response of the immune system.

- Monounsaturated fats, such as are found in olive oil or macadamia nut oil, are essential for healthy cell membranes.

Boost the immune system and protect the liver

- Antioxidants found in fruits and vegetables are essential for decreasing the potential for oxidative stress. Antioxidant and anti-inflammatory supplements can provide additional benefit. Reduction of oxidative stress allows the immune system to function optimally.

- Inflammation is a major process of disease. Natural anti-inflammatory substances such as *ginger* and *turmeric* are an important part of the protocol.

- *Vitamin C, Vitamin E, zinc* and *selenium* are essential for normal immune function. Vitamin C and E recharge a chemical called glutathione in the liver, a key component of the detoxification process. B vitamins are also key players in the detoxification process. The herb *milk thistle* is known to protect liver cells from the hazards of the detoxification process.

- There are many natural substances that augment or "tune-up" the immune system, some of which we know more about than others. The herbs *echinacea, elderberry, astragalus* and *andrographis* are well studied and appear to have very low potential for toxicity.

Remove toxic metals from the body

- Increasing the flow of bile through the liver and decreasing reabsorption of bile from the intestine is essential for toxin removal. Dietary fiber is essential for holding toxins within stool for removal. Low fiber diets allow reabsorption of many types of toxins. Vegetables and fruit provide the essential fiber for detoxification and can stimulate bile flow. *Milk thistle* is also known to stimulate bile flow.

- Exercise is essential for mobilizing toxins out of tissues and into the bloodstream, where they can be transported to the liver. A hot bath or sauna also increases blood flow.

- The skin can be a primary organ for removal of toxins. Sweating is an essential part of detoxification.

- A laxative such as *magnesium citrate*, taken during the fasting period, is beneficial for relieving the burden of abnormal bacteria in the intestinal tract. Care must be taken to generously replace fluids and electrolytes during this period.

Maintain blood pH

- Mobilization of toxins is expedited when the blood has a normal, slightly alkaline pH of 7.4. A diet consisting predominantly of fruits and vegetables provides minerals necessary for maintaining optimal pH. Diets high in processed food and meat tends to do the opposite.

Replace toxic metals with essential metals

- Heavy metals "poison" biochemical reactions by substituting for the required naturally-occurring metals in the body, such as iron, zinc, copper or selenium. As toxic metals are removed, the normal metals should be readily available for substitute. Essential metals are best obtained as natural forms found in food. Supplement therapy should follow this form.

TAKE NOTE *Mercury, cadmium, lead and aluminum are the most common toxic metals found in the environment and are strongly associated with chronic disease. All can be difficult to remove from tissues. If body stores of heavy metals are not known to be excessive, regular use of FIR sauna can be an effective method of detoxification. In cases where heavy-metal exposure is known to have occurred, detoxification should be performed only under the guidance of a healthcare practitioner who recognizes the necessity of long-term, low dose oral chelation therapy. Intravenous chelation therapy is not indicated for removal of heavy metals from the body.*

SCHEDULE FOR DETOXIFICATION

Two-day Fast (optional)

The week begins with an optional period of fasting. The fast should only be continued for one to two days. A strict fast includes water (with or without added lemon or lime) and non-caffeinated herbal teas, such as ginger tea, peppermint tea or holy basil tea. A less strict fast could include vegetable or fruit juices. Approximately two liters of liquid should be consumed throughout each day. Any type of fast should be accompanied by strict rest. This is not a time to engage in even moderate exercise. Plan to follow the fast on a weekend or during a vacation, when work-related stresses are not a consideration. *Individuals who are debilitated in any way should consult a healthcare provider before attempting any type of fast.*

Wholesome Food Choices

After the two-day fast, food is gradually reintroduced. This second phase of the protocol should last one to two weeks. Only healthy foods that do not add stress to the immune system or digestive system are allowed. All foods should be fresh. Organically produced and minimally -refined foods are preferred. ***Packaged, canned and otherwise processed foods should be avoided completely.*** Foods can be consumed raw, steamed or lightly sautéed.

Categories of foods allowed during the detoxification period

- **Vegetables** All vegetables are allowed and encouraged. Cruciferous vegetables including broccoli, cabbage, kale, bok choy, cauliflower, collards and Brussels sprouts support detoxification of hormonally active chemicals by the liver. Spinach, peas, tomatoes and potatoes are sources of glutathione. Beets provide *betaine*, a vitamin-like substance that supports detoxification. Artichoke and dandelion also support the detoxification process. Salad greens including chicory, endive and radicchio offer cleansing properties. Green leafy vegetables provide minerals such as calcium. Those with color, such as sweet potatoes, carrots and squash, provide vitamins, minerals, and antioxidants. Vegetables can be steamed, lightly sautéed or juiced. Juicing retains high levels of nutrients.

- **Fruits** Temperate fruits including berries, apples, pears, peaches, apricots and melons are preferred in quantity over tropical high-sugar fruits such as bananas and pineapples, but consumption of all fruits is encouraged. Antioxidants found in fruit are essential for detoxification. Fruit pectin augments removal of heavy metals and other toxins. Fruits may be consumed raw or added to smoothies. Dried or frozen fruit is permissible if fresh is not available. Dried dates, raisins and figs add variety and natural sweetness to combinations of foods.

- **Dairy and dairy substitutes** Rice milk is allowed from the start. Soymilk can be added later (unless soy allergies are suspected). Plain yogurt (preferably home-made and/or organic) is allowed after the first week. Make note of any gastrointestinal reactions/ changes in bowel habits when yogurt is added. (Some people do not tolerate any milk products including yogurt).

  For those who do tolerate yogurt, yogurt is easy to make and yogurt-makers are inexpensive. Homemade yogurt cultured for 24 hours is almost completely free of lactose. Individuals with known or suspected allergies to milk proteins should avoid yogurt made from cow's milk, but yogurt can also be made from goat's milk or soymilk. Strained yogurt ("Greek" yogurt) can be used like cream cheese.

  Avoid all other dairy products during detoxification, including milk, cheese, sour cream, cream cheese and cottage cheese.

- **Oils** Use unrefined, cold-pressed olive oil for cooking. Use flaxseed oil on salads or for other non-cooking uses.

  Avoid any type of processed or refined oil (including soy oil), butter, margarine.

- **Beans** Start with red lentils (see Simple Cooking for red lentil chili or look for other recipes on the internet). Hummus (which is mainly ground garbanzo beans, a.k.a. "chick peas") can be used as a vegetable dip. Tofu and edamame are acceptable soy forms at this time.

  Avoid all other beans during the first week.

- **Grains** Brown rice, basmati rice and millet are allowed during this period. Flaxseed meal can be used as an additive to uncooked food, such as yogurt, to provide texture.

  Avoid all other grains during the first one to two weeks.

- **Nuts**   *Avoid* all nuts during the first week.

- **Meats**   *Avoid* all meats during the first week.

- **Protein sources**   Protein powder can be added to smoothies. Soy or whey protein powders are complete sources of protein, but should be avoided with known or suspected allergies. Rice protein powder is an alternative. Yogurt, after the first week, is a good source of protein.

   Avoid eggs during the first week.

- **Sweeteners**   Honey (organic preferred), agave nectar, Xylitol.

   Avoid sugar, corn syrup, molasses, artificial sweeteners, foods made with sugar such as jams and jellies.

- **Condiments and seasonings**   sea salt, vinegars (apple cider, balsamic, rice, malt, etc.), wheat-free tamari or lite soy sauce, garlic, ginger, fresh herbs and all other spices.

   Avoid Mustard, mayonnaise, salad dressing, ketchup, and bottled sauces of any type.

- **Beverages**   Purified water is the best overall choice for hydration. For more flavor, add a squeeze of lemon or lime. Diluted fruit juices are allowed. Avoid fruit juices with added sugar. Non-caffeinated herbal teas and decaffeinated green or white tea are allowed. Holy basil is an excellent herbal tea to consider. It contains no stimulants, is an excellent anti-inflammatory, lowers blood pressure in hypertensive individuals, lowers blood sugar, and is soothing to the stomach. Dandelion tea with roasted barley has a flavor much like that of coffee, but less bitter. Dandelion is protective of liver function.

   Avoid Coffee, black tea, all alcohol, and soft drinks. Avoid iced drinks. (Regular caffeine users should not stop caffeine abruptly. Gradually taper off caffeine by mixing half-and-half regular and caffeinated. Green tea is an option for less of a caffeine effect.)

Sample Menu Ideas for the Detox Period

- **Beverages**   approximately 2 liters of liquid should be consumed through the day.

- **Breakfast**   Leftover brown rice, warmed, with raisins, honey and soymilk. Brown rice cakes with dried dates or figs. Any type of fruit. Yogurt with berries, sweetened with honey after week one (ground flax-seed can be added).

- **Lunch** Steamed or microwaved vegetables (see "vegetable bowls" in chapter 9). Fresh lettuce salad with salad vegetables, topped with oil and vinegar dressing.

- **Supper** Sautéed vegetables over rice (see chapter 9 for ideas).

- **Snacks** Fruit smoothie made with fresh or frozen berries, yogurt, soymilk, honey and flaxseed oil. Carrots/celery with hummus.

Supplements *Dosages as recommended on the supplement bottles should be followed.*
- **Milk thistle** This herb is possibly the most important supplement in the detoxification process. Silymarin, the active chemical in milk thistle is a potent antioxidant that protects liver cells during the detoxification process. Milk thistle also enhances the flow of bile, essential for removing toxins from the circulation. Milk thistle supplements should be taken several times daily during the detoxification protocol and can be continued thereafter.

- **Essential Fatty Acids (Omega 3 fatty acids)** These are important for decreasing inflammation and supporting optimum cell membrane function. During the first week of the detoxification protocol, essential fatty acids should come from vegetable sources such as flaxseed. Supplements containing marine sources of oil can be used once fish is incorporated back into the diet. Vegetarian supplements are available.

- **Multivitamins** This supplement provides optimal amounts of essential nutrients and minerals during the detoxification period. Look for a multivitamin with natural mixed sources of vitamin E and organic sources of minerals such as amino acid chelates. Vitamin C (500-2000mg daily), Natural vitamin E (400-800 IU daily), zinc (50mg), and selenium (400 mcg) are vital for the detoxification process. High quality multivitamins are generally taken 2-3 times daily. *Multivitamins may be continued at the discretion of the individual after detoxification is completed.*

- **Antioxidants** L-Glutathione is the most widely distributed cellular antioxidant and is essential for detoxification processes in the liver. L-Glutathione is readily synthesized in the body, but during detoxification, l-glutathione supplies can be depleted. L-Glutathione can be obtained from dietary sources and supplements, but the amount of its absorption through the GI tract is negligible. *Vitamin C and vitamin E* are known to recharge intracellular glutathione and should be taken throughout the detoxification period. *Glutamine and n-acetylcysteine,* precursors to glutathione, can be taken as supplements, but it is unknown whether they significantly increase glutathione levels.

Alpha lipoic acid is a vitamin-like substance known to have potent antioxidant properties both intra- and extra-cellularly. This unique substance is both water soluble and fat soluble and may have the ability to scavenge toxins and heavy metals from tissues. Alpha lipoic acid has the ability to regenerate other antioxidants such as vitamin C, vitamin E and glutathione. Alpha lipoic acid may play a role in glucose regulation by increasing cellular uptake of glucose.

- **Immune enhancers** Herbal supplements known to positively modulate the immune system enhance the protocol. *Andrographis, astragalus, elderberry and echinacea* are reasonable choices that have been well-studied. These herbs also have anti-inflammatory, antioxidant and antimicrobial properties.

- **Anti-inflammatory supplements** If arthritis or other anti-inflammatory conditions are present, consider taking a combined supplement with ingredients including *ginger* and *turmeric*. These ingredients are also favorable tonics for the gastrointestinal tract. Chemicals found in grape skin/seed extract, also have potent anti-inflammatory and antioxidant properties.

- **Toxin removal** Dietary fiber found in fruit and vegetables is essential for binding toxins within the GI tract and escorting them out of the body. Regular elimination (once or twice daily) is vitally important during the detoxification process. Those prone to constipation may need a fiber supplement and/or a mild laxative.

Chlorella, a freshwater algae, and tincture of cilantro are known for their mild detoxifying properties. Primarily they are effective for removal of organic toxins, but are not strong enough to hold on to heavy metals. As supplements, they can be safely used as important adjuncts during the detoxification period.

TAKE NOTE *Most over-the-counter "colon cleanse" products are nothing more than psyllium and senna (a natural laxative), usually sold for a much higher price than warranted. Some commercially-available detoxification products contain combinations of herbal ingredients, and sometimes include seaweed or algae. Use of these products may result in toxins being circulated around, but not necessarily removed from the body.* ***Products containing strong laxatives should only be used short-term. Ingredients should be carefully scrutinized. Many are best left on the shelf.***

- **Mild laxative** Magnesium is probably the best mild laxative to use during detoxification. Many individuals suffering from chronic disease are magnesium deficient. Supplementing with magnesium is safe because the body only uses as much as it needs and passes excesses into the GI tract, hence the laxative effect. Although any magnesium supplement can be used, magnesium citrate is inexpensive and easy.

- **Probiotic** Re-establishing the balance of favorable bacteria in the GI tract is an essential part of health revitalization. Some strains of favorable bacteria are known to assist in the detoxification process. Favorable bacteria can convert toxins to less toxic substances, protect the intestinal lining from toxins and facilitate elimination. Daily consumption of a fermented food such as yogurt provides some favorable bacteria, but standardized probiotic supplements deliver higher amounts of live favorable bacteria where they are needed most.

- **Systemic enzymes** Living foods provide enzymes, not only for digestion, but also for absorption into the bloodstream. Enzymes absorbed from food have anti-inflammatory properties, most probably by breaking down immune complexes and debris. For someone switching from an average American diet to a healthy diet, complete enzyme supplements can help the process go a little more easily.

Complementary Considerations

- **Removing toxins via the skin** Certain toxins stored in fat are excreted through the skin with sweating. Daily moderate exercise increases blood circulation and mobilizes toxins from tissues. Bringing them into circulation provides a perfect opportunity for removal of toxins by sweating. Working up a good sweat for 30 minutes every day should be the norm. *Exercise provides one of the most efficient methods of toxin removal possible.*

  Sauna provides another avenue for sweating out toxins. Sauna therapy is safe and relaxing. Many fitness centers offer saunas. Sauna treatments can be done several times a week, but should be avoided while fasting. Start with brief periods (10 minutes) in the sauna and stay longer as you become acclimated. Follow a sauna with a cool rinse. Remember to drink plenty of liquids before going into a sauna.

  Far infrared sauna may be the most efficient method of removing organic toxins and heavy metals known. It uses lower ambient temperature than traditional sauna. The radiant heat associated with FIR sauna penetrates deep into tissues without drying and discomfort that can be associated with convective heat used in standard saunas. FIR sauna has shown significant benefit for chronic pain, fibromyalgia, chronic fatigue, allergies, sinusitis, anxiety, insomnia, chemical sensitivities, autism, arthritis, weight control, reduction of cellulite, and many other conditions. FIR sauna is ideal for post-chemotherapy detoxification because it does not stress the body. FIR sauna is mild enough to even be considered for patients with congestive heart failure. FAR sauna is especially effective for reducing withdrawal symptoms associated with drug/alcohol rehabilitation.

If FIR sauna is available, take advantage of this extraordinary healing modality. Therapy should include at least three treatments per week. If heavy metal toxicity is suspected, testing should be performed prior to starting therapy.

A hot bath or shower also dilates blood vessels and increases blood flow, mobilizing toxins from tissues. Scandinavians use hot baths and/or sauna followed by a cool dip or rinse as a health ritual. Try it as a stimulating way to start the day or at least finish your day with a soothing bath before hopping under the sheets.

The addition of Epson salt, consisting predominantly of magnesium sulfate, to a hot bath may replenish magnesium through skin absorption and help to alkalinize tissues. Add 2 cups of Epson salt to a normal bath. Two cups in a bucket of hot water also provides a soothing foot bath at the end of a long day.

- **Seven hours of sleep every night** Sleep is essential for a healthy immune system. Good sleep hygiene and stress management practices help to ensure a good night's sleep every night.

- **"Stimulation fast"** Detoxifying your mind is as important as detoxifying your body. During the first week, try to avoid as much stimulation as possible. Turn off the TV. Turn off the radio. Avoid the paper. Avoid gossip (it's only for one week!). Take time to learn a relaxation technique or meditation. Practice yoga. Read a good book. Observe your world. Watch a sunset. Ideally, every day should begin and end with a period of relaxation, quiet contemplation, prayer or meditation.

- **Regular Medications** Prescription medications should be continued during the detoxification period, but at the lowest dose possible. Ask your healthcare provider for advice. Over-the-counter medications should be avoided if possible. Acetaminophen (Tylenol) should be avoided completely.

Reintroduction of omitted foods

Following the initial detoxification period of one to two weeks, other foods can be gradually reinstated into your diet. If food sensitivities are a concern, add foods back one at a time, allowing one to two days to observe for reactions. If reactions occur, note them in a diary, and again exclude that food. It can be reintroduced again later to see if the same reaction or symptom reoccurs. Be patient: identifying all offending foods may take one or two months.

If you are not a vegetarian, first add back lean meats, starting with poultry, and then progressing to other meats. Fish are next on the list, followed by shellfish. Reactions to shellfish are common, pay close attention here. Add several different types of beans, one type at a time. Carefully add some nightshade vegetables, including tomatoes, potatoes and eggplant. Different types of nuts should be added back individually. Allergies and sensitivities to nuts, especially peanuts are common. Eggs can be added back at this point. Dairy products are next on the list. Recognize that allergies to milk proteins and lactose intolerance are two separate problems. Finally add in grains. Start with the non-gluten grains first. Rice and wild rice rarely cause any type of reaction. Gluten grains include wheat, oats, barley, rye and spelt. Observe carefully for GI reaction at this point, as sensitivities to wheat are higher than to any other grain.

Spending several weeks on a grain-free diet is an exercise in awareness in how grain-dependent we are as a society. As a learning experience, I strictly followed a grain-free (and soy-free) diet for six weeks. I did not starve and with time adapted to it fairly well. Since going off the diet, my grain consumption is half what it used to be.

After completing the detoxification and elimination protocol, attempt to steer clear of any former bad eating habits. Aim to align your daily diet with the food guidelines as defined in chapter 8.

PILLAR III

Synchrony of the Body and Mind

Synchrony of the body and mind brings optimal health into focus.

CHAPTER 12
Left brain / Right brain

Of all the brains of all the creatures on Earth, the human brain is by far the most complex. Though we think of ourselves as having only one brain, the thinking portion of the brain is actually divided in two halves. We refer to these halves as hemispheres. It is well known to most people that the left side of the brain controls the right side of the body and the right side of the brain controls the left side of the body, but it is seldom recognized that each of these hemispheres has independent functions that are unique.

The story behind our knowledge of independent right and left brain function is interesting. Patients with intractable seizures are sometimes treated with a surgical procedure in which the areas connecting the two hemispheres of the brain are severed completely. These patients have become known as "split-brain patients." After surgery, seizures resolve completely and amazingly these patients are able to return to being normal functioning members of society with no apparent disability. Unusual "quirks" can only elicited by specially designed experiments. These experiments offer insight as to how we cope with two brain halves that function quite differently.

In the most interesting of the experiments, a split-brain patient is placed in a booth specially designed to completely separate and isolate the left and right sides of the body. In the visual field of the left eye, the patient can plainly see a spoon and a knife lying on a table in front of them. A picture of a spoon is projected onto a screen, also on the left side. On the opposite side of the booth, in the right visual field, a spoon and knife are again present; identical to the ones on the opposite side, but a picture of a knife is projected onto the screen. Both eyes were able to see a spoon and a knife on a table, but the left eye is only able to see a spoon on the screen and the right eye is only able to see a knife on the screen. If asked to name the object on the screen, the patient would confidently reply, "knife". If asked to pick up the object displayed on the screen, the patient would always pick up a spoon.

Experiments with split-brain patients illustrate that we are all a product of two brains, each functioning independently, but both contributing to who we are. Some individuals tend to be more right-brained: more creative and more abstract in their approach to life, but oblivious to time. Most others tend to be more left-brained: punctual, preferring order and planning. Life is actually somewhere in the middle, with both sides being equally important. Learning to balance the functions of the brain is important for all of us.

The right hemisphere of the brain, controlling motor function on the left side of the body, is abstract, spatial, completely nonverbal, and has little sense of time. It is our source of creativity. The left side of the brain, responsible for controlling motor functions on the right side of the body, is concrete, analytical, verbal and very conscious of time. It allows us to deal with conflict.

In our modern world, the left brain is usually dominant; however, for most of human history, this was probably not the case. The mundane chore of collecting food required little in the way of left-brain function. Verbal skills took many thousands of years to develop and written language did not show up until very late in the course of human history. Even early cave drawings definitely came from the right brain. Time schedules were dictated only by the sun, the moon and the change in seasons. Thinking was mainly in terms of being aware of the surrounding natural world—very right-brained.

Early humans did need the analytical functions of the left brain, but not nearly as much as we do today. Left-brain functions were reserved mainly for dealing with conflict. Organizing a confrontation with the clan of humans over the hill for rights to the berry patch in the valley would have required left brain function. Calculating the number of sticks and rocks to have on hand and planning the route of attack would have been beyond the capacity of the right brain. Conflict was the ingredient that propelled us toward our world today.

Left-brained functions, though only used intermittently, were a necessity for dealing with conflict. When our prehistoric man came from around a rock to find himself face to face with a saber-toothed tiger, left-brain functions immediately came into play and the two halves of the brain blended synchronously to evaluate the threat. All within a fraction of a second, rapid analysis would define any possible tools available for defense and the most acceptable escape route.

This surge in left-brain activity came with a corresponding surge of adrenaline. Adrenaline is the hormone that prepares us for conflict. Physiologically, adrenaline causes increases in visual acuity, heart rate, blood vessel constriction, muscle tension and respiratory rate, all in preparation for fight or flight. Assuming he survived the encounter, our prehistoric man would gently ease back into berry-picking mode: his heart rate and respiratory rate would slow to normal. Gastrointestinal and immune system functions, which had been placed on hold during the brief incident, would also gradually resume.

Though conflict would seem undesirable, to be avoided if possible, the feeling that occurred when the primitive man escaped death at the jaws of the saber toothed tiger must have been quite exhilarating. Very possibly he felt more alive at that particular moment than he felt at any other time in his life. The feeling that comes with brain synchrony drives many of us today. It is the feeling pursued by race-car drivers and high-level deal makers. It is often associated with conflict or risk.

At the height of intense conflict, the analytical ability of the brain functions at peak performance. Time seems to stand still. A heightened state of awareness occurs, representing optimal, synchronous functioning of the hemispheres of the brain.

Humans today are addicted to conflict. We seem to never get enough of the tiger. As a culture we thrive on it. When it doesn't come to us, we seek it out through interactions with other people, the news media, and the entertainment industry. We have, in essence, created a world of perpetual conflict, both real and imagined.

The state of perpetual conflict in which we exist today is very taxing. In the primitive man's world conflict was intermittent and could not be predicted; therefore, little anticipatory stress was associated with conflict. Today we are exposed to potential conflict around every turn. Conflict—perceived or real— causes us to constantly be on alert, always aware that the tiger is just around the corner. We can see it coming and worry about it incessantly. We exist in a state of perpetual adrenaline rush. In maintaining a perpetual state of alert, we are burning both ends of the candle at once. Our brain is constantly in the mode of dealing with conflict, creativity is suppressed, and normal maintenance functions of the body such as gastrointestinal function and immune functions are chronically placed on hold. Is it any wonder that insomnia, anxiety, hypertension, reflux and irritable bowel syndrome are the order of the day?

In addition to living in a world of perpetual conflict, we are constantly confronted with schedules, deadlines, and an almost unlimited amount of verbal and written information—all functions that depend exclusively on the left brain. One of the most obvious signs of left-brain dominance is the use of words. On a minute-by-minute basis, verbal skills are required for most everything we do. We write, talk and even think in words. Our left-brained world is a place of computers, cell phones, television monitors in every public place, schedules, deadlines and endless meetings. Being completely non-verbal, the right brain never gets a say and takes a backseat on every issue.

From an early age we are taught to use words to describe things, to be punctual, and to be very orderly. School and work tend to require a very verbal and analytical approach to life. Dawdling and daydreaming are always discouraged. *In essence, we are taught to turn off right-brain function.*

With right-brain function suppressed and the left brain always in control, the fundamental nature of brain synchrony is not possible and the brain is left in a perpetually imbalanced state. The health costs of left-brain dominance are high: anxiety, insomnia, hyperactivity, attention deficit disorder, obsessive compulsive disorder, hypertension, gastrointestinal problems, and immune dysfunction are just some of the most obvious end-results.

To rectify the problem we must achieve balance. A state of total right-brain dominance is no more desirable than that of left-brain dominance. A right-brain dominant world would be free of stress, but at the same time mundane and monotonous. Stress is not all bad. Stress can be a positive motivating factor: it moves us to get things done. Without stress we would never have goals and aspirations. For optimal health and optimal life, we need to be able to use both sides of our brain equally, shifting from one side to the other, and synchronizing them when a challenging situation arises.

The first step in shifting away from left-brain dominant behavior is practicing exercises that allow right-brain activity to flourish. This is easier for some than others, as some individuals are more naturally right-brained, but anyone who makes an effort will receive benefit.

GETTING INTO "R-MODE"

Artists will often refer to being in "R-mode." I do a bit of drawing and can relate to this concept. If you try to draw a named object such as a face in the way you think a face should look, often the outcome is not very good. The left brain, as usual, is trying to run the show and dictates that the face should be drawn according to symbols it knows—a symbol for an eye, a symbol for a mouth, etc. The left brain is verbal and does not appreciate shapes, shades and patterns, so the symbols are not representative of the actual configuration of a face. Drawing in this fashion, with the right brain suppressed, is not only frustrating but often ends with poor results.

An effective method of teaching drawing involves changing the view of the object to be drawn such that the left brain is unable to identify the object. A picture of a face, once turned upside-down, becomes a complex mix of shapes and shades of light and dark. Once left unrecognizable to the left brain, the right brain is finally allowed to take over. Sketching shapes and shades instead of defined objects, becomes timeless and relaxing, and the outcome of the drawing is always more realistic. Drawing in R-mode is one of the most relaxing pastimes I have ever known.

Recognizing the potential to suppress the stress of the everyday world by drawing, I started looking for evidence of R-mode in other activities. I typically found it where nonverbal skills were required. Sailing, an activity I have done most of my life, is extremely relaxing. Thinking is in terms of sail trim, direction, speed and location relative to land and other objects. It is very nonverbal and very right-brained. At different times when I have taught sailing, I have found it difficult to explain the concepts in words because they are so right-brained. I used to think that sailing was relaxing just because of being physically away from everything, but I now understand it is because my left brain turns off from the moment I step on the boat.

Music can be approached from either a right-brained or a left-brained perspective. I spent several years trying to master the guitar by learning to read music and then interpreting the notes and rhythm from a sheet of paper onto the fingerboard and strings. This decidedly left-brained approach ended as a frustrated failure. Had I approached the problem by listening to music and interpreting the music directly onto the frets and strings, I probably would have had a more relaxing and fulfilling experience. Many people learn better through right-brained experience and are often frustrated by the left-brained world. Very likely attention deficit disorder and hyperactivity have roots in this disequilibrium.

Mastering an instrument is not a necessary requirement for using music to achieve brain synchrony. The rhythm and beat of music predate verbal usage in human evolution by a wide margin. Listening to music is soothing and relaxing because it touches the right side of our brain as it calms the left. Of course, this is highly dependent on the type of music, as we each have our own taste. The right kind of music can help induce a state of brain synchrony during exercise, meditation, or even while at work.

Many focused nonverbal activities disengage left-brain function and at the same time disengage us from the oppressive worries of the world. Unfortunately, few of us have many opportunities to incorporate them into our daily lives. Learning some simple practices to use throughout the day can change your whole perspective on life.

TURNING OFF WORDS AND TURNING ON CREATIVITY

Using words is very left-brained. We tend to think in words. During the day we tend to get into a rhythm of thinking in words and then the words just keep coming. Turning off the flow is downright difficult, if not impossible. Breaking the cycle by incorporating right-brain activities into an average hectic day is not only relaxing but also increases productivity and creativity.

Recognizing how often you are thinking in words is not very difficult, as the left-brain pours out a continuous stream of words; the challenging part is turning it off. In our very verbal left-brained world, this practice must be cultivated. Throughout the day, make an effort to think without words. Pay attention to shapes of objects around you, especially in your peripheral vision, but without naming them.

As an exercise, pick a stationary object—an apple, ink pen, cell phone, or whatever is at hand. For several minutes, study the object intently. Without naming it or anything about it, appreciate its shape, the contours making up its margins, shades of light and dark on the surface, colors and reflections, and shadows surrounding the object. Appreciate dimensions within the object: length, width, depth and how they relate to one another. Close your eyes and imagine the object as if it were blank space, a void in the shape of the object. Notice that the flow of words, though not be turned off completely, have slowed considerably and you feel more relaxed and in control. Practice this exercise as often as you can throughout the day and especially when you are beginning to feel overwhelmed and uptight. You will be amazing at the relaxing and focusing result.

You can take the object exercise one step further by drawing the object. This type of drawing, called contour drawing, is a method of teaching drawing skills, but you do not need to draw well, or even have a desire to draw well, to receive benefit from this activity. Contour drawing is an exercise in pure right brain function that can be used by anyone, at any time, and in any place. A pen or a pencil and a scrap of paper are all the tools that are required.

The objective with this exercise is to reproduce the contours and shades of an object that is unidentifiable to the left brain on a sheet of paper in black and white. The "unidentifiable" part is accomplished by turning a picture upside-down or concentrating on the lines and shades of a very small part of the whole. As an example, you can use your opposite hand, held out in front of you, as the object to be drawn. Concentrate on the angles of the lines that make up the margins of your thumb, without identifying a "thumb." Draw in a continuous line very slowly, a millimeter at a time. Continue to draw all of the fingers. Pay attention more to the spaces between the fingers than the fingers themselves and mentally draw these shapes. Shade in light and dark *as you see them*, instead of how you think they should be.

Gradually you will find yourself slipping into R-mode. Time becomes less relevant and thought becomes more relaxed and focused. Completion of the drawing is irrelevant, as this is not the goal. The outcome of the drawing also does not matter, though you may find that you can draw better than you think. Having it framed is perfectly acceptable; I have a small drawing sitting by my computer of one of my son's tennis shoes from when he was ten years old.

Betty Edwards defined these concepts in *Drawing on the Right Side of the Brain*. Now a classic, I would highly recommend this book to anyone interested in learning how to draw and possibly anyone who just wants to learn how to relax.

DEFOCUSING

In his book *Open Focus*, Les Fehmi suggests that the anxiety and other ills associated with stress (most of the pain we experience in life) occur because our focus is too narrow, possibly as a result of left-brain dominance. He offers a solution of opening our focus to the surrounding world to diffuse concerns, defocus left-brained activity, and synchronize right- and left-brain function. Though his discussions and exercises are somewhat abstract, the principles are simple: broaden the focus of all of your senses and decrease left-brain dominance by the regular practice of exercises designed to encourage right-brain activity. Once mastered, these techniques are effective for treating everything from anxiety to chronic pain.

This experience is easy to achieve. Any place with an expansive view will suffice. It could be a mountain top in Colorado, a tall sand dune, or the roof of a tall building. Once there, take in the view with all of your senses. Pay attention to your peripheral vision as much as to the objects directly in front of you. The objects in the direct field should become secondary. Notice sounds and the direction from which they originate. Notice the smell and taste of the air. Notice the wind brushing against your skin. Notice the cool of the breeze on unprotected skin and the warmth of your toes inside your shoes. Notice an unavoidable calmness. Immerse yourself and become part of the scene.

You can actually have the same experience while sitting at your computer or reading a book. Purposefully, pay as much attention to the area surrounding the object in front of you as the object itself. Extend your concentration as far out into your peripheral vision as possible. Extend your peripheral vision to the point of being able to imagine objects behind you. Imagine any objects or shapes behind the computer screen as though the screen was not there at all. Notice any sounds and the direction from which they originate. Notice the smell and taste of the air around you. Notice any feelings such as anxiety or boredom and acknowledge them. Notice the feel of the keys against your fingers and any other sensations of touch. You have just taking a step towards synchronizing your brain and probably already feel more relaxed and comfortable than you did a few moments ago. Imagine how you would feel if you made the effort to do this several times every day. By expanding our focus we dilute out some of our dominant left-brained function and allow more right-brained activity, automatically creating balance.

Periodically breaking concentration completely can be a very effective way to decrease the tension associated with dominant left-brained thought. I call this "specific daydreaming." From an early age we are discouraged from daydreaming, and it is true that living in a fog is not conducive to getting ahead in the world, but diffusing our attention does seem to be a practical way to balance our brain function and ease tension.

These techniques are extremely effective for diffusing everyday stress, but must be practiced. The brain must be retrained to function in a different way. Throughout a busy day at work, take a moment or two to think *nonverbally* about some other place or activity. This type of thinking does not have to completely occupy your thoughts; it can be just enough to break your concentration and resynchronize the brain.

Though regular practice of right-brained activities would seem to be a waste of precious time (daydreaming, after all, is not to be condoned in our left-brained world), overall productivity generally increases. As the brain becomes more balanced and relaxed, creativity flourishes. Insurmountable obstacles seem less so. The flow of thoughts and words from the left brain gradually decrease and at the same time become less jumbled and more focused.

BRAIN SYNCHRONY

Every now and then, when we get things just right, the two halves of the brain become tuned harmoniously, and a state of heightened awareness occurs that can be associated with brain synchrony. It cannot be maintained perpetually, but we should be able to tap into whenever we desire. For the primitive man, it was being able to shift into brain synchrony by bringing in the analytical ability of the left brain when he confronted the tiger, thus preventing panic from ensuing. For us, it is shifting from a predominant left brained existence by incorporating right brain activities. The feeling of brain synchrony is like none other.

It is the classic runner's high.

It is when we are at the top of our game and on top of the world.

It is a feeling of confidence and calmness, even under the most adverse of situations.

It is being aware of everything around you, and beyond.

It may be the feeling of true happiness.

It is often the answer to depression and anxiety.

It is a powerful force of healing.

It is the state of being that many seek through meditation.

It is the place where we go just before falling into blissful sleep.

It is the feeling that many pursue through pharmaceuticals and illicit drugs, but quickly find that this shortcut is short-lived and fades into the misery of withdrawal and addiction.

The state of brain synchrony can be measured by a device called an EEG machine. An electro-encephalogram (EEG) is a tool that measures the electrical activity of the brain. This activity is quite dynamic and changes from minute to minute and even from second to second. Patterns of brain wave activity reflect the particular state of awareness an individual may be experiencing at any given moment.

The erratic and irregular waves produced by a brain functioning as left-brain dominant are termed *beta waves*. Most of us exist in this less- than-desirable state on a daily basis. When the two sides of the brain are synchronized, mental acuity and brain performance are optimal. This wave is represented by a smooth and regular wave called an *alpha wave*. An alpha pattern is where we would like to be more of the time than we actually are. Deep meditation causes further smoothing of the wave into a *theta wave* and deep sleep rounds out the pattern even further into a *delta wave*.

Brain synchrony not only bodes well for mental performance and a strong sense of well-being (even during life's most extenuating circumstances), but also relates to good health in general. Production of alpha, theta, and delta waves is associated with optimal healing and optimal immune function. Regular practice of right-brained exercises, relaxation techniques, and meditation all promote optimal healing.

Just as left-brained desynchrony is a learned behavior (many bad habits are learned behaviors), consistent production of alpha waves, associated with brain synchrony, is also a learned behavior. Breaking old habits and learning new ones does take some effort, but anyone willing to practice can achieve this goal. Consistently being able to achieve a state of brain synchrony can be accelerated through a discipline called biofeedback.

There are different modalities for conducting biofeedback. An instrument called an EMG can be used to measure muscle tension, allowing the patient to more effectively relax muscle groups. A simple thermometer can be used to measure finger temperature, providing feedback on adrenaline release, which causes constriction of blood vessels and the classic cold hands of anxiety. In one of the most effective forms of biofeedback, brain waves can be measured with an EEG machine, allowing the patient to learn brain synchrony directly. This is referred to as neuro-biofeedback.

As we progress further into the electronic age, biofeedback will become more available on an individual basis. Once relegated to a clinical or laboratory setting, inexpensive instruments of different types are becoming available for "home" biofeedback. At some point in time, biofeedback may become the preferred treatment for any stress-related disorder.

With or without the advantage of biofeedback training, brain synchrony exercises are effective for treatment of almost any stress-related disorder, with positive benefit noted for anxiety, attention deficit disorder, hypertension, reflux, irritable bowel syndrome, migraines, insomnia, and menopausal symptoms. Brain synchrony is also an avenue toward higher brain performance in general. Whether your goal is improved job performance, heightened athletic ability, or just feeling more in tune with the world, the concept of synchrony of the body and mind should be explored.

CHAPTER 13
An Active Body

The top of this dune has the best view around. At approximately fifty feet above sea level, it is the highest natural point in the county. On a clear fall day you can make out the lighthouse at the cape several miles down the shoreline to the east. To the west are piers, condominiums, and beach houses. The inlet and port are in plain view. Boats of various shapes and sizes are always coming and going to and from different directions. Through them, it is easy to feel a connection with all of the rest of the world. This particular spot is a midway point on a hike that I regularly follow during the cooler months of the year. It is a good spot to take in the whole world and take a break from it, at the same time. The experience is certainly one of healthful defocusing.

The trail meanders along a narrow pathway around and over a couple of miles of sand dunes. The sand and the dunes provide m-re than just scenery. Unlike walking on pavement, the sand cushions stress on joints, but at the same time strengthens foot, calf and thigh muscles. The up and-down trek over dunes varies the level of exercise, without adding stress to the body. The trail is never quite the same. It changes from day to day and season to season, with the weather, the foliage, the tide, the birds, and the ocean. After a good workout, the beach offers a leisurely stroll back to the parking lot. If timing is right, this usually coincides with the sun setting on the horizon. The full route takes about an hour, and the last thing that I have on my mind is "having to do exercise."

Regular vigorous physical activity is a necessity of good health, but the concept of "doing exercise" is a fairly new. Prior to the petroleum age, daily vigorous physical activity was simply part of life. Mobility, sustenance, and most everything else in life required physical labor. There was no reason to exercise. Today, obtaining food is a simple matter of driving to the store, and our jobs and lifestyles have become much more sedentary. Because physical labor is no longer a requirement for survival, doing enough physical activity to stay healthy is a matter of choice—a choice that seems to be difficult for many individuals.

When we start tallying up the reasons why we should be more physically active, the consequences of *not* being so become quite apparent. Vigorous physical activity is associated with an automatic increase in heart rate. The heart pumps harder to move more blood and carry more oxygen to active muscle fibers. Exercise causes blood vessels to dilate, or open up, allowing blood to flow more freely. The resulting increase in blood flow removes carbon dioxide and waste products from tissues. The rush of blood also washes out toxins and equilibrates hormones. In effect, exercise "blows out the pipes."

Vigorous physical activity mobilizes glucose and fat stores and allows the entry of glucose into cells even *without* insulin, an important factor in decreasing the incidence of insulin resistance and diabetes. The increased blood pressure and increased heart rate that occur with exercise are associated with chemicals that cause *dilation* of blood vessels, allowing blood to flow more freely. This is why regular exercise can alleviate hypertension, often without the use of drug therapy. The resulting increased blood flow reduces toxic buildup and atherosclerotic plaque formation, thus decreasing the risk of stroke and heart attack.

The benefits of exercise go beyond the physical. In our confrontation-filled world, stress stays "pent up" inside with no outlet. Exercise offers release that normalizes elevated levels of adrenaline. It is the normal endpoint of the "flight or fight" response. Regular exercise offers an outlet to diffuse and moderate stress in our lives.

With the benefits of physical activity being so obvious, you would think we would be stepping all over each other trying to get out and run around the block. Instead, it seems that most people have an aversion to exercise. Exercise, with the movement of muscles and ligaments over bones and joints, precipitates pain. Because it hurts to move, human nature would suggest that moving less is a good plan. This is actually the opposite of how it works. Regular exercise is associated with an *increase* in endorphins. These powerful chemicals not only decrease pain, but also are also associated with an increased sense of well-being. This is why drugs like morphine and heroin that mimic these natural chemicals are so profoundly addictive. The more regularly you exercise, the more liberally these chemicals are generated internally, and the better you feel.....naturally.

We would all be perpetual couch potatoes if it were not for natural pain-fighting endorphins floating around in our bodies. These "feel good" chemicals allow us to go about our normal daily activities without excessive discomfort, even though we have a baseline level of pain that is always there. Fortunately for most of us, the level is very low and easy to ignore, but it is there just the same. As we grow older the baseline pain level gradually creeps upward, and for individuals with conditions such as arthritis or fibromyalgia, the pain can be completely debilitating.

With exercise there is an initial increase in pain followed by a gradual, but corresponding increase in endorphins. It takes about 15 minutes for endorphin production to catch up. Many people never get past that first 15 minutes and relate exercise only to pain and discomfort. Why do something if it doesn't feel good? Sometimes in life you have to push past the pain to get the gain.

ADOPTING AN ACTIVE LIFESTYLE

A sedentary lifestyle is associated with a lower baseline level of endorphins, a higher baseline level of pain, a lower sense of well-being, and an aversion to exercise. An active lifestyle is, of course, associated with the opposite. How do we get from one to the other? Getting past that initial pain is challenging, and maintaining a comfortable flow of endorphins means doing some sort of exercise every day.

The focus of exercise should always be pleasure and never drudgery. The inevitable pain that comes with exercise can easily be diffused by the pleasurable aspects of exercise. Long ago I left behind the practice of doing exercise for the sake of doing exercise.

The key to making it work is raising the energy level of the body by becoming more active in every aspect of life. There are many ways to accomplish this goal, well beyond just working out at the gym.

How you go about becoming physically active is a matter of personal choice. For my college-age children, a trip to a fitness center is an essential daily affair. They enjoy the social aspects and gain support from other people. For me, the thought of being confined to a stale-smelling room with forty other sweaty people working out on whining machines while twelve televisions flash is next to torture. I like variety, space and solitude. Exercise is a part of my daily routine, but it varies from day to day. Whether hiking sand dunes, kite surfing when the wind is right, or biking to work or the grocery store, I can generally find something active to do.

Staying in good physical shape does not necessarily mean following a standard exercise routine. My wife sometimes participates in exercise classes at a fitness center, but the main source of her physical fitness comes from gardening and other yard work. She also walks a lot. On a similar note, my parents, who are in good shape for being in their seventies, remain so by being physically active. They do much of their own home maintenance by choice and are constantly painting, repairing stutters, pulling up fence posts, and putting in new gardens. I have rarely known them to sit idle.

YOU HAVE TO START SOMEWHERE

Probably the biggest impediment to becoming more active is inactivity itself. Another common roadblock is excessive weight. Obesity is commonly associated with back, joint, and foot problems, aside from just having to move the extra mass. It takes perseverance, but the cycle can and must be broken. Overcoming this hurdle will undoubtedly involve a little pain, will probably cause some embarrassment, and at times will be boring. But if you persist, even before the weight comes off, stamina will improve, the pain will lessen, and a larger variety of activities will be possible. *Regular physical activity is essential for good health and losing weight.*

Start slowly with activities that are comfortable and safe, but make the most of them and try to do just a little more each day. Walking is good, but even better if up an incline like hills or sand dunes. Biking and swimming are easy on joints. Kayaking and rowing are affordable water sports that are excellent for including the upper body in a workout routine. *Any type of regular exercise raises the energy level of the body and burns more calories.*

Take advantage of supports for joint protection and special shoes to eliminate foot pain. A personal trainer or exercise counselor can be of real benefit. Trained individuals can guide you and keep you focused, even when you are ready to throw in the towel.

Being physically active should never seem like drudgery. It is truly one of the gifts of life. The reward of regular physical activity is being able to do things that you never thought possible. This is when exercise becomes fun.

It may lead you to develop a passion for some type of recreational activity.

It means not being just a spectator.

Beyond exercise just for the sake of exercising, it means taking on an active lifestyle.

It doesn't matter how you do it, but you need to work up a good sweat at least once a day...everyday!

Look for ways to be more active in everyday life. Go outside every chance you get. Make a habit of walking places instead of driving whenever you can. At the very least, park further from your destination and walk a bit more. Buy a bike! Take a hike! Join a fitness center and really use it. Become associated with active people. Spend your weekends being active. Build something. Create something. Grow something! Turn your yard into a garden. Working a shovel into the soil or even using a rake is great exercise.

Turn off the television! TV sucks the life out of you. It hypnotizes you into doing absolutely nothing – sometimes for hours. Obesity and television are intimately tied together. There are so many interesting things to do in life. Don't spend your time watching other people live their lives while yours is slipping by! If you have children, by all means limit their TV-watching, too.

Or use the television more wisely. Interactive computer games have come a long way since Pacman. The latest systems include wireless devices that detect body movements. Both motivational and instructional, these systems will guide you through a wide variety of complete workouts right in your own living room!

Learn a new sport. There are plenty of choices: tennis, hiking, basketball, swimming, walking, biking, racquetball, golf (without the cart, of course), mountain climbing, mountain biking, horseback riding, sailing, surfing, windsurfing, kite surfing, skiing, skating and many more. Take dance lessons. Go bowling. Becoming active recreationally and pursuing an activity to a certain level of skill builds confidence and positive feelings about life in general.

Try out an exercise ball. For an under-$20 piece of exercise equipment, the Swedish exercise ball offers one of the best options for strengthening and toning muscles of the entire body. The ball can be used in a variety of ways, from stretching to total workouts. Used correctly, the exercise ball is excellent for back rehabilitation. The simple act of sitting on an exercise ball properly aligns the spine and tones the muscles of the body. Many people confined to sedentary jobs have found benefit from using an office ball in place of an office chair. Take an exercise ball and a couple of hand weights to work for brief workouts during the day.

Exercise balls can be purchased through the Internet or at your local fitness store. Make sure you get the correct size ball for your height. *Exercise Balls for Dummies* by LaReine Chabut is an outstanding resource for beginners.

Rev up your energy level during the day. That feeling of lethargy, loss of "pep," and lack of enthusiasm are signs of a decreased energy level. Sometimes low energy is a result of not eating properly during the day, not drinking enough liquids, or not sleeping well during the previous night. It can also have a physical cause, such as declining thyroid function. But often it is a result of everyday stress, monotony, and standing or sitting in the same position all day. Bringing your energy level up is actually easy to do. A couple of trips around the parking lot at a brisk pace can raise energy levels. Even ten minutes of stretching can help. The right kind of music can definitely have a positive effect. At the end of a long hard day, a 15- to 20-minute session of deep relaxation followed by 30 to 40 minutes of vigorous exercise can change your entire outlook on life.

An active lifestyle is not limited to the young or those who are already physically fit. I know an individual who at age 92 is still passionate about tennis and stays in good physical condition for his age because of it. There are scores of handicapped individuals who are passionate about a recreational activity that requires physical fitness. Passion for physical activity is the distinguishing factor between exercising regularly and following an active lifestyle. Those who try to exercise regularly but don't enjoy it generally give it up. Those who adopt an active lifestyle often find it addictive!

Fitness centers can be a valuable resource and generally are worth the investment. Beyond being just basic exercise and recreational outlets, these centers offer a wide assortment of programs for improving health and physical fitness. Individuals with young children often find daycare and children's programs are available. Fitness centers can be extremely valuable not only in the pursuit of losing weight but also to become more health-oriented in general. Use the gym to remain motivated and stay in shape for other activities that you enjoy.

Don't let kids or your spouse be an impediment to being more active. Take them with you. Pick activities they can do also. Sports programs for children are great, but *don't just be a spectator.* Become involved in their activities and involve them in yours. You'll be a closer and happier family for it.

Take advantage of "free" exercise. Use physical labor to complete tasks that could otherwise require a machine or hiring someone. There are so many different ways to take advantage of this concept. Tilling and hoeing your own garden is a full body workout. Wash your own car. Walk or bike to work or to the store if you can. It requires a little extra planning and attention to the weather, but it can take some of the "ho hum" out of the day. Biking is excellent transportation and is easy on joints.

My sand dune hike lies within a state park that is only a ten-minute drive from my house. Search for places like this near where you live and whenever you travel. It adds a whole new dimension to the concept of staying in shape.

DOING EXERCISE RIGHT

Although the benefits of regular exercise are profound, there is a downside. Exercise causes wear and tear on joints and ligaments. The habit of performing a stretching routine prior to starting exercise reduces the potential for injury. Taking care of joints with proper supports in the event of strain or mishap is also very important. Practicing disciplines such as yoga keeps ligaments and muscles loose and improves balance. Proper nutrition keeps bones, ligaments, muscles, and joints healthy.

If you are over fifty, consider giving up your running shoes for a bike. Your joints are too precious to be pounded into the pavement.

The sun can be intense. Protect your skin with clothing and/or moderate use of sunscreen before outdoor activities.

When pursuing recreation activities, set reasonable limits, follow good nutritional habits and drink plenty of water.

The intensity of exercise should be considered less important than the regularity of it.

There is always some discomfort when first beginning an exercise routine. In fact, the first 15 minutes of exercise is downright painful, even for those who exercise regularly. We call this the warm-up period. Breathing is faster and labored, muscles and joints are stiff, and it is just not pleasant. Gradually, breathing slows to a regular pace, everything kind of settles in, and it begins to actually feel pretty good. This "good feeling" is the result of endorphins and other chemicals being generated by exercise. Things stay like that for a while, and then as energy stores run low, fatigue begins to set in. The amount of time between warm up and exhaustion depends on the fitness level of the individual and the intensity of the activity. The sense of feeling good can last for hours after exercise is over.

When you take the step from being sedentary to becoming more active, the sense of feeling good associated with exercise may seem elusive at first, but don't give up: it will come, and your effort will be worthwhile.

HOW MUCH EXERCISE IS ENOUGH?

Official recommendations vary, but in actuality the correct answer is highly dependent on an individual's work requirements and lifestyle. Someone who regularly spends his or her days sitting behind a desk probably needs a good solid hour of formal exercise every single day, whereas a carpenter may need no formal exercise at all. Most of us probably fall somewhere in between. In my profession I may work inside an office, but find that I rarely sit still. Walking up and down halls, standing up, sitting down and constantly moving around is a necessity. Outside of the office I enjoy many types of recreation and am, in general, a very active person. This is the point.

Stay active. Never slow down. When you do is when you will grow old.

See your healthcare provider for personal guidelines before making the step toward an active lifestyle. Regular exercise is often an important part of recovery from significant stress or illness, but the intensity and frequency of exercise should be adjusted according to the degree of debility. An overzealous exercise program in a stressed individual can be very disabling in itself and can worsen the individual's condition.

THE NEGATIVE SIDE OF EXERCISE

Weight-lifting can be beneficial, it but should not make up the majority of your exercise routine. The repetitive motion associated with weight-lifting is hard on ligaments and tendons. It is a common cause of tendonitis. If weight-lifting is part of your exercise routine, stay within reasonable limits and incorporate lifting along with other forms of exercise to achieve a whole body workout. Excessive weight can cause long term or permanent damage to ligaments and muscles. Lightweight hand weights are much safer and tone just as effectively.

Bulking up may add to your looks, but will not add to your lifespan!

One concerning aspect of exercise is the increase in oxidative stress and toxin production caused by the elevated metabolism from energy production. Antioxidants found in healthy diets help protect tissues from damage. Negative effects can be minimized by exercising regularly to stay in shape and building up to higher levels of exercise gradually. This is especially true if you have not exercised in a long time and/or have a history of atherosclerosis or other health problems.

Passions can sometimes carry exercise to an unhealthy extreme. Individuals who pursue competitions such as triathlons, long-distance running, and other extremes often place undue stress on the body. For some individuals, however, endurance training and extreme athleticism are an important part of getting the most out of life. Measures to protect the body during intense recreational activity include training, healthy diet, and brain synchrony exercises. Important dietary considerations include slow-release sources of glucose found in whole grains (especially barley and oats) and beans, healthy fats found in a variety of nuts and healthy sources of protein. Antioxidant protection should come from regular consumption of fresh vegetables, fresh berries, and citrus.

SYNCHRONY OF MIND AND BODY

In order to escape the tiger, the primitive man's brain and body had to be optimally synchronized. This state of being goes beyond simple physical activity. Often referred to as the "runner's high," it is associated with a feeling of being super-human. Many athletes find the feeling addictive and spend their lives pursuing it. Though this feeling can be achieved with any type of vigorous, focused physical activity, it is typically accentuated by the level of skill involved. Fortunately, you do not have to pursue extreme athleticism to enjoy the benefits.

DEFINING THE INTENSITY OF EXERCISE

Breathing defines how excited or relaxed we are at any given moment. Breathing is also the key to optimal exercise, because *how* you breathe during exercise very much influences the experience you will have.

When we're anxious, we breathe through our mouths. Such breathing is quick, shallow, and expands only the upper portion of the lungs. This is how most of us breathe when we exercise, huffing and puffing away and in doing so sending a message to the brain that we are excited. Excitement causes release of adrenaline. Adrenaline prepares the body for a sudden escape from danger, not a long haul. Adrenaline mobilizes glucose stores as the primary source of quick energy. Exercise is less efficient and less comfortable. Glucose stores found in the liver and muscles are burned up in about 20 minutes and are easily replaced by a Snickers bar on the way out of the gym. Net loss in calories equals net gain.

When we are relaxed, we breathe through our noses. Breaths are automatically slower, deeper, and expand the lower portion of the lungs. By shifting to nose-breathing during exercise, we send a message to the brain that we are relaxed. The body settles in for the long haul and fat is burned more readily, while glucose is conserved. Waste products are removed more efficiently. Stamina is increased. Synchronization of the body and mind happens naturally. Exercise becomes meditative and relaxing.

Many long-distance runners use this technique quite effectively. Try it the next time you exercise vigorously. Use mouth-breathing during the warm-up period and then switch over to nose-breathing as soon as possible. Set your level of exercise to your ability to maintain nose-breathing. When you lose the ability to hold on to nose-breathing and have to revert to mouth-breathing, back off on the level of exercise for a couple of minutes until nose-breathing can be resumed. In the beginning, the intensity of exercise may be lower than you are used to, but will gradually build back to normal. With this method you will find exercise to be more effective and enjoyable. Also, it is also hard to hurt yourself with exercise if you stick with nose-breathing.

The concept of controlled breathing as a way to balance the body and mind has been around for ages. The ancient practices of tai chi, Qi gong (Chi gung), yoga, Pilates, and karate all use breathing to improve body fitness and, at the same time, synchronize the body and mind.

The mind and body are separate, but inseparable at the same time. Synchronization of the mind and body through exercise is a way to achieve this higher state of being necessary for optimal health.

CHAPTER 14
A Calm Mind

It is possible to seemingly do everything right from a health point of view and still be unhealthy. Even with a healthy diet, regular exercise and avoidance of toxins, without the last (and most difficult-to-achieve) piece of the puzzle in place, good health is not assured. In modern society, emotional stress may be the largest overall threat that we face. Learning effective tools for minimizing and managing stress is an absolute and essential part of maintaining good health.

The feeling of being "stressed out" is something that we have all experienced and something that some individuals live with every day. Being overly stressed is a symptom of not having control of life's situations, of the behavior of others, of work schedules, and of time itself. Sometimes this feeling is real and sometimes it is the way we perceive life to be. This sense of loss of control contributes to a feeling of hopelessness, the root of depression. Anxiety and depression rob the body of vital energy. Emotional stress affects the hormone systems of the body, suppresses the immune system, and in doing so increases the risk of almost every known disease.

On a biochemical level, emotional stress affects the hormones of the adrenal gland ("stress" gland). We actually have two adrenal glands, located at the top of each of our kidneys.   The middle portion of the gland secretes the hormone epinephrine, better known as "adrenaline." Adrenaline is the hormone that raises our heart rate, heightens our senses, quickens our reflexes, and makes us more alert when we are confronted with a threat. A surge of adrenaline can be life-saving when we are confronted with emergencies. It was the driving force that often kept our primitive man alive when he was confronted by a saber-toothed tiger.

The outer portion of the adrenal gland produces several hormones, with the most important one being cortisol. Cortisol is the "life giving" hormone, for without it we would quickly perish. Cortisol prepares the systems of the body for stress. During times of emotional stress or perceived threat, we secrete more cortisol so the systems of our body will be ready to meet the challenge. Increased cortisol shifts the resources of the body away from everyday concerns such as digesting food and repairing cumulative damage toward handling any immediate threat. *When we have the perception that a threat is always imminent, cortisol secretion remains higher than normal.*

Some stress is a normal part of life and the hormones adrenaline and cortisol allow us to deal quite well with this everyday stress. Stress only becomes a problem when it is overwhelming and, in particular, chronic.

Maintaining persistently elevated levels of adrenaline and cortisol "burns both ends of the candle at once," causing us to age faster and have a higher susceptibility to disease. In shifting the resources of the body away from everyday maintenance and repair, cumulative damage starts to add up and eventually the body starts to deteriorate.

Chronically high levels of cortisol and adrenaline adversely affect all of the hormone systems of the body including the other adrenal hormones controlling fluid balances, the chemical messengers controlling the neurological system, the messengers and hormones of the immune system, the hormones of the gastrointestinal system, and the reproductive hormones. In addition, since people often respond to stress by overeating, there is the added problem of excessive consumption of glucose with associated increased insulin secretion. What a mess! Expect a forecast of high blood pressure, fluctuating blood glucose levels with episodes of hypoglycemia, agitation and irritability, insomnia, gastrointestinal problems, increased risk of heart attack and stroke, infertility, abnormal periods, allergy symptoms and/or many other conditions.

Adrenaline and cortisol secretion are under direct control of the higher brain by way of the HPA axis and autonomic nervous system (see chapter 4). Time schedules, verbal interactions with other people and tedious analytical tasks—all functions of the left hemisphere of the higher brain—are the primary driving force behind stress intolerance. A concerted effort to shift behavior toward right-brain functions is one way of alleviating the perception of stress.

Regularly incorporating right-brain exercises into daily life reduces the perception of being overly stressed and allows stress to be a motivating factor instead of a detriment.

ANXIETY

Adrenaline is useful when it comes in controlled spurts. Adrenaline propels us toward the level of brain synchrony that allows us to deal with everyday stress. But often the stresses of life surpass everyday worries and concerns. Job changes, financial worries, challenges with raising children, personal illness, illnesses of loved ones and negative interactions with other people can be overwhelming. When the stress of life builds to the point of becoming oppressive, anxiety is the result. You can feel it building like a storm. Adrenaline levels start to rise—first as a small cloud, then a squall, and sometimes on to a raging tempest, difficult to control. Once established, it can take days or even weeks to dissipate.

The storm of anxiety depletes the calming neurotransmitters of the brain, leaving the nervous system in an agitated state. Anger, fear, irritability, worry and poor concentration are some of the most typical symptoms of anxiety. Physical manifestations of anxiety can often include gastrointestinal symptoms, chest pain, palpitations and difficulty breathing. Once a person becomes susceptible to anxiety, spontaneous episodes of anxiety known as panic attacks can occur. Sleep disturbances are often associated with anxiety, as dysfunctional fluctuations of adrenaline and cortisol keep the mind abnormally alert.

Recognizing when adrenaline production is getting out of control and defusing the storm before it starts to build are keys to controlling anxiety.

INSOMNIA
Approximately 25-50% of the population suffers from insomnia at some point in their lives. Insomnia is not actually a disease, but a symptom of disease. Insomnia can have many causes. For some people it is chronic pain, for others it is a periodic disruption of normal breathing at night that we call "sleep apnea." Many medications cause disruption of sleep. Food allergies and gastrointestinal dysfunction can cause insomnia. Most commonly, though, it is a reaction to chronic stress, causing disruptions in the normal hormonal and neurotransmitter pathways associated with sleep.

The same chemicals that keep us calm during the day also keep us asleep at night. The main calming neurotransmitter of the brain is gamma amino butyric acid, called GABA for short. There are different GABA receptors in the brain; some keep us calm but awake during the day and others maintain sleep at night. The exact mechanism by which all this happens is not completely understood; in simple terms, it appears that stress, anxiety, worry and even pain "use up" GABA and leave the brain in an excited state. An alert mind is associated with increased adrenaline secretion. Cortisol follows adrenaline and keeps the brain alert as well. A vicious, self-perpetuating cycle is created. Sleep is next to impossible in states of increased adrenaline and cortisol production.

There does seem to be a genetic predisposition for insomnia. Perhaps the distant ancestors of today's poor sleepers were the easily-roused survivors who alerted the others when danger was near. In our hyper-stimulated world, however, being such a light sleeper can become an unhealthy aggravation. Stressful lifestyles, stimulants such as caffeine, artificial lighting, computers, televisions, and odd work schedules are just some of the contributors to disruption of the normal hormones involved with sleep. On top of it all, it seems to worsen as we age.

For me, insomnia has always been the most obvious outward manifestation of stress. By age 45, burning both ends of the candle balancing a busy obstetrical practice with the rest of life caught up with me. Even with improved dietary habits and regular exercise, my health slowly began to deteriorate. At first I turned to the world of conventional medicine for help, but quickly found that my body and synthetic medicines are not compatible. (Retrospectively, there is little doubt that medical therapy hindered and prolonged recovery.) Ultimately, I took matters into my own hands and set forth on a self-directed course of rehabilitative therapy. A complete (and more sensible) lifestyle change, carefully chosen natural therapies, and years of practicing relaxation techniques gradually brought me back to a level of normal health and a regular good night's sleep.

The nature of sleep is very complex. For most mammals, cycles of sleep are obviously tied to cycles of night and day, but they are also a product of how a certain animal evolved. Dolphins, horses, rabbits, and tigers all have very different sleep cycles from those of humans. In most animals, episodes of deep sleep are necessary to allow the resources of the body to be focused totally on healing.

In humans there are four different stages of sleep as defined by brain wave patterns and another type of sleep, defined by rapid eye movements, that we call "REM" sleep. In terms analogous to a computer, REM sleep is the time when we put all of our files back in order for the next day. You can think of dreams as your screen saver. Stages one and two are lighter stages of sleep. Healing occurs most intensely when people are in stages three and four of sleep, at which point they are very hard to arouse. We tend to spend less and less time in stages three and four as we age.

Humans typically go in and out of the different cycles of sleep throughout the night, spending only a few hours in stage three and four sleep during an eight-hour rest period. In our world today this would seem to be quite inefficient. Certainly diving directly into three or four hours of intense deep sleep and being done with it would be practical, but this is not how we evolved. In distant times, becoming almost comatose for several hours at a time would have been an almost certain invitation to be eaten by something large; for survival purposes we learned to catch short intervals of deep sleep here and there. This seemingly inefficient sleep pattern is the one that we must live with today.

The good news is that insomnia really is just a symptom and will resolve if all of the causes are removed. Imbalances in neurotransmitters rectify themselves if given the right opportunity. Sometimes proper diagnosis involves a trip to a sleep clinic for disorders like sleep apnea, restless legs syndrome or narcolepsy, but for the everyday type of insomnia most common in our fast-paced world, the treatment is a matter of normalizing hyper-stimulated adrenal and nervous system functions. Interestingly, the key to a good night's sleep hinges mainly on how effectively we manage stress during the day.

A good night's sleep is an essential component of good health. Sleep is the time when the operating systems of the body are being fine-tuned, general maintenance functions are being performed and the immune system is functioning at peak level. Without sleep, all systems of the body suffer and the incidence of disease increases.

CHRONIC FATIGUE

When you push the stress button hard enough or for long enough, it all adds up. This situation can occur at any age, but is more common after forty. With chronic or excessive stress, adrenaline keeps pushing the body, even when it cannot be pushed any further; however, at some point, the resources of the body become taxed to the extent that a normal response to stress is impossible. Having lost the ability to keep up, the normal rhythmic fluctuations of cortisol become dysfunctional. Without normal cortisol secretion, the body loses the ability to appropriately manage day-to-day functions.

When fatigue regularly reaches a certain level it becomes known as chronic fatigue syndrome. Though fatigue is the most obvious symptom, chronic infections, anxiety, sleep disturbances, weakness and depression are typical. When accompanied by muscle and ligament pain, the condition is called fibromyalgia. Usually there is an inciting factor such as traumatic physical stress, prolonged emotional stress, severe work stress, or possibly a viral or bacterial illness; nevertheless, once established, adrenal dysfunction is always part of the picture. All systems of the body are adversely affected, including (and especially) the immune system. Many chronic conditions including pain syndromes and autoimmune diseases may be related to this same mechanism.

Chronic fatigue is, as much as anything else, a manifestation of imbalances within the entire hypothalamic-pituitary-adrenal axis. As you remember from chapter 4, the HPA axis allows us to respond to change. Without this balance, all systems in the body are affected. Adrenal dysfunction and fatigue always go hand in hand. Thyroid dysfunction is commonly associated with chronic fatigue. Chronic fatigue is common in menopausal females. Effective therapy for chronic fatigue always includes support of hormonal function and reducing all stress factors, such that normal balance can return to all functional systems of the body.

DEPRESSION

Mood is normally a pendulum swing between happy and sad, a natural reflection of life's ups and downs. Mood becomes depression when life's pendulum becomes hung on the down side. This happens to all of us from time to time, with some people being more susceptible to depression than others. The downside of life is often a matter of perception: is the glass half full or half empty?

Depression can be defined in chemical terms. Sadness, in reaction to life's events, affects the balance of neurotransmitters within the brain. Many neurotransmitters are involved, but *serotonin*, the so-called "mood hormone," is the most often considered. Hormone imbalances associated with depression can usually be related to a specific cause—intense or prolonged anxiety, exhaustion from severe insomnia, a tragic occurrence, prolonged illness or hormonal changes associated with menopause, for instance—but occasionally depression seems to happen even in the absence of such inciting factors.

The causes of depression may be present but not readily obvious. Diets high in sugar and processed starch are associated with higher rates of depression. It is also noteworthy that toxins produced by abnormal strains of bacteria in the GI tract have shown ties to depression. Exposure to toxins in general may adversely affect the hormone systems of body enough to contribute to depression.

Some individuals have a genetic predisposition toward depression and are therefore more apt to feel depressed even in the absence of inciting factors. For them, the glass is always half empty. Genes cannot be altered and this is a situation where properly administered medicinal therapy can be life-changing. Another situation where pharmaceutical therapy may be indicated is in the case of individuals having wider "pendulum swings" than average. Referred to as manic-depression or bipolar disorder, this condition is also a function of genetic susceptibility.

Regular exercise, avoidance of processed foods, appropriate counseling and support groups are as important as drug therapy for management of depression.

HORMONE-DRIVEN STRESS INTOLERANCE

The normal cyclic reproductive cycle that a woman experiences each and every month is closely tied to all other functions in the body. Dysfunction or abnormal fluctuations of hormones within this cycle can cause stress intolerance, fatigue, mood changes, anxiety, depression and swelling, a collection of symptoms commonly known as premenstrual syndrome. Though some individuals do seem to have a genetic predisposition, symptoms are often tied to poor nutrition, exposure to hormonal active toxins, poor sleep habits and poor stress management skills. Improvements in health habits and stress modification are often associated with resolution of symptoms.

Cessation of reproductive function, referred to as menopause, is a natural part of a woman's life, but the hormonal changes that occur during and leading up to menopause can be the trigger for stress intolerance, anxiety, insomnia, fatigue, depression, or all of the above at the same time. Most of the symptoms will pass with time, but appropriately administered hormone therapy or alternative therapies can ease symptoms and help to save a job, a relationship, or even a life.

Though less well defined, a gradual decrease in normal male reproductive hormones with age can be associated with symptoms fatigue, stress intolerance and mood changes. Poor nutrition, exposure to hormonally active toxins, poor sleep habits and poor stress management skills can often be defined as inciting factors. Hormone function often normalizes along with symptoms when these inciting factors are removed.

DEFUSING EVERYDAY STRESS

The anticipation of stress is usually worse than stress itself. To get rid of stress, or at least the perception of it, we must periodically turn-off the very verbal, analytical and time-conscious left brain (as was discussed in Chapter 12). In doing so, we connect with the all-important hormone regulatory system in a calming way. Adrenaline production is decreased and the rhythms of cortisol secretion are normalized.

Turning off the left side of the brain is not necessarily an easy task in our very left-brain dominant world. Effectively suppressing the left brain and allowing right-brain functions to flourish takes practice and effort, but there is a reward: reconnecting with the creative, calmer side of your mind not only reduces stress but also balances life and allows you to reach your full potential as a human being.

Wandering off into the right side of your brain every now and then is a perfectly acceptable way of achieving lasting mental health. Some people do it in a big way, such as by casting off for a three-year cruise around the world, but such drastic steps are rarely necessary. Many hobbies (drawing, needlepoint, woodworking, fishing, sailing and gardening are just a few examples) require skills that originate from the right side of the brain.

If you do not have a hobby, consider adopting one. If you already have a hobby, consider making it a more prominent part of your life.

There are many different ways of dealing with stress, from simple to complex. Any of the right-brained exercises found in Chapter 12 can be beneficial. Your approach to life—how you deal with people and situations—does matter, and a positive attitude is more important than anything else. Though we cannot control all of life's variables, we do have choices. Choices that reduce personal stress have the potential to improve not only our own lives but also the lives of everyone around us.

Listen to your body. The tension associated with the building storm of stress and anxiety can rise rapidly. Recognizing the early signs of tension is the first step in learning how to defuse stress.

RELEASING MUSCLE TENSION

One of the most obvious effects of built-up stress is muscle tension. Whether due to an injury or just from walking outside on an extra cold day, we all tend to brace against pain by reflexively tightening up the muscles of the back, neck, and shoulders and breathing in a rapid, shallow fashion. We brace against the building discomfort of stress in the same way, except that muscle tension becomes a normal state of being instead of just a transient phenomenon. Chronic back, neck, and shoulder pain, as well as tension headaches, can be the result of built-up muscle tension.

Do a tension assessment. At any given moment you are probably more tense than you realize. Learn to recognize the feeling of your body bracing against stress.

How is your breathing? Is it shallow and quick or deep and slow? Are you breathing just within the upper part of your chest or down into the deeper chest and abdomen?

How cold are your hands and feet? Adrenaline causes constriction of peripheral blood vessels. A relaxed state is associated with warm feet and hands.

What is your focus of attention—intensely narrow or more diffuse?

How tense are the muscles of the shoulders and neck?

Every time you feel stress building, resist the urge to tighten up.

As much as an uptight posture is a sign of tension, maintenance of a relaxed posture makes it almost impossible to be uptight.

Relax your abdomen and roll your shoulders. Loosen them up and let them fall until limp. Breathing will automatically slow down and become deeper.

Remind yourself a hundred times a day if necessary:
Relax the shoulders and breathe deeply.

This simple little exercise is amazingly effective. Every time you remind yourself to relax the shoulders, also get in the habit of taking three deep breaths through the lower part of your abdomen. Not only will you feel more relaxed but you will also ward off tension headaches and neck pain.

Movement is another effective method of diffusing tension. If you have a sedentary job, do not sit in one place anymore than necessary. Move around. Walk everywhere you can. During a lunch break, make a habit of going for a walk or doing some kind of physical activity. Activity gets blood flowing and diffuses the focus of concentration. Try an exercise ball (see Chapter 13).

Stretching is an excellent way to diffuse stress and relieve tension. The discipline of yoga is the most commonly practiced form of stretching found today. Though formal classes are very beneficial for beginners, the stretching poses can be done nearly anywhere. Once several basic poses are learned, they can be incorporated into daily routines.

ESCAPE FROM THE STORM

Much of stress has more to do with how we <u>perceive</u> the world to be than how it actually is.

There are people who have endured greater stress than you or I will ever know and lived to tell about it.

Life is synonymous with challenge and conflict. How we <u>deal</u> with challenge and conflict involves learned behaviors. As much as life teaches us to be anxious, we can also learn to be calm, even in the face of great adversity.

Even the most anxious individual has moments of absolute calmness. Learning how to cultivate moments of calmness in the face of stress is an essential skill for overcoming anxiety and gaining control over stressful situations. Individuals who regularly practice relaxation techniques handle any type of stress better.

The issue of overcoming stress and anxiety is about regaining control. Sometimes even the perception of regaining control is enough to defuse stress and anxiety. Learning effective tools for diffusing stress is essential for maintaining good health.

Moments of complete calmness interspersed throughout the day are important not only for reducing anxiety but also for regaining control of life. Methods for mastering spontaneous relaxation have been around for most of eternity. Meditation, yoga, and prayer are time-tested activities that all induce a relaxed state. Newer and more defined techniques such as progressive relaxation, autogenics, self-hypnosis, and brain synchrony exercises focus specifically on relaxation.

The common denominator for all relaxation techniques lies in producing a shift from the analytical thought of the left brain to the more abstract thought processes of the right brain. The most notable feature of an over-excited mind is the constant stream of verbal thought. All effective relaxation techniques block or slow the flow of verbal thought from the left brain. In doing so, the body relaxes and adrenaline levels decrease. The functions of the body normalize and the healing potential of the body increases. Attention to breathing is a good place to start this process.

LEARNING HOW TO BREATHE

Attention to breathing synchronizes many of the functions of the body. Our breath flows as life-giving oxygen into the blood, which carries it to every part of the body, where it provides a critical part of energy production in cells.

The first step in learning how to relax spontaneously is learning controlled breathing. Breathing is unique in that it is an "autonomic" or automatic response that can also be controlled with voluntary actions. When we control our breathing it ties into other autonomic responses. Slowing the rate of breathing is associated with a decreased heart rate, decreased blood pressure, and—very importantly—decreased adrenaline levels. Slowed breathing also is associated with increased production of endorphins, those wonderful internal chemicals that improve our sense of well-being.

Most of us breathe with our chest muscles. The more uptight we are, the shorter and shallower the breath becomes, and the more tension there is in the shoulders and neck. When relaxed, we use abdominal breathing: instead of using the chest wall muscles, we are then using mainly the diaphragm.

Observe this by first lying comfortably on your back. Control and slow your breathing to an easy rhythm. Place one hand on the abdomen, close to the belly button. As you breathe, try to keep the chest wall still and pull air into the lungs by expanding the abdominal muscles. Your hand should rise and fall with each breath. Breathing should be done through the nose, not through the mouth. Ideally, each inhalation (inspiration) should be shorter than the exhalation (expiration). Expiration should be long and drawn out.

It takes a little practice. Relaxation happens quickly, even after only a few minutes. Focused concentration on breathing by itself is a simple and profoundly effective relaxation technique that can be done nearly anytime you have a few minutes—while waiting at a stoplight, during a break at the office, or while waiting for water to boil.

Try this simple breathing exercise. Using abdominal breathing, try to extend your breath for as long as possible without holding your breath. Inspiration and expiration should be equal. At first attempts, your inspiration and expiration will be about 5-7 seconds each, but your goal is to extend each to 15 seconds, resulting in only 2 complete breaths in one minute. Don't strain. Make it easy and comfortable. Work up to 15 seconds slowly. You can practice this one anywhere, even at a stoplight.

Another simple breathing exercise is sequential count-to-ten. Using abdominal breathing of normal length, begin counting each breath. Count first to up to 2 and then start over, 1-2-3. Next 1-2-3-4, starting over with a higher number with each sequence up to 10. It takes more concentration than you can imagine. Completion of two sequences of 10 often results in deep relaxation with lowered pulse rate and normalized blood pressure.

RELAXING THE BODY

We tend to take the functions of the body for granted. Becoming more attuned to the functions of the body is a very important step in synchrony of the body and mind. Awareness of muscle tension and learning how to relax the different muscle groups of the body is a way to monitor how the body is doing overall. Assessing muscle tension and responding by relaxing muscles can be done on a limited basis throughout the day. Progressive muscle relaxation, a formal technique, requires more time but is a powerful tool for health.

The basic goal of this technique is complete relaxation of each of the muscle groups in the body. Start in a supine position (i.e., on your back) with support of the head and legs. Establish controlled, relaxed abdominal breathing. Progressively concentrate on each area of the body independently. Work up from the feet to the calves to the thighs, hips, back, and abdomen. Progress to the chest, shoulders, upper arms, lower arms, and then finally to the hands. Don't forget the neck, ears, face, and cheeks. Last of all, imagine your forehead becoming as smooth and flat as possible. It is helpful to imagine a feeling of warmth and heaviness.

If relaxing muscles seems difficult or if you are particularly uptight and tense, another technique makes use of progressive tightening of each of the muscle groups independently—as tightly as possible—and then relaxing. In the beginning, it may be helpful to purchase an audio tape or CD on progressive relaxation. With practice, muscle relaxation will become almost spontaneous.

RELAXING THE MIND

Now that the body is relaxed, it's time to work on relaxing the mind. The practice of calming the mind is most often referred to as meditation.

Meditation is an oasis that is always there, always within reach, but sometimes hard to grasp. It can free you of worry and the constant stream of intruding thoughts. It does not have to involve odd positions, weird music, or chanting. It can be anything you want it to be.

There are a number of different forms of meditation and many different perspectives on how to meditate. There is nothing magical or mystical about meditation. Simple daydreaming is a form of meditation. The most intense form of meditation is when all attention is focused on nothing. Clearing the mind of *all* thoughts, however, is extremely difficult and requires a great amount of practice. Most of us need to focus our attention on something. This can really be anything: our breathing, counting sheep, a candle flame, a monotonous sound, a mental image, or even a thought. Again, the common denominator is slowing or stopping the flow of words, such that a shift from left-brain dominance to right brain function occurs.

The most frustrating part of meditation, especially for beginners, is making the shift happen and knowing when it occurs. The most effortless way I have found to achieve this goal is through the techniques of "Open Focus" as described by Dr. Les Fehmi. Dr. Fehmi is one of early pioneers of neuro-biofeedback; with thirty years of experience in practice and research, he has refined these techniques quite well. They can be discovered through his book *Open Focus Brain* or through resources at his website: *www.openfocus.com* or *www.openfocus.biz.* Not only are these methods effective, but, more importantly, they are easy to master.

Open focus is a good place to start for many people, but it should be noted that there are many forms of meditation or spontaneous relaxation, and you have to find the one that works best for you. Meditation can involve formal techniques, but it also can be very informal. Monotonous activities or tasks, such as knitting or woodworking, can consume the mind enough to push unwanted thoughts away and encourage a relaxed state of mind. Simply focusing on something calming is also effective. A favorite CD of mine is of ocean waves crashing on a California beach. It's easy to focus on the waves and imagine actually being there.

During meditation and relaxation, outside thoughts often try to intrude. How much they intrude depends on the complexity of life and the stress level at that particular time. When thoughts intrude, recognize them, gently push them away or just notice them without allowing them to be the dominant thought, and refocus on the topic of concentration. If thoughts are overwhelming, stop, get up, and walk around. Get a snack or a drink and then start all over again.

THE REGULAR PRACTICE OF MEDITATION

Sages, monks and some spiritual leaders may meditate for five hours every day, but their goals are very different from yours and mine. From a health point of view, preventing excessive flow of adrenaline is our main objective. Some days, life is not very challenging and the need to meditate may not be there at all.

On other, more stressful days we may desperately need a full five hours of meditation. Here lies the rub: on the most stressful days we tend to have the least time to step away. This is why incorporation of spontaneous relaxation into our daily lives and the regular practice of meditation are so important.

In an overly stressful world, individuals with any significant anxiety maintain a hypersensitive adrenal gland. Even the thought of a stressful situation sends adrenaline levels soaring. For health and happiness, this over-active gland needs to be tamed and the most positive way to do it is through regularly practiced meditation or self-relaxation. As with any skill, the body and mind respond to training. With training, the gland becomes less hypersensitive and stressful situations are better-tolerated.

Training means daily practice. It may require getting help from others. This can be in the form of audio/video resources or it can be direct training from an experienced individual. At the very least, make a pledge to sit quietly and simply focus on breathing for 10 minutes two times daily for eight weeks. Don't try too hard. Let it come naturally. If you stay with it, this simple pledge will change your life. As meditation becomes more comforting and comfortable, connecting with your inner self will become an essential part of your daily life.

RESOURCES FOR MEDITATION

Meditation should be comfortable and something to look forward to. It should not be thought of as a chore and should not have special requirements for time and place. Peace and quiet are helpful, but not essential; I have had some success with meditation in the middle of a busy airport.

Position is also less important than some sources would have you think. The classic "lotus" position works well for some people, but any sitting or lying position is acceptable. This can be in a lounge chair, lying on the floor, lying in bed, or even sitting on your porch steps.—anywhere that is comfortable for you. Remember, the primary purpose of meditation is relieving stress and therefore it should not be a stressful experience.

There are many excellent resources in book, CD and DVD formats for help in mastering these techniques. An Internet search for "spontaneous relaxation" or "meditation" will bring up a plethora of choices. These guided sessions will help your practice become more regular and effective. Another very useful and novel adjunct is special music with brain waves super-imposed. This work was pioneered by Dr Jeffrey Thompson and can be readily found on the Internet. He has composed a variety of different formats for encouraging concentration, meditation, and even sleep. I have found them to be very effective tools and use them regularly to arrive at a deeper state of relaxation more quickly. An MP3 player is another tool I have found to be helpful. A large number of relaxation CD's can be loaded into these portable devices.

Find yourself a special place.
The concept of a special place is an important one. For some it is an icy mountain top in Patagonia; for others, it is a quiet garden in the back corner of a yard. Generally it is a place of peace and solitude, away from everything and everyone. You can have more than one. Going there frequently can help maintain your sanity even during stressful times. Traveling to special places can be a lot of fun also. Some people spend entire vacations seeking out special places in natural areas such as our national parks. Sometimes just knowing that these places exist is enough to give you a sense of peace. A special place can be the object of meditation even if you cannot go there.

Why are gurus always pictured sitting on a mountain top? The symbolism is not lost on those who meditate regularly. The mountaintop represents being above all worry and stress. It is a place where you can go at any time.

Don't miss the "moments in-between."
Have you ever looked back at the end of a particularly busy day, with feelings of being stressed-out and fatigued, only to realize that the day was filled with minimal accomplishments? Part of the problem was that you missed the "moments in-between." So often we spend so much of our time rushing from one thing to the next that we spend a lot of time waiting. Waiting for stop lights, waiting for appointments, and waiting for other people seem to be functions of modern life, but this has the potential of being the most valuable time of the day. Most of us spend it anxiously anticipating where we want to go or what we want to do, but it could be used for planning some other important part of our lives or, possibly more importantly, just meditating.

When life gets to be a bit too much, take time to pay attention to this particular moment. If you can, sit down and look for the good in this moment. Every moment of every day has something good about it. Let all other concerns slip away and for this brief period of time just appreciate being alive. Try to get in the habit of going through this simple thought process several times each day. If each moment is cherished for the good that it has to offer, then your outlook on life in general can only be positive.

HEALING MEDITATION

This special type of meditation has the potential of being one of the most powerful forms of healing. Emotional stress is a common part of chronic disease and cancer. This is true especially of conditions that cause pain. Regaining that sense of control is profoundly important in healing. Support from friends, family, and positive interactions with caregivers can increase control. Meditation, even in a basic form, is a very powerful tool for regaining a sense of control and decreasing the stress response associated with disease. Regular meditation provides an escape from pain, outside stressors, suffering, and discomfort. Having the ability to escape provides an increased sense of control over the situation. As an added benefit, adrenal function is improved and the immune system gets a boost.

The focus of healing meditation becomes the illness itself. This may be an injured part of the body or an area of pain. It may be a place in the body where cancer exists or it may be the body as a whole as in the case of a disease such as chronic fatigue or multiple sclerosis. Prayer can be included as a very important part of this meditation.

On a deeper level, healing meditation takes on a more spiritual quality. Beyond food, beyond exercise, beyond medications, beyond supplements, beyond herbal therapies and beyond simple relaxation, deep meditation is the key to healing. A deeper understanding of life and "self" must happen before true healing can occur. This understanding must reach a point where love of life goes beyond fear of losing it. Seek out an experienced individual to use as a guide when pursuing this level of meditation.

THE SPIRITUAL SIDE OF MEDITATION

Life is difficult and bad things happen. Meditation can be an avenue for escape from the difficulties of life, but it can be more. Anyone who meditates regularly will admit that there is something else; something that is beyond who we are. Describing it any further is difficult. The religions of the world have been trying to do so for all of time. It may be best to just accept that it is so and take comfort in the fact that we are never truly alone. Peace and comfort are always at hand, even in the most adverse of situations. Meditation, done without so much as a word or a thought, is the way to touch this concept most deeply.

A GOOD NIGHT'S SLEEP

The key to sleeping well at night is consistently having stress-controlled days. Regularly practicing methods to maintain low adrenaline levels during the day is very conducive to falling asleep normally at night and not waking in the middle of the night. Beyond stress reduction, here is some sound advice for restoring normal sleep cycles:

Avoid caffeine and other stimulants completely. Most beverages are available in caffeine-free versions. Look for hidden stimulants in supplements and foods. Be aware that many if not most medications disrupt stage 3 and 4 sleep. Avoid alcoholic beverages in the evening. Alcohol itself is a sedative, but its metabolites are stimulants. Expect to be wide-eyed and awake about 3 to 4 hours later.

Be very particular about bedtime routines. Try to set a pattern of going to bed and getting up at the same time each day. Respect normal day and night cycles as much as possible. If you work an odd shift, use darkening shades to completely darken the room where you sleep.

Avoid excessive light stimulation in the evening. Use low lights and turn off televisions and especially computer screens after 8 pm. This will help stimulate natural melatonin levels. Try reading before bedtime or practicing relaxation techniques.

Always sleep in a very dark room.

Avoid exercise after 8 pm except for relaxing yoga routines.

Sleeping pills would seem like the simplest solution to insomnia, but there is absolutely no substitute for natural sleep. Sleep-inducing medications are often useful for transient insomnia, but are never ideal for long-term therapy. Taking sleeping pills will quickly prevent your body from returning to a natural rhythm of sleep. If you use sleeping pills chronically, be prepared to "pay the piper," as all sleep-inducing medications suppress natural sleep mechanisms of the body and tolerance develops. At some point you will have to stop taking the sleeping pills and it may not be easy.

When searching for solutions to chronic insomnia, look for a healthcare practitioner who is skilled in evaluating and treating different forms of insomnia without using potent pharmaceuticals. Supplements are available that are not only safe but also effective, if combined with the proper lifestyle modifications.

SOMETIMES YOU HAVE TO ROW YOUR OWN BOAT

Life is hard. Life is hard, not for just a few but for each of us. The difficulties of life are different for each individual—we each have our own boat to row. Good or bad, our destiny shapes who we are. We must learn to accept our destiny and make the absolute best out of it. Lamenting what could have been and might have been only makes suffering worse.

Stress seems to always be pushing us. Often the push is uncomfortable, but the direction of the push is a matter of outlook. Those who are able to find a silver lining generally end up with a positive outcome. Following the push of stress to a positive end requires vision, acceptance, tolerance and sometimes humility.

Being caught up in the vicious pace of a rat-race lifestyle often causes suffering. Relaxation techniques and meditation are effective tools for dealing with emotional stress in the short term, but an overly stressful lifestyle needs a long-term solution. The first order of business in this regard is putting things into perspective. Often our life situation is not as bad as we perceive it to be. The second is recognizing that we have more control over our life situation than we often allow. Simple changes in the way we go about life can dramatically reduce daily stress.

Learn to accept your own pathway in life, even though it may be different from those around you.

THINGS THAT SEEM TO BE THREATENING, BUT ARE NOT

Anxiety is synonymous with fear—fear of the unknown, fear of things that seem beyond our abilities, fear of losing control; it all adds up. Be reassured that obstacles are rarely as big as they seem and things are rarely as bad as your mind makes them out to be.

Think of all the obstacles you have overcome in your life. You will overcome the ones before you just as well. Our abilities are always greater than we give ourselves credit for. Remind yourself of this every day.

STRESS CAUSED BY OTHER PEOPLE

Interacting with other people can certainly be a source of stress. When it comes to negative interactions with bosses and co-workers, make sure that your own fears, anxiety or arrogance are not contributing to the problem. In dealing with someone whose behavior you deem unacceptable, recognize that though your paths are presently intertwined, your destinies may be quite different. Things will inevitably change over time.

No matter how hard you try, you will never please everyone.

Responding negatively to negativism can only make a bad situation worse.

Make the best of the present and prepare for the future. If your present work situation is unacceptable, use it as a platform for learning about people in general and yourself and move toward change in the future. Use the techniques found in this chapter for dealing with stress to make the best of the situation until change can happen. Who knows, one day you might be running the company.

Stand up for what you believe in, but pick your battles well. Much stress and anxiety is created over trivial matters. Some things need to just roll off your shoulders. Before acting on a matter, ask yourself whether it is significant enough for the bother. Does action have the potential to cause more grief in the long run? If the matter is significant, look for positive avenues for resolution, such that everyone wins in the end.

Do not let others pull you down. Accept that you only have so much influence on those around you. Emotionally unstable individuals tend to drain energy from the people closest to them. In certain situations distance is required. It is also impossible for you to help someone else unless you are emotionally stable. When it comes to children, know that the greatest influence you have is by the example you set. If you have set a poor example, be willing to tolerate the consequences.

Stress is often caused by having to deal with illness in a loved one. It is draining, both physically and emotionally, to care for someone who is very ill, especially if that person is in pain. That person may not be able to change his or her situation and may become increasingly dependent on you. Do whatever you can to help out, but remember to reserve some time and space for yourself. Get help from others whenever possible. You do not have to do it all yourself. Keeping up your strength is essential for helping someone else.

SELF-IMPOSED STRESS

Sometimes we voluntarily impose stress on ourselves. Stress is often required to "get ahead" and improve our standing in life, but the vicious cycle of working harder to gain more can become self-defeating. It is better to have a well-defined plan with specific and reasonable goals in mind.

The soccer mom (dad) syndrome. Many kids follow a schedule that would challenge the CEO of a major corporation. Many parents live vicariously and follow an equally demanding routine. Even "down time" is a scheduled event.

We are teaching our kids not only to be competitive, but also to be anxious and uptight. In the process, we are making life, in general, overly structured and uncomfortable.

Typically, when I counsel patients suffering from mental stress, I often find that an overly structured life is contributing to their misery. They are caught up in a vortex, and breaking free is nearly impossible. When I suggest a less structured lifestyle, meditation, or casual exercise, they quickly insist that they lack time.

Outside of normal sleep, unstructured time is the most health-friendly time of the day. Adrenaline decreases and contentment increases. Exercise is much more beneficial and enjoyable if not relegated to a time slot. Unstructured does not necessarily mean nonproductive. It just means not *having* to produce or to follow any particular time schedule. Any type of activity is more meaningful if not constrained by time limits and necessity.

Build space into your life for unstructured time. It can be used to accomplish a goal, such as better health, but sometimes it can best be used to accomplish nothing more than to take time to reflect on life.

DEALING WITH TRAUMATIC STRESS

If you have been through a harrowing experience, first you must stabilize your life by eliminating as many stress factors as possible and then rebuild slowly from there. Gather all resources at your disposal. Lean on others you can trust as much as you can without being an imposition. Get help with the kids. Take time off from work, if possible. Manage only absolute necessities and let everything else go.

Your daily goal should be to keep your adrenaline levels as low as possible. With time, the chemical imbalances in the brain that cause anxiety and depression will resolve. Moderate exercise is important, but activities should be pleasant and positive. Walking for 30 minutes is a simple but surprisingly effective antidepressant.

Avoid news media so that you can focus on recovery. The Middle East and Brittany Spears' latest exploits are not your primary concerns. Read books and watch movies or television only if the topics are uplifting or positive. Above all, avoid associating with negative people; instead, seek out individuals with positive outlooks.

Practice the exercises found in this chapter and make them part of your life. Fill your life with as much positive thought and feeling as possible.

LETTING GO OF STRESS

The feeling of letting go of all stress and all negative emotions is like none other. You may have felt it after walking away from a difficult exam (especially if you felt good about it) or maybe at the beginning of a vacation, as you distanced yourself from the regular responsibilities and work. It may have occurred after intense exercise, with the buildup of natural endorphins in your system. You may have also felt it just after the first beer on Saturday night (but less so with each additional bottle). Release from stress and anxiety can occur with a dose of Xanax or Valium, but in an artificial kind of way. The effects are transient and each subsequent dose provides less and less of a response.

Being able to feel this kind of release is a very important part of health. Unfortunately, having a feeling of total release does not happen spontaneously very often. All of the suggestions and exercises found in this chapter are designed to reduce stress, but sometimes you just have to let go. As a summary and a reminder, I will leave you with the following inspiration. Read it daily, if you like. If you follow it and believe in it, it will become a powerful force in your life.

I will look for the positive in every moment of every hour of every day, for negative emotions are a waste of precious time.

I will work to negotiate a better situation for myself in life, but at the same time I will not take advantage of others or cause others ill will.

I will set reasonable goals for myself and work every day to accomplish those goals, recognizing that some days will be better than others. I am only human.

I will let go of things that I can do nothing about, because I know that worrying about things beyond my control is very destructive.

I will look for the good in every individual, but I will not allow myself to be abused or taken advantage of.

I will let go of negative people in my life. I will either help them change or leave them behind.

I will let go of stress, for it can only do me harm.

CONCLUSION, and a new beginning...

Change is part of the mystery of life. About the time you decide that life is not worth living, change happens and everything falls into place. Looking backwards, you realize that the positive change that finally occurred would never have been possible without the pain that preceded it.

Controlling all of life's variables is impossible. We do, however, have control over many aspects of our lives, often more than we realize or take advantage of. Choices are as much a part of life as change. The choices we make when confronted with change will greatly influence our total life experience. Pursuing choices that positively influence our chances for good health influence our life experience more than any other factor.

YOU are the only one who can change your life.

Time's wasting.

Start making a plan now!

CREATING YOUR OWN ISLAND

It is possible to create your own "island" within the world in which you live. You may already have some ideas about how you would like yours to be. Creating an island within your own world is a matter of making choices— choices about the types of food you are willing to purchase, the amount of time you are willing to devote to work, the type of job you are willing to have, and how much personal time you set aside for your own health and well-being.

It is a material world and your island will require certain material things, but priorities are important. Things that you cannot do without—food, water, companionship, shelter and money—can be considered essentials. Your world should be structured such that these essentials are safe from most threats, but they also should be maintained at a level that does not cause stress. In other words, if you are working three jobs to afford something, then maybe it is time to reprioritize. Luxury items should always contribute to your life in a positive way, but should never cause significant stress, even if lost completely.

THE CONCEPT OF WORK

Work (paid or unpaid) can help define who we are. There is something to be said for a job well done. Though it can define you, it also can consume you. Too many people struggle in jobs they do not enjoy to be able to afford things they do not really need. Find a job that you can enjoy. Job satisfaction can help to elevate your mood, reduce your stress and improve your health.

MATERIAL THINGS: PUTTING YOUR WANTS INTO PERSPECTIVE

There is nothing wrong with getting ahead in life, but always keep your priorities in order. The first priority for happiness is health, for without good health nothing else really matters. The second priority is happiness in love and relationships, for which devotion and self-sacrifice are required. Well behind the first two, a third priority includes material things. Such "wants" are often a source of misery instead of pleasure when not placed into proper perspective.

When an object of desire is sought for the positive experiences it may provide, the outcome is generally good.

When an object of desire is coveted just for the sake of having it, the repercussions are generally negative.

Ask yourself, does the object you desire have the potential to enrich your life?

An object of desire does not necessarily have to be material. You may desire a higher position in your employment for improved status and better pay; but is the increased stress worth it? Will it have a positive or an adverse effect on other aspects of your life?

Keep your financial concerns simple. If frugality has not been your practice, consolidate all of your debts into one loan and make a pledge to never to become over-extended again.

Much of life's misery arises from the never ending pursuit of unrealistic goals and perpetual dissatisfaction with the present moment.

In the long run, strive for realistic goals and be willing to accept some compromises.

The game is always changing. Learn to accept change and to change with change.

Contentment means not wanting for anything.
True happiness is wanting everything you have.

IT'S A MATTER OF TIME

We each have twenty-four hours in every day, but rarely does it seem to be enough. At least eight hours should be allotted for sleep and many of us are obligated to eight hours of work. If work consumes more than eight hours on most days, then it may be time to reevaluate your concept of work. After work and sleep, about eight hours are left for all of life's other activities.

Of those eight hours, a certain amount of time will be necessary for preparing food, paying bills, caring for spouses/children and other life concerns, but some of it should be left as unstructured time. Unstructured time is not the same as wasted time. Unstructured time is your personal time for activities such as exercise, meditation, reading, writing or other hobbies. Unlike sitting in front of a television, these activities are productive and contribute to your health in a positive way.

Unstructured time is the most important time of the day. It is your time to gain on life instead being beaten down by it. Health and happiness are often directly related to the amount of unstructured time allowed each day. When planning priorities, unstructured time should always have a place near the top.

LIVING WITHIN YOUR GENES

For health, the limiting factor is often our genes. Our genetic makeup defines our tolerance to foods, our threshold for disease, how we deal with stress and, to a certain extent, our outlook on life. Going against your genes will only get you into trouble. Listen to your body and do what feels right. If certain foods make you feel bad (even if they taste good), it's time to let them go. The same goes for many other aspects of life. Pursue activities that make you feel alive. Some people are born to dance and others express themselves through painting. Find your own niche, and go where life leads you.

IT'S A SMALL WORLD AFTER ALL

Part of creating your own island is making your world smaller and simpler. So much of what comes through the news media is sensationalized and does not have a direct impact on your life. Filter your news intake if it tends to cause you anxiety. Consider taking periodic vacations from news media. You will be surprised at how little you will miss. If you want to know more about the world, read a travel novel or *National Geographic* for a less sensational approach. Reading about history is reassuring; you will note that humans have not changed very much in all of recorded time and the world is probably no worse off than it has ever been.

Making your world smaller extends to your relationships with other people. To some extent, you can choose who you allow on your island. Look for meaningful relationships that pick you up instead of dragging you down.

Another part of creating your own island is having a positive outlook on life. Try to see the good in other people and overlook the bad. Remember that you are only human and others around you are the same. Tolerance is, indeed, one of the most important virtues we can achieve as human beings. Smile more often, even if you don't feel like it. Also remember that every day is not going to be a "great" day, but tomorrow could be the best yet. It is amazing how quickly life can turn around with the right outlook.

THE FOUR YEAR PLAN

"Creating your own island" is not something that happens overnight. I think anyone who has been caught up in a rat-race lifestyle has been tempted to just walk away, but life is never quite so simple. Loyalty to a hard-won career, even if it is a major source of stress, is hard to give up. A spouse's career, kids in school, and dependence on those material things that seem so important tend to get in the way. A real change in lifestyle takes time, effort, and, most importantly, a plan.

Think ahead as to what kinds of changes you would like to make in your life over the next four years. Four years seems to be a realistic time interval for most people to make real change. Take stock of what you really need to be content. Are you at the point in life where you could consider some type of retirement or choose a less stressful job that gives greater contentment? Down-sizing your home and living expenses may be a part of the plan. Taking better care of your health by taking more time for relaxation, exercise, and cooking better food should be an essential part of the change. As you make a plan, decide what stage you would like to be at in one year, two years, three years, and ultimately in four years. The stress of change may be part of the picture, but ultimately you will be more relaxed, content, and healthier.

OVERCOMING AND RECOVERING FROM ILLNESS

Sometimes a change in lifestyle is forced by a significant illness. The above considerations apply, but must be followed more intensively. While trying to regain health after a serious illness, you should be especially conscientious about how you live life. All potential stress factors that may contribute to maintaining a state of chronic disease must be reduced or eliminated. After healing has occurred and health is recovered, a more normal life can be resumed and more stress can be tolerated.

The concept of threshold is very important in understanding chronic disease. Chronic disease does not happen suddenly; rather, it occurs insidiously. The forces that cause disease are present and causing subtle but cumulative damage long before symptoms arise. A state that could be defined as "pre-disease" occurs, with the patient asymptomatic and unaware, until a certain threshold defined by our genes is crossed and suddenly a cascade of symptoms ensues. Symptoms gradually increase and coalesce into a well-defined disease process.

The time between onset of symptoms and absolute diagnosis is often quite protracted; by then, more than one diagnosis may be present. Any point along this continuum is the time to act, but the earlier the better, of course. Even if a diagnosis has been made, most chronic disease processes can be reversed if the pressures are released. Recognize that chronic disease does have well-defined causes, but the causes are multi-factorial. Stress factors must be reduced to below threshold levels and kept there long enough for healing to occur. Basic guidelines for optimizing your healing potential include the following:

If you suffer from a chronic disease, take control of your own situation. Spend more effort searching for reversible causes that have contributed to your disease than worrying about your diagnosis.

If your condition has not yet been firmly diagnosed, you may still benefit from some of these suggestions.

The recommendations for healthy food and eating are extremely important. Avoid almost all meat and processed food while recovering from an illness. Meat, dairy, processed corn, and processed wheat are the primary inflammatory foods. Especially avoid any processed sugars and starches. A healthy daily allotment of vegetables and fruit are essential. Fresh, organic food is essential. Avoid foods containing any types of chemical additives. The healthiest way of cooking food is steaming. Avoid grilled or fried foods and overly-cooked food.

To gain extra nutrients, consider juicing organic fruits and vegetables daily.

Drink plenty of clean, pure water.

Nutritional supplements can be beneficial for the transition toward better health. Pursue the advice of a qualified healthcare provider in choosing an appropriate regimen of supplements. (See Appendix C as well as the last page of the references.)

Take medications as directed by your healthcare provider, but be aware that sometimes side effects from medications can impede healing. Many medications suppress the immune system and/or have the potential to induce vitamin and mineral deficiencies. As you become healthier you may be able to reduce the dosages of some medications. Try to avoid becoming over-medicated.

Have your thyroid and other basic labs checked. Abnormal thyroid function often accompanies chronic disease. (See Appendix B for basic recommended labs.)

Manage insulin resistance and diabetes aggressively. High insulin levels adversely affect other hormone systems of the body, and baseline (fasting) blood glucose levels in the 95-110 range (even though considered normal) impede healing functions of the body. Normalize insulin and blood glucose levels by whatever means necessary.

Become acutely "toxin aware" and avoid exposure to toxins as much as possible. Hidden or unrecognized toxins can be an underlying factor in any chronic disease. An appropriately designed detoxification protocol can often improve your energy and augment healing. Review the recommendations in Chapter 11.

Try far-infrared sauna treatments. Some experts consider this to be an essential part of detoxification. Define a treatment protocol with your healthcare provider.

Alcohol and caffeine should be avoided until you are well.

Regular exercise is essential for overcoming chronic disease. Even if the extent of your ability is walking around the living room three times, do it regularly until you can do more. Work up gradually. Though exercise is beneficial, it is important not to over-tax the body. The regular practice of yoga can be very beneficial for a healing body.

Make your world as "small" and stress-free as possible. You may have to rely on other people you can trust and cut back on your day-to-day needs and living expenses. You will likely discover a "stress threshold" that precipitates symptoms. Try to maintain stress below the threshold. Remember, adrenaline is the enemy when trying to recover from chronic disease. Anything you can do to consistently lessen your adrenaline levels is beneficial. As your health improves, you will be able to tolerate more stress and enjoy a little more freedom.

Avoid becoming upset about things that you have no control over. This is extremely counter-productive because it detracts from your focus on healing and recovering.

Meditation is the most powerful healing tool I know of. Become familiar with techniques of meditation or self-relaxation and practice them as often as you can.

Pray regularly.

Rest often. Make sure you are getting plenty of sleep. I would recommend seven or more hours every night. Natural and pharmaceutical sleep aids may be indicated, but use them cautiously and wisely. Avoid medications known to suppress the immune system or cause habituation.

Establish a relationship with a healthcare provider who is willing to listen and offer guidance, without dictating therapy. A thorough evaluation is sometimes indicated to uncover hidden threats that may respond to targeted therapy.

The start of each day provides a new opportunity to renew your health. Take advantage of it. Concentrate all of your efforts on that goal.

Look for the positive moments in every day and try to generate as much of a positive outlook on life as you can. Smile, even when you do not feel like it. I cannot tell you how important this is in overall healing.

Absolutely anything can be improved with motivation and a positive attitude. You can become well again.

BRIEF EPILOG

With persistent effort my health has rebounded, but I recognize the need for continual vigilance–good health is not something to be taken for granted. Stress and genetics probably played a significant role in the insomnia and fatigue I experienced throughout my forties, but a tick bite and a test indicating possible exposure to the bacterium that causes Lyme disease may have also been a factor. I may never know for sure–at present I remain happily free of a diagnosis.

I am content with my life and my health for right now, but I recognize the need for periodic change. My next four year plan may be to look for that perfect island. I am sure it actually exists somewhere, possibly in the Caribbean or the Greek Isles. I probably wouldn't stay, but it sure would be a pleasure to go and look around!

SCHEDULE FOR COMPREHENSIVE HEALTH INTENSIVE

If you are not satisfied with your life or your health, isn't it time to make a change?

Anyone can change his or her health for the better and gain more out of life at the same time.

You could go off to a world-renowned spa for an extended period and have someone else do it for you, but is the time and expense really necessary?

You can make changes gradually or more intensely, depending on what works best for your situation—but progressive change is essential.

PRACTICAL CONSIDERATIONS FOR THE PROGRAM

For optimal results, set aside two to four months to complete the program. Ideally, one to two hours should be devoted each day toward achieving your goals. Changes made during the program should be complimented by permanently improved health habits after the program is completed.

Let everyone know of your plan and how important it is to you.

A couple of months off from work is ideal but probably impractical; use vacation time and any other influence you might have to reduce work stress and make work less of a priority during this period. If significant illness is present, consider taking limited disability. The payoff to you and your workplace will be worth it.

If childcare is an issue, get help from friends or family, or considering hiring someone short-term.

Set reasonable goals and try to achieve them. At the same time, do not become discouraged about not achieving goals or not being able to follow every recommendation in the book. This is a learning experience—any effort is acceptable. The skills learned will be valuable for the rest of your life.

The more effort you put into the program, the greater improvement you can expect in your immediate health and wellbeing.

FIRST OFFICE VISIT

Introduction to the program. Review health assessment questionnaire. Order indicated lab studies.

Section 1 (first 2-4 week period)   Core information for the program is provided in *Health First!*. During this first period, the patient should read chapters 1 through 4. The first step in overcoming chronic disease is to understand the factors that cause disease. The information in the first four chapters will define these important concepts and lay a foundation for making real change in your life.

Detoxification   Removing toxins from the body is an essential part of regaining health. Begin the detoxification/elimination protocol as defined at the end of chapter 11. The two-day fast is optional; if chosen, it should be followed during a weekend or vacation period.

Over the course of the revitalization program consider undergoing far infrared (FIR) sauna therapy. FIR sauna is one of the most effective and safest methods of removing toxins from the body. Most symptoms of chronic disease will show improvement with regular sauna therapy. Removing toxins is the quickest way to start feeling better.

Exercise   Regular exercise is essential for the program to work. If regular exercise is not a part of your life, consultation with your healthcare provider and an exercise therapist is recommended. At the very minimum, begin walking for at least 30 minutes every day. If you already exercise regularly, continue with your regular routine.

Stress management   Stress is a normal part of life, but anyone can learn better ways of managing stress. One important aspect of stress management is teaching the body and mind how to relax spontaneously. Obtain an audio CD on spontaneous relaxation (many are available) and listen to it at least once daily or at night before going to bed—this is essential and really takes very little time. A peek at chapter 14 offers specific references. Instruction in yoga, Tai Chi, Qigong or a similar discipline is very beneficial, as is time spent with a meditation instructor or hypnotherapist. One session a week with a professional can keep you moving in the right direction.

Goals   Consider and define goals to be achieved during the program. Set reasonable short-term goals that can be achieved during the two months of the program and then long-term goals to strive for after the program is completed. Goals can be personal or health-oriented. Placing them in writing is important for the program to work. You may desire to improve indicators of health, such as lowering cholesterol or improving high blood pressure. For many people, weight loss is a concern. Anxiety or insomnia may be a significant problem, in which case mastering relaxation techniques may be your primary goal. Reducing medications or learning how to manage an illness without conventional medications may become a goal. Improved physical stamina and exercise tolerance is important at any level of health.

SECOND OFFICE VISIT

Review goals and define reasonable expectations. Review lab results. Review concepts from part one of the book and ask questions. Briefly discuss dietary and eating habits.

Section 2 (second 2-4 week period) During this time period, immerse yourself in the topic of food and eating. Have some fun with it. Try different foods. Chapters 5 through 9 are devoted to all aspects of this important topic.

> **Diet** Progress from the detoxification/elimination diet to the guidelines offered in chapters 7 and 8. Evaluate your pantry and refrigerator as recommended in chapter 8. Chapter 9 offers specific ideas about converting to a healthy diet. Steps to stock your kitchen with healthy alternatives are provided. Recipe ideas that are easy and tasty are also provided in chapter 9 and in Appendix D "Simple Cooking." During this two-to-four week period, try to follow only the meal suggestions provided in this resource.

> **Exercise** Follow recommendations provided by healthcare provider and your exercise counselor. If you are just beginning, you might consider purchasing an exercise ball at any fitness store. *Exercise Balls for Dummies* is an excellent resource. Continue walking at least 30 minutes per day or following your regular exercise routine.

> **Stress management** Listen to a spontaneous relaxation audio CD at least once daily. Practice the same routine often enough that the body responds effortlessly. The more you practice, the easier it becomes.

THIRD OFFICE VISIT

Ask any questions you have about nutrition. Review goals and expectations for the program. Briefly discuss toxin awareness.

Section 3 (third 2-4 week period) This section will be devoted to toxin awareness. By now you should appreciate how much synthetic toxins contribute to disease. You probably feel better after completing the detoxification protocol. Now you will learn how to minimize exposure to specific sources of toxins and how to maximize the detoxification capacity of the body. Read chapters 10 and 11.

Toxin awareness After reading chapter 10, follow the recommendations at the end of the chapter to limit toxin exposure within your personal environment. Chapter 11 is focused on the role the gastrointestinal system plays in detoxification and elimination of wastes. Individuals suffering with gastrointestinal problems will find great benefit by following the recommendations included here. Previous dietary guidelines should be continued.

Exercise Working up a sweat at least once a day is an essential part of detoxification. Follow your regular exercise routine. At this point you should be increasing the level of intensity and deriving more pleasure from being active.

Stress management Spontaneous relaxation should be happening easily with a guided audio CD. Shift your practice to using relaxing music only. Extend your practice of spontaneous relaxation to periods of time that would be otherwise wasted—such as waiting in an airport or sitting in the doctor's office.

Diet At this point you should be improvising with recipe ideas of your own and gradually bringing family members into the circle of healthier food. Search the Internet for new ideas about new foods. Join the many smart people across America who are enjoying the benefits of healthy food!

FOURTH OFFICE VISIT

Ask questions about toxins. Review goals as related to your new diet. Review health goals and evaluate progress. Discuss medication adjustments and any need for other lab studies. Discuss the remaining chapters. Set future goals.

Section 4 (fourth 2-4 week period) In chapter 12 you will learn about principles of mind and body synchrony and how they apply to achieving optimal health and well-being. Chapter 13 is devoted to helping you push past the daily grind of mundane exercise toward enjoying an active lifestyle. Chapter 14 deals with the last and most challenging hurdle for many people—overcoming stress.

Exercise Your regular routine should be getting boring by now. It is time to add variety and rev up the intensity. Try out some new forms of exercise. Take a water aerobics class or join an organization such as a cycling club or a rowing club. Start enjoying your new-found energy every day!

Stress management   Stress can disrupt all aspects of life, especially health. Stress can also be a positive motivating factor. Being able to always see the positive side of any situation is the ultimate key to stress management. The last chapter in this book offers practical tools and advice for making this happen.

FIFTH AND FINAL OFFICE VISIT (OPTIONAL)

Review all goals and expectations of the program. Discuss continued care for specific indications.

SCREENING LABS FOR THE HEALTH PROGRAM

LEVEL 1 BASIC ASSESSMENT

- **CBC with diff** Count of red blood cells and inflammatory cells. Measures hemoglobin for detection of anemia.

- **Metabolic panel** Measures basic blood chemistry, liver function and kidney function. Includes fasting blood glucose.

- **Lipid profile** Measures triglycerides and cholesterol. Shows total cholesterol as well as the breakdown by particle types HDL ("good") and LDL ("bad") cholesterol. Satisfactory screening for individuals under age fifty with no risk factors. Includes C-reactive protein as a screen for inflammatory risks associated with atherosclerosis.

- **Thyroid screen** Thyroid stimulating hormone (TSH) is used for basic screening purposes in individuals with a positive family history or asymptomatic women over age fifty.

LEVEL 2 OVER AGE 50 OR WITH RISK FACTORS

- **Advanced atherosclerosis screening** For all individuals over age fifty and individuals under fifty with any risk factors. Includes complete lipoprotein particle profile (substitutes for basic lipid profile) and C-reactive protein. More specialized panels reveal specific LDL remnants that are the source of atherosclerosis. Fasting insulin levels are often included.

- **Hemoglobin A-1-C and fasting insulin** Screening for insulin resistance and early onset diabetes.

- **Essential fatty acids (AA/EPA ratio)** The ratio of omega-6 to omega-3 fatty acids can be measured by special testing. The ideal ratio for a low inflammatory response is 4:1. This ratio is commonly found in the traditional Japanese population who demonstrate the greatest longevity and lowest risk of cardiovascular disease in the world. The ratio of most average Americans is closer to 11:1. Inflammatory conditions and neurologic disorders are common at 20:1. (Metametrix Labs). Determining the body saturation of omega-3's may prove to be one of the most sensitive indicators for predicting stroke and heart attack.

- **Micronutrient profile** Testing for deficiencies in specific vitamins and minerals. Assays for vitamin D and vitamin B-12, and minerals including calcium and magnesium, can be ordered through standard labs. Types of testing can be defined by a qualified healthcare provider.

- **Complete hormone profile** DHEAS, testosterone, estradiol, estrone, and progesterone. Blood testing is most accurate, but only offers a snapshot in time. Salivary hormone testing offers a broader analysis, but is much less accurate. Salivary testing is best for guiding hormone replacement therapy. (Indicated if fatigue or hormonal dysfunction are present.)

- **Complete thyroid testing** Includes thyroid stimulating hormone (TSH) and free (active) thyroid hormones, T-3 and T-4. Thyroid antibodies may be ordered in certain situations when symptoms consistent with hypothyroidism persist despite normal hormone levels. Thyroid antibody testing includes thyroid peroxidase (TPO) and antithyroglobulin antibody. (Indicated if fatigue is present.)

- **Risk of thrombosis** A small percentage of people are "hyper-coagulators" and are at risk of thrombotic events (blood clots). Screening labs for genetic susceptibility include Leiden factor V, homocysteine, protein C deficiency, protein S deficiency and antithrombin. These tests should be considered in anyone with a family history of thrombotic events, especially if estrogen products are being considered.

- **Estrogen metabolites** Evidence suggests that different individuals metabolize estrogen in the body by different pathways. Measurement of different metabolites may help define risk of hormonally-dependent cancers. 16-alpha-hydroxyestrone metabolites are associated with increased estrogen receptor stimulation and 2-hydroxyestrone/2-hydroxyestradiol metabolites are associated with the opposite. Urine samples for measurement of the 2-OHE/16-alpha OHE ratio may be an important biomarker for defining high risk individuals. While this test is still considered investigational, it may be helpful for guiding dietary modifications in both female and male patients.

LEVEL 3 HISTORY OF CHRONIC DISEASE

- **3-hour glucose tolerance test with insulin levels** Indicated when insulin resistance or diabetes is suspected.

- **Food sensitivity testing** Food sensitivities are often an underlying factor in chronic disease. This can be a beneficial adjunct to an elimination diet. Different panels are available for food and airborne allergies.

- **24-hour cortisol levels** Salivary hormones are tested at four different times during the day. (Cortisol concentrations are much higher than other adrenal and reproductive hormones, so salivary levels are valid for testing.) (Quest labs) Indicated primarily in cases of chronic fatigue that are refractory to therapy.

- **TB skin test.** Recommended if lung disease or possible exposure has been present. (In debilitating chronic situations where there is a history of TB exposure/positive test, previously treated, a chest x-ray may not be enough to rule out chronic TB. The gold standard is **Quantiferon TB Gold**, run by Quest labs.)

- **Heavy metal testing** Heavy metal toxicity can be a factor in chronic disease. Total RBC concentration can be used as a screen. If toxicity is strongly suspected, the best measurement involves 24-hour urine collection after stimulation with DMSA. (Hair samples are not always accurate because detergents in daily shampoo can add to or wash out toxic substances.)

- **Lyme disease testing** Indicated when chronic fatigue and arthritis are present.

- **Rheumatoid factor / ANA titer** Indicated when arthritis or suspicions of autoimmune disease are present.

- **HIV, Syphilis and Hepatitis** If sexually transmitted disease suspected.

Specific recommendations for laboratory evaluation should be defined by a qualified healthcare provider.

EVERYDAY SUPPLEMENTS FOR OPTIMAL HEALTH

An optimal diet should provide all the nutrients necessary for optimal health, but few individuals are able to follow a perfect diet every day. Also, many foods that should be considered healthy now have health concerns, such as mercury in fish or deficiencies present in non-organic foods. Nutritional supplements can safely provide an optimal complement of nutrients, especially as the need becomes greater with age and nutritional requirements change.

Taking supplements specifically for the purpose of health enhancement or improving longevity of life is, however, tricky business. The human body is quite complex and identifying specific dietary deficiencies is not straightforward. Many products on the market are poorly balanced, contain synthetic ingredients or are in a form that the body cannot readily assimilate. Using dietary supplements in anything but a natural form can actually do more harm than good.

The key to using dietary supplements appropriately is letting Mother Nature be the ultimate guide. Sometimes this requires as much common sense as science. The best supplements are actual food substances or collections of nutrients from natural sources, presented in a form that is as readily absorbed and assimilated as are natural foods.

Nutritional supplements come in many forms, with tablets, capsules and tinctures being the most common. Most often the form is a matter of personal preference, but sometimes it can make a difference. Probiotics and some enzyme preparations need to be enteric coated for protection against stomach acid. Others, such as melatonin and vitamin B-12 are best delivered under the tongue as a sublingual preparation. Liquid tinctures are the most rapidly absorbed herbal supplements.

Fillers often matter to individuals with sensitivities and allergies. Always scrutinize the non-active ingredients before purchasing a supplement.

THE TOP THREE

For anyone over 40, the first three listed categories — essential fatty acids, antioxidants and liver protection—should be considered indispensable for achieving optimal health. Other categories can be considered on an individual basis.

Essential Fatty Acids (Omega-3 fatty acids) *Essential fatty acids (EFA)* are important for decreasing inflammation in the body and supporting optimum cell membrane function. They also prevent oxidation of cholesterol and platelet aggregation, important factors in reducing the risk of atherosclerosis. An optimal supplement contains a balance of both marine (*fish oil*) and vegetable sources of essential fatty acids. For individuals desiring to avoid fish products completely, vegetable supplements are available. *Organic flax oil* is also an adequate substitute (two tablespoons daily mixed with food).

There are many "fish oil" supplements on the market. Freshness is the key to quality. Oxidation (spoilage) can occur during the manufacturing process or if the product sits on the shelf too long. A better quality supplement should not have a "fishy" smell or taste. EFA supplements should be taken as a single ingredient supplement, because spoilage is more likely if they are combined with other ingredients. EFA supplements should be refrigerated when purchased and stored in the refrigerator at home. Only buy EFA supplements that are labeled as pharmaceutical grade.

Natural Antioxidants and Anti-inflammatory Substances Cumulative damage from oxidative stress and inflammation are major contributors to aging and disease. Arthritis, Alzheimer's, atherosclerosis, and even diabetes have close links to inflammation and damage induced by exposure to free radicals. Fruits, especially berries, are loaded with antioxidants and natural anti-inflammatory chemicals that combat these powerful forces of disease. Consuming large quantities of fruits would make sense, but this is not always practical. Quality supplements can provide most of the benefits of fruits and berries on a daily basis.

There are many different types of antioxidant/anti-inflammatory supplements, but if you were to choose only one type, *grapeseed/grape-skin extract* would be the best choice. The skins and seeds of grapes (especially Muscadine grapes) contain *ellagic acid, resveratrol,* and other potent anti-oxidant with anti-inflammatory chemicals.

Liver Protection We are literally bombarded with toxins every day. Over a lifetime, the liver takes quite a beating. The detoxification process conducted by the liver produces high levels of damaging free radicals. For protection, the liver cells generate an anti-oxidant called glutathione, but this is not always enough. Dietary anti-oxidants are beneficial, but certain herbal substances are known to offer additional protection specifically for the liver. As much as our health depends on healthy liver function, taking a protective supplement is probably not a bad idea. The most well-known of the liver protectants is *milk thistle*, containing the active chemical *silymarin*. Other substances known to protect liver function include dandelion, licorice, artichoke leaf, and grapeseed extract.

Joint and Cartilage Support   Arthritis and joint pain is common enough in individuals over fifty to be considered almost ubiquitous. Cumulative damage from various factors of disease result in excessive inflammation, with the main culprit being a dysfunctional immune system. Though the problem is best addressed by pursuing a healthy diet and lifestyle to counteract the underlying causes of disease, supplements can often be beneficial.

There are many natural anti-inflammatory supplements available, with *essential fatty acids* and *grapeseed extract* leading the roster. *Glucosamine* and *chondroitin* help support healthy cartilage, but there is some question as to whether chondroitin is absorbed very well. MSM and SAMe are known for joint support. Other natural anti-inflammatory supplements commonly available include *ginger, devil's claw, turmeric, boswellia, yucca,* and *holy basil,* just to name a few. Natural anti-inflammatories have a great advantage over pharmaceuticals in that they promote healing and have few potential adverse effects.

Osteoporosis Protection   A well-balanced, healthy diet generally provides enough of important minerals including calcium to maintain healthy bones, but supplements provide insurance. Calcium supplementation, however, must be administered properly. Most calcium supplements are supplied as inorganic salts, to be taken in large doses; there is evidence that this may do more harm than good.

Though standard calcium supplements are associated with decreased fracture risk in the short term, large doses of calcium may "burn out" bone remodeling cells, worsening osteoporosis in the long run. Inorganic calcium is also known to precipitate out in other tissues, including atherosclerotic plaques, increasing "hardening of arteries" and the risk of associated maladies.

Ideally, calcium should be administered in small doses with food several times daily. The *citrate and malate forms of calcium* are the best absorbed. Total daily dose of calcium, with dietary sources and supplements combined, should be around 1200 mg. If dietary sources are satisfactory, supplemental calcium may only need to be 500 to 750mg and no more. Calcium supplementation should be accompanied by other bone-healthy minerals including boron (2mg) and magnesium (400mg). Few supplements on the market meet these qualifications.

When it comes to bone health, adequate *vitamin D* is essential. Vitamin D is important not only for the maintenance of healthy bones, but also for a healthy immune system. Direct, unprotected sun exposure to the face and arms for 20-30 minutes three times per week provides adequate vitamin D. Sunscreen typically blocks 95% of vitamin D production. Individuals not receiving satisfactory sun exposure should consider supplementation. Whether from fortified foods or from supplements, Vitamin D is especially important in winter when we have decreased sun exposure. Post-menopausal females, especially, need at 1000 to 1500 IU of Vitamin D daily.

Prostate Disease   Prostate disease is common in males over fifty and all too often progresses to cancer. Though heredity appears to play a role (highest in African-American males), high consumption of animal fat, low intake of fruits and vegetables, obesity and physical inactivity are also closely associated with increased risk of prostate disease. Toxins in the environment almost certainly play a role in prostate cancer.

Symptoms of urine dribbling, urgency, weak stream and frequent urination at night are early signs of changes in the prostate gland. Symptoms should be evaluated by a qualified health provider and routine screening with the PSA test and prostate exams are indicated.

Beyond a shift to a healthy diet and practice of regular exercise, several herbal substances have been associated with improvement in symptoms and shrinkage of the prostate gland. Early use of appropriate supplements may prevent progression of disease. Supplements associated with prevention of prostate disease include *saw palmetto, pygeum* and *stinging nettle*. The minerals zinc and selenium are also important.

The Basic Multivitamin   The question of whether to take a broad-spectrum multivitamin is quite controversial. On one hand, information suggests that our requirements for vitamins and minerals go up as we age, even beyond that provided by a healthy diet, and that many disease processes are associated with vitamin deficiencies. On the other hand, some clinical studies have consistently shown no benefit and even possible detriment from taking a multivitamin. Most studies, however, have been done with synthetically-derived vitamins, suggesting that essential vitamins and minerals should be obtained only from natural foods.

A perfect diet is the answer, but even individuals who strive for this goal admit that eating the perfect diet every day is challenging. A multivitamin could fill dietary voids, but special care must be taken in choosing the correct formulation. The basic "once a day," composed of synthetic vitamins "dumped" into the system at one time, is clearly not the best option. Consumption of synthetically-derived vitamins and inorganic forms of minerals may do more harm than good. Scrutiny of the many multivitamins on the market yields only a limited number that may be worth considering.

Tips for getting the most from your multivitamin:

Vitamin A Though essential for many functions within the body, too much vitamin A is toxic. A multivitamin should not contain more than 10,000 units of vitamin A by itself. Children should not take vitamin A at all. Natural carotenes (such as beta-carotene) are converted to vitamin A in the body and are a safer route for supplementation. Look for natural carotenes in your multivitamin. Carotene supplements may include the well-known carotenoid chemicals beta-carotene, lycopene and lutein.

B vitamins B vitamins are easy to acquire through a healthy diet, but obtaining extra B vitamins via a multivitamin is acceptable. B-vitamins are water soluble and toxicity by over-supplementation is rare. Strict vegetarians, elderly people, and individuals with gastrointestinal conditions should take supplements of B-12. Individuals with compromised gastric function or gastric bypass should take B-12 by the sublingual route or weekly injection.

Folate Naturally occurring folates are preferred over the more commonly found folic acid. Folic acid is readily absorbed, but it is an inactive form of folate that must be enzymatically converted to active folates within the body. This process happens more readily in some individuals than others. Excessive, inactive folic acid has potential for toxicity. The vast majority of multivitamins (even some that are very high in price) contain synthetic folic acid. Look for natural folates in your multivitamin. Active folates commonly found in quality supplements include *folinic acid* and *l-5-methyltetrahydrofolate.*

Vitamin C Extra vitamin C is important in times of stress, but an everyday supplement should not exceed about 750mg.

Vitamin D Becoming recognized as one of the most important vitamins for supplementation, vitamin D actually serves as a hormone in the body. The current USDA recommendation is 1000 IU daily. A multivitamin should contain at least 400 IU. Individuals over the age of fifty, especially postmenopausal females and anyone who seldom gets sun exposure, should be thinking about vitamin D supplements.

Vitamin E There are eight different forms of vitamin E, all with different uses within the body. The "gamma" form is the most common in the heart. Loading up the body with one form (namely synthetic d-alpha tocopherol, as found in most supplements) makes little sense. Look for mixed natural tocopherols in your multivitamin.

Iodine   This is important for normal function of the thyroid gland. Recent evidence suggests a link between low iodine levels and breast cancer.

Minerals   In general, minerals are best assimilated by the body when introduced in organic forms, such as amino acid chelates, rather than the more commonly found inorganic forms. Eating vegetables is probably the best way to get your daily minerals.

Herbal ingredients   If your multivitamin gives you a "lift" shortly after taking it, it probably contains stimulants. Many herbal ingredients are beneficial, but companies often adulterate multivitamins with herbal stimulants that offer no health benefits, just to sell more vitamins. Be careful of herbal ingredients added to general supplements. Even when herbs are well chosen, the dose is usually too small to make any difference. Even some beneficial herbal substances are not tolerated by certain individuals.

Immune Modulators   One focus of supplement therapy has always been immune enhancement. Improved ability to fight off microbial infection, prevent cancer, and decrease the incidence of autoimmune diseases is very desirable. Substances known to positively affect immune function include multivitamins, vitamin C, zinc, and selenium. Vitamin D is also essential for normal immune function.

In the herbal world, there are many substances that positively affect immune function, with elderberry and *Echinacea* being the most widely recognized in this country. There is some evidence that these substances may limit the duration of a viral illness, such as a common cold. Most interesting is an herb from India called *Andrographis*, which has shown more benefit in shortening the length of a viral illness than any other. A growing body of evidence from studies in Europe suggests that *Andrographis* is one to consider during cold and flu season. (Use of these products should be confined mainly just to cold and flu season.)

In a world where external threats from microbes are common and internal threats from factors causing immune dysfunction are ever-present, immune enhancement on a daily basis is worth consideration. With this goal in mind, the ideal substance would be one that affects a continual "tune-up" rather than constant stimulation of the immune system. One product that may fit that description goes by the trade name *Epicor*. Derived from baker's yeast, *Epicor* appears to influence all aspects of the immune system in a positive way. Chemically, it contains potent anti-oxidants and natural immune-enhancing substances. To date, *Epicor* has been the subject of numerous laboratory studies, animal trials, and human trials. All studies have shown positive efficacy and very low potential for toxicity.

When taken regularly, *Epicor* appears to decrease the incidence of viral, bacterial, and parasitic invaders. *Epicor* may also have positive benefit in the management of autoimmune disorders.

While the concept of immune enhancement is still very new, these products are proving to be very effective for preventing or shortening common viral illnesses such as colds and flu.

Prevention of hormonally-active cancers Regular consumption of cruciferous vegetables is associated with decreased risk of breast, uterine and prostate cancer. This group of vegetables, including broccoli, cabbage, kale, Brussels sprouts and cauliflower, are rich in *indole* compounds. This unique family of chemicals expedites clearance of estrogen and estrogen-like compounds.

Though various types of indole and cruciferous vegetable supplements are available, the value of such supplements has yet to be defined. Taking a supplement should not be considered equal to the real thing. That being said, supplements may be better than nothing at all for individuals who cannot being themselves to eat cabbage or broccoli on a regular basis.

Lignans, found in beans and seeds, offer protection from hormonally-active cancers. Whole flax seeds have the highest levels of lignans.

Co-enzyme Q-10 CoQ-10, as it is often called, is a necessary chemical component of the energy production systems of the cell. Though each cell has the ability to manufacture it, we lose some of this ability as we age and CoQ-10 becomes more like an essential vitamin. Supplementation should be considered when low energy level is a concern. CoQ-10 is especially important for generation of energy within the heart and should be considered as a daily supplement for an individual who has a heart condition or high blood pressure. CoQ-10 supplements are also advised for individuals taking cholesterol-lowering medications (statins), as these medications lower CoQ-10 levels. This may be a contributing factor to muscle pain commonly occurring as a side effect with statin medications.

Glucose-modulating supplements Half the American population over age forty is on the way to becoming insulin resistant and many already have Type II diabetes. Dietary changes are definitely indicated, but do not repair damage already done. Supplements to help preserve the body's ability to manage blood glucose levels are worth considering. Anyone with fasting blood glucose consistently over 100 but below the level of established diabetes should consider taking a supplement.

Many non-toxic substances found in nature positively affect glucose metabolism. Supplements with combinations of ingredients including *chromium, gymnema, fenugreek, bitter melon, cinnamon, vanadium, banaba,* and *alpha lipoic acid* are available. Blood glucose should be monitored and additional medical therapy should be considered if fasting blood glucose is over 130 or other indications of diabetes are present.

Probiotics   Constant replenishment of favorable bacteria in the gastrointestinal tract is an essential component of good health. Daily consumption of yogurt is an ideal source of favorable bacteria, but many individuals do not tolerate any milk products. If gastrointestinal dysfunction is a factor, a probiotic supplement should be strongly considered. Choose a supplement under the guidance of a qualified healthcare practitioner.

Ocular support   Anti-oxidants in general help protect the retina and lens of the eye, but the carotenoid *lutein* is a natural part of the pigment of the macula. The yellow color of lutein is found in a wide array of fruits and vegetables, but high-risk individuals should consider a supplement. Individuals with a family history of macular degeneration, individuals having light skin and blue eyes or individuals with high sun exposure should consider a lutein supplement. Lutein is found in some but not all multivitamins. *Bilberry extract* is another supplement known to be important for vision health.

Garlic   Garlic has a number of beneficial effects that have been clinically documented. Garlic is a natural blood thinner or anticoagulant and has effects of lowering cholesterol and blood pressure. Also it has antibacterial, antifungal, and antiviral properties and may have immune-enhancing and anti-cancer properties. Unfortunately, it loses its potency with cooking or processing. Freeze-dried, enteric-coated preparations on the market are much more palatable than eating raw garlic. Some people have GI upset even with coated preparations. Specially-aged garlic supplements are the best-tolerated. The normal daily dose of garlic includes 10mg of alliin or an allicin potential of 4000mcg (the equivalent of one to two raw cloves per day).

Mental acuity and cognition   Health of mental function is closely tied to good health practices in general. A healthy diet, well-managed blood glucose levels, regular exercise, stress moderation and especially plenty of sleep are supportive for preserving healthy mental function well into later life. B vitamins and antioxidants are particularly important for maintenance of normal mental function.

Medicinal herbal supplements associated with improved cognition in dementia patients include *DMAE*, *ginko*, *vinpocetine* and *huperzine*. These supplements should be reserved for individuals with documented mental decline and used only under the guidance of a healthcare practitioner.

The above guidelines are very general. Individual needs may vary according to diet and health status. Consult a healthcare provider with knowledge in wellness-based medicine for choosing the best regimen of everyday supplements.

For a more specific and up-to-date guide in choosing supplements, please visit **www.FDNHhealth.com**. This website offers high quality supplements and other products at reasonable prices. It is designed to reflect the concepts I have defined in this book.

An opinion on aspirin

A daily dose of enteric-coated aspirin, 81mg is recommended by many providers. Aspirin reduces inflammation and inhibits platelet aggregation (decreases clotting). There is good evidence that aspirin reduces risks of stroke caused by blood clots, heart attacks and colon cancer. Aspirin has, however, been associated with increased incidence of hemorrhagic stroke (stroke caused by rupture of blood vessels in the brain.) This is not surprising, because aspirin does nothing to strengthen the integrity of blood vessels; in fact, it may do the opposite.

Virtually all the daily supplements, with essential fatty acids leading the way, have blood thinning properties. Unlike aspirin, essential fatty acids and the anti-inflammatory supplements actually improve the integrity of the vascular system. The supplements recommended would be expected to provide all of the benefits of aspirin (and more), without the risk.

MORE SIMPLE COOKING

QUICK SUPPERS

Healthy shrimp and grits (with quinoa instead of grits)

Try this version and you will never be satisfied with anything else. Shrimp are high in protein, calcium, vitamin B-12, and selenium, but very low in food energy. Shrimp are high in cholesterol, but tend to raise favorable HDL cholesterol more than LDL cholesterol. Because they are low in fat overall and high in omega-3 fatty acids, consumption of shrimp actually lowers the risk of atherosclerosis.

   Shrimp, ½ to 1 lb. (depending on the number of people)
   Onions, chopped
   Red bell peppers, chopped
   Celery, chopped
   Garlic, minced
   Hummus, a couple of large spoonfuls
   Low-fat sour cream or yogurt, a couple of large spoonfuls
   Old Bay (or similar) seasoning, a good shake
   Hot red chili paste, ½ teaspoon
   Salt to taste
   Quinoa, several cups, precooked (1 cup quinoa, 2 cups water, salt; cook for
      15 minutes)

Sauté the shrimp, onions, pepper, celery and seasonings in olive oil with garlic and seasonings. Add in the hummus and sour cream. Stir in the quinoa and serve. A baked butternut squash goes well with this dish.

Beef, barley, and cabbage rolls

Barley is an underutilized grain. It works well when included in many varieties of dishes and can also be prepared and eaten as a hot breakfast cereal, similar to oatmeal. Barley is very good for the digestive tract, lowers cholesterol, aids in the removal of toxins from the body, and slows the absorption of glucose for 10-12 hours after it is consumed!

   Small free-range steak, sliced into small cubes
   ½ onion, chopped
   2 cups cooked hulled barley
   Several large steamed cabbage leaves
   ½ can pizza or tomato sauce

Barley cooks like rice. Add 1 cup hulled barley to 2 cups of water. Heat the water to boiling and then reduce to simmer. Cover and cook for about 40 minutes. Cook a double batch to use in other dishes or for breakfast.

While the cabbage leaves are being steamed, sauté the steak and onion in olive oil until brown. Add in the barley and sauce. Scoop the mixture into the cabbage leaves, roll, and place back into the same pan. Cover and simmer on low for a few minutes. This should be enough to serve 3-4 people.

Quick and Easy Turkey Dinner
  2 boneless turkey breasts (free range)
  4 large sweet potatoes
  Several stalks of broccoli

Grill or bake the turkey breast for about 30 minutes (medium-low on the grill, 350 degrees in the oven). A good marinade is olive oil, fresh lemon, and allspice-based seasoning. (Save one of the breasts for the wild rice and turkey casserole recipe found in the casserole section.)

Peel the sweet potatoes and slice into smaller pieces. Place in a pot, cover with water, and boil until tender. Remove from boiling water and drain. Mash with a large fork. Mix in 1 to 2 tbsp. margarine and 1 to 2 tbsp. brown sugar. Transfer to a baking dish and smooth out. Bake at 350 for about 20 to30 minutes.

Steam the broccoli and sprinkle with your choice of cheese.

Spinach and sausage
  Fresh (or frozen) spinach or Swiss chard
  Soy sausage (or regular, if you insist)
  Chopped onions
  Chopped mushrooms
  One or two eggs
  Soy sauce
  Cooked brown rice (or quinoa)

Sauté the onions, mushrooms and sausage in macadamia nut oil. Add the spinach (or chard). When the spinach is wilted, crack the eggs and stir them in until cooked. Season with soy sauce and serve over brown rice.

Tempeh sauté
Tempeh is a very healthy source of protein made from cultured soybeans. Properly prepared, tempeh is quite tasty. Tempeh keeps well in the refrigerator and is quick and easy to prepare.

One package tempeh
Sliced brown button mushrooms (any mushrooms can be used)
Grated garlic
Grated ginger
Soy sauce
Olive oil

Sauté all ingredients together over low to medium heat, covered part of the time, until the mushrooms are tender.
Serve with rice and steamed greens.

Black rice, black beans
Black rice sounds exotic enough that I had to try it. After minimal searching, I found it at a local grocery on the rice and pasta aisle. Supposedly this heirloom rice was once reserved for the emperors of China.

2 cups black rice—cooked
1 can black beans
1 stalk celery—sliced
1/3 onion—chopped
Handful of raisins for sweetness
½ - 1 teaspoon cumin
Splash of white wine
Slivered almonds or cashews
¼ c. shredded cheese—any white cheese (Romano, fresh parmesan, or Monterey jack)
Sea salt to taste
Olive oil

Cook the black rice as per directions on the package in a 1½ - 2 quart pot. When cooked, the rice actually has a deep purple color and gives off a wonderful nutty aroma. Sauté celery and onions in olive oil. Add in cumin, salt, black beans, and wine; simmer covered for several minutes. Stir this sautéed mixture in with the rice. Add in the raisins, almonds, and cheese. Serve with a steamed vegetable such as Swiss chard and a glass of white wine—a truly sophisticated meal that takes no time at all to prepare.

Salmon and Greens
1/2 to 1 lb. fresh salmon
Bottled red pepper vinaigrette dressing (any brand)
1-2 bunches (more than you think) of fresh greens (collards, kale, Swiss chard)
1-2 cups sliced mushrooms
½ cup chopped green onions

1-2 tsp. minced garlic
1-2 tsp. rice vinegar
2-3 tbs. olive oil
1-2 tsp. sesame oil
salt, paprika, and cayenne pepper to taste
sliced fresh plums
Yellow squash, chopped
Sweet onions, chopped

Steam the salmon (coated with the roasted red pepper dressing) for 5-10 minutes. Grilling also works well.

Chop the greens. This is done by laying the leaves on a chopping board and cutting cross sections about 1-inch thick with a large knife. In a deep pan, sauté the greens in olive and sesame oil with the mushrooms, onions and garlic. Throw them in, all at once, until the pan is packed to overflowing, and cover. Stir every minute or two until the greens are steamed down and soft.

Microwave or steam the squash and onions for about 6 to 8 minutes and top with your choice of cheese.

Serve the salmon and greens side-by-side, with the plums as a garnish. The squash is a side dish.

Cilantro Shrimp Pasta
1 lb. shrimp
1 thinly sliced orange bell pepper
1 thinly sliced tomato
2 tbs. (about) fresh minced cilantro
1-2 tsp (about) minced garlic
Paprika to taste
Cayenne pepper to taste
Salt to taste
1-2 tbs. olive oil
½-1 cup grated parmesan or Monterey Jack cheese
Splash of soy milk
Whole wheat pasta

Sauté shrimp, peppers, tomato, cilantro, garlic, spices in olive oil. Add cheese and soy milk. Mix until cheese is completely melted. Serve over whole wheat pasta. Serve with baked winter squash and hot tea to drink.

Back porch summer supper
Fresh bluefish with salt, pepper and olive oil, grilled on low for about 15 minutes.
Steamed corn on the cob with just a pat of butter.
Sliced tomato grown in the backyard.
Fresh green salad with walnuts, blueberries, and blackberry vinaigrette dressing.
This dish takes less than 30 minutes to prepare and 5 minutes to wash dishes.

Pineola chicken
Boneless chicken breasts – one per person
Sweet onion, sliced into round sections
Pesto: (Grind together in food processor)
1 cup fresh pine nuts
½ cup freshly grated parmesan cheese
1-3 tablespoons minced garlic
Fresh minced or dried herbs (basil and oregano work well)
Squeeze of fresh lemon

Pesto is most commonly found combined with pasta, but it has many uses in cooking. There are many different types and combinations of pesto, but a common ingredient is often pine nuts. Do not shy away from pine nuts when you see the fat content, as they are favorable fats. Pine nuts are rich in anti-oxidants and have a reputation as a natural appetite suppressant. Once you make your pesto, freeze the extra (in an ice-cube tray) for use with a pasta and vegetable dish at another time.

For this dish place the chicken breasts on top of the sliced onions in a glass baking dish. Cover the chicken with the remaining onion slices. Bake at 350 degrees for 30 minutes. Remove the top layer of onions. Spread pesto over the top of the chicken and bake for another 20 minutes.

Baked red potatoes or sweet potatoes and steamed sweet peas complete the meal.

Stuffed Quinoa Peppers
Cooked quinoa, about 2 cups
Red, green, or yellow bell peppers (1/2 to 1 per person), seeded
Half of a sweet onion, chopped
6-10 mushrooms, sliced
Minced garlic
1 package of frozen spinach (or fresh, but remember it takes a lot)
½ can diced tomatoes
Bottled salsa
Teaspoon vinegar

Tablespoon chili powder
Hot chili sauce to taste
Salt to taste

Originating from South America, the grain quinoa is high in quality protein and fiber, but is gluten-free and also is low in starch. Quinoa is considered the least allergenic of all grains.

Steam the spinach until soft. At the same time, prepare the quinoa as per instructions on the box. Sauté onions, mushrooms, and seasonings in olive oil. Mix in the cooked quinoa, spinach, tomatoes, and salsa. Fill a whole or a half pepper (depending on the size of the pepper) with the mix and place in a baking dish. Sprinkle freshly grated parmesan cheese on the top and bake at 350 degrees for about 20-30 minutes. This can be a meal in itself, but also can be served with another vegetable or a salad.

Chicken/Zucchini Teriyaki
2-4 chicken breasts cut into small pieces
2-4 cups of zucchini squash cut into small pieces
onion
1-2 cups of mushrooms
1-2 tbs. olive oil
½-1 cup plain or garlic hummus
1-2 tbs. strained or plain yogurt
1-2 cups of teriyaki sauce

Cut the zucchini squash and mushrooms into small pieces. Chop up the onion. Steam the vegetables until tender. In a wok, stir-fry the chicken in olive oil. Add the steamed vegetables and mix together. Stir in the teriyaki sauce, hummus, and sour cream/plain yogurt. Heat until bubbling and serve.
Serve with steamed green beans and whole-grain bread.

Seafood Steamer
Steam unpeeled shrimp, clams, and fish or scallops seasoned with "Old Bay" or similar spices. Serve with baked red potatoes and slaw.
Slice little red potatoes in half and bake for 20 to 30 minutes with salt, pepper, a little olive oil and/or other spices on top. The potatoes can also be cooked in the lower pot of the steamer.
Slaw—any recipe will do. Here's how I make mine: Shred a bowl full of cabbage and carrots. Add enough (not too much) mayonnaise to stick it together. Add 1 to 2 tsp. of vinegar, salt, pepper, and a little mustard.

SOUPS AND CHOWDERS
Chicken vegetable stew
   2-3 boneless chicken breasts
   1-2 tbsp. olive oil
   raw mushrooms (about 2 cups, chopped)
   onion (1-2 cups)
   minced garlic
   other assorted vegetables
   vegetable or chicken broth
   1 cup uncooked brown rice
   2 tbsp. freshly minced herbs – thyme, oregano, rosemary
   salt and pepper
   1 large can crushed tomatoes
   1 can tomato puree

In a large deep stew pot, sauté 2-3 chopped up chicken breasts (free range) in 1-2 tbsp. olive oil along with the mushrooms (any kind) and the chopped onion. Add 1-2 tsp. of fresh minced garlic.

Add other vegetables to your liking. I toss in about a cup of each of the following: chopped cabbage, chopped carrots, green beans, peas, corn, a stalk of chopped celery, and 3 medium zucchinis.

Add enough water to cover all of the vegetables and several cups of organic vegetable or chicken broth for flavor. Add one cup of uncooked brown rice. Season with 2 tbsp. of fresh minced thyme or an herb of your choice (oregano, rosemary, marjoram, and basil work well), 1 tsp. of salt, and pepper.

Bring the mixture to a boil and then reduce to a simmer for about an hour. Toward the end add the crushed tomatoes and tomato puree.
This is enough for a crowd or for several meals, and it freezes wonderfully.

Easy Vegetarian Chili
There are almost an unlimited number of chili recipes and many of them can be made without meat. The following is a recipe for a rich and healthy chili that can be made in about 10 minutes. You won't miss the meat.
   Carrots, onions, zucchini, and cabbage, chopped (2-3 cups total)
   Olive oil
   Minced garlic
   1 can of organic crushed tomatoes
   1 can of dark kidney beans, rinsed
   1 can of black beans, rinsed

Spices include chili powder, cayenne pepper (freshly mince preferred), cumin, and salt

Secret ingredient: 1 tablespoon of cocoa powder

Chopped prunes and sundried tomatoes are a nice addition

Mashed tempeh and/or cauliflower are excellent for thickeners

In a medium pot, sauté chopped carrots, onions, and garlic in 1 to 2 tbsp. of olive oil. Cook until the carrots are tender. Mix in one can of crushed tomatoes (look for fire roasted organic tomatoes), one can of dark red kidney beans, and one can of black beans. Add in one bay leaf, 1 to 2 tbsp. chili powder, cayenne pepper to taste, salt to taste, and 1 to 2 tsp. of cumin. Simmer for about 10 minutes.

Serve with whole grain bread and a salad.

Moroccan Vegetable Chili

This is a very healthful dish. It is meat-free, gluten-free, and dairy-free, but the combination of flavors and spices creates a very flavorful meal.

Vegetables--broccoli, cauliflower, carrots, onions, and red bell peppers

Red lentils

Macadamia nut oil (or olive oil)

Light vinegar (such as rice wine vinegar)

One can of diced tomatoes or tomato sauce (organic)

Spices including: chili powder, hot chili sauce, curry paste, cumin, and salt

Grated ginger

Minced garlic

First prepare the red lentils. Red lentils are best if thoroughly washed until the water is clear. This usually takes four to six washings. A cup of dry lentils will absorb about 1 ½ to 2 cups of water. Bring to a boil and then simmer for about 10-15 minutes. Save the leftovers for lunch the next day.

Stir-fry or sauté about 2 cups of diced onion and peppers in 1-2 tablespoons of oil. Meanwhile, steam or microwave a handful of carrots, 1-2 sticks of broccoli and an equal amount of cauliflower.

Returning to the onions and peppers, add in the spices to your tastes. This is usually about 1-2 tablespoons of chili powder, ½ teaspoon of chili paste, a teaspoon of cumin, a tablespoon of curry paste, 1-2 teaspoons of vinegar, salt to taste, and a full teaspoon each of grated ginger and minced garlic. Stir in the lentils and the vegetables and the dish is complete. Serve alone or over brown rice.

The Best Beef Stew
1 small sirloin steak (free range preferred) - diced
2 cups mushrooms – sliced in half
1 whole onion – diced
2 tbsp. olive oil
4 small red potatoes - diced
3-4 stalks of celery cut in pieces
1 bag of peeled carrots
1 bag frozen or fresh green beans (or green peas, corn, or butterbeans)
1-2 tsp. garlic
2-3 tbsp. minced herbs – rosemary, sage, & thyme
2 tbsp. garbanzo bean flour (optional)
2 tbsp. balsamic vinegar or red wine
1 small can of tomato paste (organic)
1 can diced tomatoes (organic)
1 cup barley grain

In a stew pot sauté the steak, onions, garlic, and mushrooms in olive oil until brown. Sprinkle in the bean flour if you desire a thicker stew. Toss in everything else and cover with water. Bring to a boil and then lower to a simmer for 40-60 minutes. Serve with whole grain bread and red wine.

Something for a Cold January Night
1-2 large acorn squash (any winter squash)
1-2 cups soy milk
½ cup cream (optional)
½ tsp. nutmeg
½ tsp powdered ginger
salt and pepper to taste

Peel and half the squash. Remove the seeds. Cut into smaller pieces and boil in water until soft. Drain the water and blend the squash in a food processor. Transfer back into the pot and add soy milk, cream, and spices. Cook briefly on medium heat until bubbling.

For variation try using Garam Masala (coriander, black pepper, cumin, cardamom, and cinnamon) as the spice and add in a couple of tablespoons of coconut milk for flavor.

Serve with a fresh greens salad, whole grain bread with thinly sliced Swiss cheese and a glass of Pinot Grigio.

Root Stew

A rich creamy stew that will make anyone like beets—but you can leave them out if you insist.

   Assorted roots such as carrots, parsnips, turnips, sweet potatoes, red potatoes,
      beets, leeks (or onions) – chopped into small pieces
   Several stalks of celery, chopped
   2-3 tbs fresh minced cilantro
   1-2 tsp curry powder
   1-2 tsp cumin
   ½ tsp cinnamon
   Salt and pepper
   1-2 cups soy milk
   (Light cream 1/2 -1 cup on special occasions)

Toss all the ingredients into a large pot. Add water until the vegetables are covered. On the stove bring to a boil and then lower to a slow simmer for about one hour. The sweet potatoes will break apart and thicken the stew. Serve with a salad and fresh bread.

STANDARD AMERICAN FARE

Gingered butternut squash

This dish starts with ginger tea. Peel a piece of fresh ginger a little larger than your thumb. Slice it into thin slices and place in a tea strainer. Immerse in small pot of water and bring to a boil. When the water is barely boiling, turn off the heat and allow the tea to steep for about ten minutes. You can add in a couple of bags of regular tea if you like. Sweeten and serve hot or with ice. Take the ginger left over from making the tea and mince finely with a knife. Mix with 1-2 tablespoons of butter and 1-2 tablespoons of brown sugar.

Split a butternut squash in half, clean out the seeds, and place with the cut side down in a baking dish with water covering the bottom. Bake at 375 until soft (30-45 minutes). Flip the squash and make several cross-ways slices into the meat of the squash with a knife. Spread the ginger mixture across the surface of the squash, pushing it down into the slices. Bake for 5-10 more minutes and serve.

Kale and beans

   A large bag full of fresh kale, washed
   Half an onion, chopped
   Red bell pepper, chopped
   Minced garlic

Minced fresh thyme and/or rosemary
One can of red beans (or any other beans)
1-2 cups of cooked rice
½ - 1 cup of vegetable broth
1-2 heaping tablespoons of apricot jam
1-2 tablespoons of balsamic vinegar
Olive oil
<1/2 teaspoon of red pepper paste or fresh-minced hot red pepper

Sauté the onion, red pepper, garlic, red pepper paste and thyme in olive oil in a large pan on medium high heat. When the onions are brown, add in the kale. Cover the pot, but open it frequently to stir. When the kale is wilted, add in the vegetable broth and all of the other ingredients. Lower the heat and simmer covered for about ten minutes. Serve.

Other greens can be used. Try it with collards or Swiss chard. This dish goes well with the gingered butternut squash.

Mashed cauliflower
Steam a head of cauliflower until soft. Chop it up in a large bowl and add in butter and soymilk. Use a food processor or hand mixer to blend until thick and smooth. Salt to taste.

Steamed vegetables
Any kind, in any combination. Try various seasonings and sauces.

Rice and beets
Okay, so I'm one of those odd individuals who liked beets from the beginning, but you can develop a taste for them and this dish will help. Peel about four fresh beets. Boil until soft. Dice into small cubes after cooling. Mix with cooked brown basmati rice, salt (to taste) and 1-2 teaspoons of balsamic vinegar.

Quinoa as a side dish
Quinoa has a texture and taste mildly reminiscent of grits. The flavor stands alone, but can be dressed up. Start with two cups of water to one cup of grain. Cook on low, covered, for about 15 minutes. Spice it up with a sauté of onions, red bell peppers, celery, garlic and fresh oregano in olive oil.

You can just use half of the quinoa for the dish and refrigerate half for breakfast. The next morning, reheat the quinoa with butter, milk (soy milk), maple syrup and raisins for a really tasty breakfast cereal.

Sweet potatoes

Wash sweet potatoes thoroughly. Stick them with a fork several times before placing in the oven. Bake them at about 375 until soft. This usually takes about 35-45 minutes.

The potatoes can also be cut into chunks and steamed or boiled until soft. Drain the water. Mash with a fork and add a little butter. At this point, you can go the usual route by adding brown sugar and cinnamon, or you can get creative: try a sprinkle of cocoa or cumin, instead.

Slaw

There are probably more different kinds of recipes for slaw than for any other single dish. It can be made in a food processor or chopped by hand. Raisins and apples add sweetness without sugar. Use a large bowl and chop enough cabbage and carrots to fill it about half full. This makes it easier to mix. The exact amount of the ingredients does not matter, but use less mayonnaise and oil than you would think necessary, just enough to coat the vegetables.

  Chopped cabbage—green, red or Savoy—or a mix of all three
  Chopped carrots
  One chopped apple
  One cup raisins
  A teaspoon of mustard
  A spoonful of mayonnaise
  A dribble of macadamia nut oil
  A hint of vinegar
  Salt and pepper to taste

Mix everything together and serve. Try other variations with other spices, such as cumin and a dash of cayenne pepper.

Bahamian peas and rice

Peas and rice is a staple dish found all over the Caribbean with many derivations. Most of them contain bacon, but here is a vegetarian version. Red beans, black-eyed peas or lima beans can be used, but most commonly this dish is made with Crowder peas. There are so many variations of this recipe, that missing ingredients are never a problem.

  brown basmati rice, cooked (2-3 cups)
  Small sweet onion, diced
  2-3 stalks of celery, diced
  Olive oil.
  1 can Crowder peas, rinsed

1 can diced organic tomatoes
2 tablespoons of tomato paste
2-3 tablespoons fresh minced thyme
1-2 teaspoons minced garlic
Small amount of hot chili paste or chopped hot pepper
½ -1 5.5 oz. coconut milk
½ cup (or less) vegetable broth
½ lime
Salt to taste

In a 2-3 quart pan, sauté the onions, celery, garlic, thyme and hot pepper in a small amount of olive oil until the onions are brown. Add in all of the other ingredients and then the rice. Stir over low heat until all of the ingredients are well-mixed.

Baked fish

Any large fish such as grouper, ocean trout, or snapper will do. Place the whole fish (headed, scaled and gutted) in a large baking dish. Cut slices along the body of the fish into the flesh to allow flavors to blend. Surround the fish with sliced vegetable such as onions, celery, tomatoes, small red potatoes, red or yellow bell peppers and mushrooms. Spread minced garlic and fresh minced herbs such as oregano, thyme or rosemary on top of the fish. Dribble olive oil over the top of everything. Cover with foil. Bake at 425 for about 45 minutes, depending on the size of the fish.

Ranch beans

This recipe will make you never want to open another can of regular baked beans again.

1 can each of white beans (cantanoli), pinto beans, and kidney beans (organic preferred), washed in a colander and drained.
1 bell pepper, chopped (red, orange, yellow, or green)
½-1 sweet onion, chopped
Minced garlic
¼- ½ cup of sweet BBQ sauce
1 tablespoon chili powder
½ teaspoon cumin
½ teaspoon Mexican oregano
Cayenne pepper to taste
Salt to taste
Olive oil

Sauté the peppers, onion, and garlic in olive oil until soft. Stir in all the beans and all the spices. Serve as is or bake at 350 for 15 minutes.

CASSEROLES AND BAKED DISHES

Casseroles generally require more prep and kitchen time, but the tradeoff is being able to store them in the refrigerator or freezer. I never make just one lasagna—there are always two, one for dinner and one for the freezer. Casseroles are perfect to serve a crowd.

As with other dishes, do not worry about specific ingredients or the amounts of ingredients. Feel free to add or subtract items according to your particular tastes. That is what cooking is all about.

Grouper Moussaka

This is a light and healthy version of what is traditionally a heavy meat dish. Grouper is used here because it is a less oily white meat fish with few bones and it soaks up all the flavors of the Moussaka. Other fish such as flounder or halibut work just fine, too. This recipe can also be made vegetarian by omitting the fish and substituting tempeh.

1-2 lbs. of fresh grouper, preferably in one filet
1 large or 2 medium eggplants
1 medium sweet onion, sliced and chopped
1 package of fresh mushrooms, sliced
3 medium tomatoes (sliced into small chunks) or one can crushed tomatoes
1 yellow or red bell pepper
1 6oz. can of tomato paste
1 handful of fresh basil, oregano, and a little rosemary, minced
1 teaspoon cinnamon
½ teaspoon tumeric
Lots of minced garlic
Shredded parmesan cheese
2-3 tablespoons olive oil
Salt to taste

Béchamel sauce

2-3 tablespoons olive oil
4 tablespoons of garbanzo bean flour (Found in most health food stores, this is a tasty flour substitute. Hummus can be used if this is not available.)
2 cups of soy milk
½ cup shredded parmesan cheese

Dash or two of nutmeg

Peel and slice the eggplant into ½ inch thick slices. Lightly salt the pieces and lay them into a colander for about 20 minutes. Everyone says this is to allow the bitter juices to sweat out, but I have never noticed much difference when I cook eggplant without this step. Place the eggplant on a baking sheet and bake for about 20 minutes in an oven pre-heated to 375.

While waiting on the eggplant, prepare the Béchamel sauce. In a saucepan, whisk the garbanzo bean flower and olive oil together on medium heat until bubbly. I sometimes add a teaspoon of butter. Set aside to cool completely. Add the soy milk and slowly reheat, stirring constantly. Continue until thickened. Stir in the cheese and nutmeg, and set aside.

Sauté the mushrooms, onions, and peppers in olive oil until tender. Add in the tomatoes, tomato paste, garlic, herbs, and spices. Simmer for about 10-15 minutes.

Place the fish in the middle of a large baking dish. Slice the eggplant into smaller sections and layer around the fish. Layer the mushroom mixture over the top of the fish and eggplant. Pour the béchamel sauce across the top. Bake covered with foil for about 35-45 minutes. During the last 10 minutes remove the foil and sprinkle parmesan cheese over the top. Serve with a lettuce salad.

Wild rice and turkey
   2 cups of cooked brown rice
   2 cups of cooked wild rice
   2-3 cups baked turkey or chicken, chopped into small chunks
   1-2 tbsp. of garbanzo bean flour or unbleached flour
   2 tbsp. olive oil or macadamia nut oil
   Chopped celery, onion and mushrooms
   1 cup soymilk
   1 cup vegetable or chicken broth
   broccoli, several stalks chopped into small pieces
   1 egg
   lemon
   1-2 tbsp. mayonnaise or hummus
   salt and pepper
   fresh rosemary, minced.

In a saucepan, sauté 1 to 2 tbsp. of garbanzo bean flour in a couple of tbsp. of olive oil. Cook about one minute, cool, and then stir in one cup of soy milk and one cup of chicken or vegetable broth. Cook on medium heat, stirring continuously, until thickened.

Meanwhile, lightly steam or microwave the broccoli and sauté the onions, celery and mushrooms in oil.

Lightly beat one egg yolk with a little fresh lemon. Slowly mix in a spoonful of the broth/soymilk mixture and then pour it all back into the saucepan. Add in 1 to 2 tbsp. of either mayonnaise or hummus and heat through.

Mix this sauce with the turkey, broccoli, vegetables, brown rice and wild rice. Salt and pepper to taste. Rosemary is also a nice spice for this dish.

Transfer to a casserole dish. Grate fresh parmesan cheese on top. Bake at 350 for 20 to 30 minutes, or until brown.

Prepare more than one dish at a time and freeze the extras for later use.

Three-layer Vegetable Lasagna
  1 box whole wheat lasagna noodles
  1 eggplant
  Several cups of vegetables—zucchini, onions, mushrooms, spinach, broccoli,
    carrots (any combination)
  1 tsp minced garlic
  1 tbs minced fresh oregano
  1 tsp fresh minced basil
  1 jar pasta sauce
  Filling
    ½-1 cup low fat cottage cheese
    ½-1 cup low fat ricotta cheese
    1 egg
    ½ cup mozzarella cheese
    ½ cup parmesan cheese

Slice eggplant into ½ inch slices and place in a colander to allow the slices to "sweat." Pat dry with a paper towel. This removes some of the bitterness. Lay the eggplant on a cooking sheet seasoned with cooking spray. Bake at 350°F for about 15 minutes, or until lightly browned. Boil the noodles until tender and drain. (Add about one tsp of olive oil to the water to prevent the noodles from sticking together.) At the same time, steam or microwave (6 minutes on high) all of the vegetables, basil, oregano, and garlic until tender. In a separate bowl, mix the cottage cheese, ricotta, cheese, egg, mozzarella cheese, and parmesan cheese.

For the layering process use a deep baking dish roughly 9 x 11. Most commonly three layers of noodles are used, but this recipe can be made lighter with less filling and fewer layers of noodles. Also less mozzarella and ricotta cheese can be used. Layering goes like this: Start with a layer of noodles on the bottom. Add a layer of eggplant slices (or ½ eggplant and ½ browned ground beef). Thinly spread eggplant with the cheese mixture. Drizzle with some of the sauce. Add another layer of noodles. A layer of vegetables comes next. More sauce goes on top of the vegetables. Top with the final layer of noodles and the rest of the sauce. Sprinkle with mozzarella and parmesan cheese. Cover with foil and place in the oven at 350° for 30 min. Remove the foil during the last 15 minutes to allow the cheese to brown.

This dish can be prepared and then kept in the refrigerator for several days or frozen prior to baking. Make two lasagnas and freeze one for later use.

Sweet Potato Burritos
4 cups sweet potatoes, cooked and mashed
Can of black beans, rinsed and drained
Can of kidney beans, rinsed and drained
1 onion, chopped
1 T. minced garlic
3 T. soy sauce
3-4 tsp. prepared mustard
1-2 T. chili powder
2 tsp. ground cumin
Just a dash of cayenne pepper
Whole wheat tortillas
Shredded cheese (optional)
Salsa (optional)

Sauté onions and garlic in 1-2 tbsp. of olive oil. In a large bowl, mash beans slightly and mix with the spices, onion and garlic. Add a bit of water if stiff. Mix in the mashed sweet potatoes.

Spoon mixture into tortillas, fold, and place in casserole dish. Spread salsa on top. Bake at for about 15-20 minutes.

These freeze quite well. Wrap them separately and place into a freezer box for quick meals.

Sweet and Sour Winter Roasted Vegetables
The aromas in the kitchen and the warmth of the oven while this dish is cooking are enough to melt away any cold winter night.
  Beets
  Carrots

Brussels sprouts
Mushrooms
Red onions
Sweet potatoes
Cauliflower
Prunes (secret ingredient)

Olive oil—about ¼ cup
Maple syrup—about ¼ cup
Apple cider vinegar—about ¼ cup
Ground sage
Fresh or dry minced thyme
Salt and pepper

Cut vegetables into chunks—enough to fill a 2 quart container. Steam the vegetables for about five minutes. Place them into a large baking dish and drizzle olive oil across the vegetables. Sprinkle sage, thyme, salt and pepper across all of the vegetables. Bake at 400 degrees for 20 minutes, covered. Mix the vinegar and maple syrup well and pour over the mixture. Bake for another 20 minutes. Take off the cover for part of the time to allow the vegetables to brown slightly.

ACKNOWLEDGMENTS

First and foremost, I would like to thank my patients for all they have taught me over the years.

I would like to thank Leslie McCombs-Porter who edited my rewrites more times than I would like to remember. Her comments and guidance have been beyond value.

I would like to thank my wife for her exceptional editing talents and for putting up with years of rewriting and weekends waiting and watching, while I slaved over a computer. Her professional insights and input have been invaluable. Having someone close at hand with training in science has helped me stay on the straight and narrow.

I would also like to thank Dawn Brock, whose eye for detail and originality has been essential for formatting the book into readable form.

Jill Miller deserves my full appreciation for her down-to-the-wire efforts in creating an outstanding cover.

My thanks to staff members present at my office during the time the book was written. Each of them contributed in positive ways. A special thanks to Christie Fulcher, R.N., who also helped proofread on several occasions and provided input and feedback on a daily basis while the health program was being created.

REFERENCES

Some writing is the result of specific research with the primary purpose of conveying information. This type of writing is essential in a book of this sort and should be backed by specific references. The primary references cited were used to research factual information.

Secondary references provided factual information as well as opinions or theories worth considering. Some information, such as the theories about alkalinity and osteoporosis, is less absolute but helps guide the reader toward a specific goal and provides food for thought.

Much of the writing in the book happened spontaneously—often as a result of searching for better ways to explain concepts to patients. During the time I was immersed in writing the book, ideas would often come while on a long walk or in the shower and would end up scribbled on snips of paper, later to be included. This type of writing generally does not result from well-defined references, but is the consequence of years of accumulated knowledge, synthesized through common sense into a workable form.

Toward the end of writing the book, well after the sections on toxins were complete, a friend gave me a copy of *Detoxify, or Die*, by Sherry A. Rogers, M. D. This became a vital reference on the subject and was used to fill in deficiencies and complete loose ends.

In many places in the book, reference is made to specific web sites or specific books and authors. These resources are listed here in hopes that readers will use them to pursue greater knowledge.

Primary references
Harper's Biochemistry, 25th Edition, A Lange Medical Book
    Robert K. Murray, M.D., PhD., Daryl K. Granner, M.D.
    Peter D. Mayes, PhD., DSC, Victor W. Rodwell, PhD.
    McGraw-Hill, Copyright 2000, 1996, 1993, 1990, 1988
    ISBN 0-8385-3684-0

Review of Medical Physiology, 20th Edition
    William F. Ganong, M.D.
    Lange Medical Books, McGraw-Hill 1999
    ISBN 0-8385-8282-6

Advanced Nutrition and Human Metabolism, 3rd Edition
James L. Groff, Sareen S. Gropper
Wadsworth, Copyright 2000
ISBN 0-534-55521-7

Textbook of Functional Medicine
David S. Jones, M.D., Editor in Chief
Institute for Functional Medicine
Copyright 2005
ISBN 0-9773713-0-1

Modern Nutrition Health and Disease, 9th Edition
Editor Donna Bulado
Williams and Wilkins
Copyright 1999
ISBN 0-683-30769-X

The Relaxation and Stress Reduction Workbook, 5th Edition
Martha Davis, PhD.
Elizabeth Robbins Eshelman, MSW
Matthew McKay, PhD.
New Harbinger Publications, Inc.
Copyright 2000
ISBN 1-57224-214-0

Modern Concepts in Biochemistry, 3rd Edition
Robert C. Bohinski
Allyn and Bacon, Inc.
Copyright 1979
ISBN 0-205-06541-X

The Relaxation Response
Herbert Benson, M.D.
Avon Books, Inc.
Copyright 1975
ISBN 0-380-81595-8

Meditation for Dummies
Stephan Bodian
Wiley Publishing Company, Inc., Indianapolis, Indiana
Copyright 1999

The Open Focus Brain
  Les Fehmi, PhD., Jim Robbins
  Trumpeter Books
  Copyright 2007
  ISBN 987-1-590301-376-4

Drawing on the Ride Side of the Brain
  Betty Edwards
  G. P. Putnam's Sons
  Copyright 1987
  ISBN 0-87477-513-2

The Healthiest Diet in the World
  Nikki and David Goldbeck
  Penguin Putnam, Inc., Dutton Books
  Copyright 1998
  ISBN 0-525-94282-3

Estrogen Metabolism and the Diet-Cancer Connection: Rational for Assessing the Ratio of Urinary Hydroxylated Estrogen Metabolites
  Richard S. Lord, PhD, Bradley Bongiovanni, ND, and J. Alexander Bralley, PhD, CCN.
  Alternative Medicine Review, Volume 7, Number 2, 2002

Foods to Fight Cancer, Essential foods to help prevent cancer
  Richard Beliveau, Ph.D. and Denis Gingras, Ph.D.
  DK Publishing, New York, New York
  Copyright 2007
  ISBN 978-0-7566-2867-3

Detoxify or Die
  Sherry A. Rogers, M.D
  Sand Key Company, Inc.
  Copyright 2002
  ISBN: 1-887202-04-8

Breaking the Vicious Cycle
  Elaine Gottschall, B.A., M.Sc.
  The Kirkton Press, Baltimore, Maryland
  Copyright 2004
  ISBN 0-9692768-1-8

Biofeedback, A Practitioner's Guide, 3rd edition
Mark S. Schwartz and Frank Andrasik, editors
The Guilford Press, New York, New York
Copyright 2003
ISBN-13: 978-1-57230-845-9

Laboratory Evaluations in Molecular Medicine
J Alexander Bralley, PhD, CCN and Richard S. Lord, PhD
The Institute for Advances in Molecular Medicine, Norcross, Ga.
Copyright 2001
ISBN-10: 0-9673949-1-0

Secondary references

Healing with Whole Foods, Asian Traditions and Modern Nutrition, 3rd Edition
Paul Pitchford
North Atlantic Books, Berkeley, California
Copyright 1993
ISBN 1-55643-430-8

Staying Healthy with Nutrition
Elson M. Haas, M.D.
Copyright 1992
Celestial Arts, Berkeley, California
ISBN 0-89087-481-6

Overcoming Thyroid Disorders, 2nd edition
David Brownstein, M.D.
Medical Alternatives Press
Copyright 2008
ISBN 978-0-960882-2-9

Foods That Fight Pain
Neal Barnard, M.D.
Three Rivers Press   New York, New York
Copyright 1998
ISBN 0-609-80436-7

The Natural Testosterone Plan, for sexual health and energy
    Stephen Harrod Buhner
    Healing Arts Press   Rochester, Vermont
    Copyright 2007
    ISBN 978-1-59477-168-2

The Lyme Disease Solution
    Kenneth B. Singleton, M.D., M.P.H.
    Brown Books, Dallas, Texas
    Copyright 2008
    ISBN-13: 978-1-934812-00-6

Cruising World
    October 2008 "Skimming the Sands of Sable"

National Geographic
    November 2005 "The Secrets of Living Longer"

Diet, Life Expectancy, and Chronic Disease–Studies of Seventh Day Adventists and Other Vegetarians (reference for the Heidelberg Vegetarian Study)
    Gary Fraser
    Oxford Press
    Copyright 2003

Website references
Toxins:
www.pollutioninpeople.org
www.chemicalbodyburden.org
www.ourstolenfuture.org

Gastrointestinal disorders:
www.breakingtheviciouscycle.info

Alkaline water:
www.hightechhealth.com

FIR sauna:
www.hightechhealth.com

Healthy food:

www.barleyfoods.org *recipes using barley grain*

www.quinoa.net *recipes using quinoa*

www.sunnylandfarms.com *resource for fresh nuts*

www.eatwild.com *resource for finding local free-range meat*

www.oceansalive.org *resource for finding healthy seafood*

www.organicconsumer.org *resource for finding organic food*

www.whfoods.com *extensive resource for information about food*

www.localharvest.org *resource for finding locally harvested foods*

www.bobsredmill.com *resource for organic grain products*

Healthy products:

www.realgoods.com *resource for many environmentally favorable products*

www.seventhgeneration.com *"green" household products*

www.shaklee.net *non-toxic cosmetics and skin products*

Relaxation:

www.TheRelaxationCompany.com *source for Dr. Jeffrey Thompson's CD's*

www.openfocus.com

Nutritional supplements:

www.naturaldatabase.com *paid source for scientific data about nutraceuticals*

For a more specific and up-to-date guide in choosing supplements, please visit **www.FDNHhealth.com**. This website offers high quality supplements and other health products at reasonable prices. It is designed to expand on the concepts I have defined in this book and to be a continuing resource for individuals who desire to improve their health.